Lupus Erythematosus

Peter H. Schur · Elena M. Massarotti
Editors

Lupus Erythematosus

Clinical Evaluation and Treatment

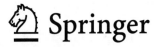 Springer

Editors
Peter H. Schur
Division of Rheumatology,
Immunology, Allergy
Brigham and Women's Hospital
Boston, MA, USA

Elena M. Massarotti
Division of Rheumatology,
Immunology, Allergy
Center for Clinical Therapeutics
Brigham and Women's Hospital
Boston, MA, USA

ISBN 978-1-4614-1188-8   ISBN 978-1-4614-1189-5 (eBook)
DOI 10.1007/978-1-4614-1189-5
Springer New York Heidelberg Dordrecht London

Library of Congress Control Number: 2012941092

© Springer Science+Business Media New York 2012
This work is subject to copyright. All rights are reserved by the Publisher, whether the whole or part of the material is concerned, specifically the rights of translation, reprinting, reuse of illustrations, recitation, broadcasting, reproduction on microfilms or in any other physical way, and transmission or information storage and retrieval, electronic adaptation, computer software, or by similar or dissimilar methodology now known or hereafter developed. Exempted from this legal reservation are brief excerpts in connection with reviews or scholarly analysis or material supplied specifically for the purpose of being entered and executed on a computer system, for exclusive use by the purchaser of the work. Duplication of this publication or parts thereof is permitted only under the provisions of the Copyright Law of the Publisher's location, in its current version, and permission for use must always be obtained from Springer. Permissions for use may be obtained through RightsLink at the Copyright Clearance Center. Violations are liable to prosecution under the respective Copyright Law.
The use of general descriptive names, registered names, trademarks, service marks, etc. in this publication does not imply, even in the absence of a specific statement, that such names are exempt from the relevant protective laws and regulations and therefore free for general use.
While the advice and information in this book are believed to be true and accurate at the date of publication, neither the authors nor the editors nor the publisher can accept any legal responsibility for any errors or omissions that may be made. The publisher makes no warranty, express or implied, with respect to the material contained herein.

Printed on acid-free paper

Springer is part of Springer Science+Business Media (www.springer.com)

Preface

Most physicians, regardless of their area of expertise, will encounter a patient with lupus during the course of their careers, or must consider the diagnosis when evaluating a patient with a particular complaint. Often considered the prototypic autoimmune disease, it is characterized by protean manifestations and affects a wide range of organ systems. Despite the widespread availability of antinuclear antibody testing and other technological diagnostic advances, the diagnosis of lupus can be elusive, difficult, and inexact. Treatment of the disease can also be challenging, and focused upon the immune system and the specific organ system affected. Advances in immunology and biotechnology have led to a burgeoning world of new therapies in development that offer patients the real possibility of new therapies, and physicians and scientists insights into the pathogenesis of this complicated immunological disease.

This textbook summarizes the clinical aspects of lupus facing the general clinician in the twenty-first century. The reader will find introductory chapters regarding general diagnostic and treatment principles, followed by chapters addressing the lupus-specific organ manifestations. Special topics regarding pregnancy and comorbidities are also presented. All these chapters were written by highly experienced physicians with special expertise in lupus.

We hope you will find this text to be a valuable, single source, "go-to" reference for the common and not so common problems affecting patients with lupus that you may confront in your practices.

Boston, MA, USA   Peter H. Schur, M.D., F.A.C.P.
                                                     Elena M. Massarotti, M.D.

Contents

1 **SLE Epidemiology: Epidemiologic Subtypes and Risk Factors for Development** 1
   Julia F. Simard and Karen H. Costenbader

2 **The Immunopathogenesis and Immunopathology of Systemic Lupus Erythematosus** 13
   David S. Pisetsky

3 **Diagnosing and Monitoring Lupus** 27
   Elena M. Massarotti and Peter H. Schur

4 **Recommendations on How to Monitor the Patient with Systemic Lupus Erythematosus in the Clinic or at the Bedside** 41
   Vivian P. Bykerk

5 **The Treatment of Lupus: General Principles** 53
   Elena M. Massarotti and Peter H. Schur

6 **Cutaneous Manifestations of Lupus Erythematosus** 67
   Henry Townsend and Ruth Ann Vleugels

7 **Musculoskeletal Manifestations of SLE** 95
   Simon M. Helfgott

8 **Cardiac and Vascular Disease in SLE** 107
   Robert A. Sands

9 **Pulmonary Manifestations of Systemic Lupus Erythematosus** 115
   Hilary J. Goldberg and Paul F. Dellaripa

10 **Hematologic Manifestations of SLE** 127
   Ami S. Bhatt and Nancy Berliner

11	**Lupus Nephritis**..	141
	Mary Anne Dooley	
12	**Gastrointestinal Manifestations of Systemic Lupus Erythematosus**..	153
	R.S. Kalman and J.L. Wolf	
13	**Neuropsychiatric Aspects of Lupus**......................................	169
	S. Khoshbin	
14	**Systemic Lupus Erythematosus and Pregnancy**	183
	Bonnie L. Bermas	
15	**Antiphospholipid Syndrome**	197
	Bonnie L. Bermas	
16	**Lupus-Like Syndromes Related to Drugs**............................	211
	Joseph F. Merola	
17	**New and Emerging Therapies**..	223
	Elena M. Massarotti	
18	**Co-morbidities in Systemic Lupus Erythematosus**............	229
	Mary Gayed, Chee-Seng Yee, Sasha Bernatsky, and Caroline Gordon	

Index.. 251

Contributors

Nancy Berliner, M.D. Division of Hematology, Brigham and Women's Hospital, Boston, MA, USA

Harvard Medical School, Boston, MA, USA

Bonnie L. Bermas, M.D. Division of Rheumatology, Director, Lupus Center, Brigham and Women's Hospital, Boston, MA, USA

Harvard Medical School, Boston, MA, USA

Sasha Bernatsky, Ph.D. Royal Victoria Hospital, Montreal, QC, Canada

Ami S. Bhatt Harvard Medical School, Boston, MA, USA

Clinical Fellow in Hematology and Oncology, Brigham and Women's Hospital and Dana Farber Cancer Institute, Boston, MA, USA

Vivian P. Bykerk, M.D. Hospital for Special Surgery, New York, NY, USA

Karen H. Costenbader, M.D., M.P.H. Lupus Center, Brigham and Women's Hospital, Boston, MA, USA

Harvard Medical School, Boston, MA, USA

Paul F. Dellaripa, M.D. Division of Rheumatology, Brigham and Women's Hospital, Boston, MA, USA

Interstitial Lung Disease (ILD) Clinic, Brigham and Women's Hospital, Boston, MA, USA

Mary Anne Dooley, M.D., M.P.H. Division of Rheumatology and Immunology, University of North Carolina at Chapel Hill, Chapel Hill, NC, USA

Mary Gayed, M.B.Ch.B. Rheumatology Department, City Hospital, Sandwell and West Birmingham Hospitals, NHS Trust, Birmingham, UK

Hilary J. Goldberg, M.D., M.P.H. Division of Pulmonary and Critical Care Medicine, Brigham and Women's Hospital, Boston, MA, USA

Harvard Medical School, Boston, MA, USA

Caroline Gordon, M.D. Rheumatology Department, City Hospital, Sandwell and West Birmingham Hospitals, NHS Trust, Birmingham, UK

Rheumatology Research Group, School of Immunity and Infection, College of Medical and Dental Sciences, University of Birmingham, Birmingham, UK

Simon Helfgott, M.D. Division of Rheumatology, Brigham and Women's Hospital, Boston, MA, USA

Harvard Medical School, Boston, MA, USA

R.S. Kalman, M.D. Beth Israel Deaconess Medical Center, Boston, MA, USA

Harvard Medical School, Boston, MA, USA

S. Khoshbin, M.D. Division of Neurology, Brigham and Women's Hospital, Boston, MA, USA

Harvard Medical School, Boston, MA, USA

Elena M. Massarotti, M.D. Division of Rheumatology, Center for Clinical Therapeutics, Brigham and Women's Hospital, Boston, MA, USA

Harvard Medical School, Boston, MA, USA

Joseph F. Merola, M.D. Department of Medicine, Division of Rheumatology and Department of Dermatology, Brigham and Women's Hospital, Boston, MA, USA

Department of Medicine, Harvard Medical School, Boston, MA, USA

David Pisetsky, M.D., Ph.D. Department of Medicine and Immunology, Duke University Medical Center, Durham, NC, USA

Medical Research Service, Durham VA Hospital, Durham, NC, USA

Robert A. Sands, M.D. Division of Rheumatology, Brigham and Women's Hospital, Boston, MA, USA

Harvard Medical School, Boston, MA, USA

Peter H. Schur, M.D., F.A.C.P. Division of Rheumatology, Brigham and Women's Hospital, Boston, MA, USA

Harvard Medical School, Boston, MA, USA

Julia F. Simard, Sc.D. Clinical Epidemiology Unit, Karolinska University Hospital, Stockholm, Sweden

Henry Townsend, M.D. Division of Clinical Immunology and Rheumatology, Department of Medicine, The University of Alabama at Birmingham, Birmingham, AL, USA

Ruth Ann Vleugels, M.D., M.P.H. Connective Tissue Disease Clinic, Brigham and Women's Dermatology, Boston, MA, USA

Harvard Medical School, Boston, MA, USA

J.L. Wolf, M.D. Beth Israel Deaconess Medical Center, Boston, MA, USA

Harvard Medical School, Boston, MA, USA

Chee-Seng Yee, Ph.D. Rheumatology Department, City Hospital, Sandwell and West Birmingham Hospitals, NHS Trust, Birmingham, UK

Rheumatology Research Group, School of Immunity and Infection, College of Medical and Dental Sciences, University of Birmingham, Birmingham, UK

Chapter 1
SLE Epidemiology: Epidemiologic Subtypes and Risk Factors for Development

Julia F. Simard and Karen H. Costenbader

Epidemiology

While the etiology of systemic lupus erythematosus (SLE) is still enigmatic, epidemiologic research is continuously informing our understanding, with new insights into environmental risk factors and gene–environment interactions that play a role in disease susceptibility. SLE is a heterogeneous multisystem autoimmune disorder characterized by organ system manifestations which vary over time and autoantibodies that target mainly intracellular constituents. Antinuclear antibodies (ANA) are observed in over 95% of patients, while other characteristic autoantibodies [anti-double-stranded DNA (anti-dsDNA), anti-Smith (anti-Sm), anti-Ro, and anti-La antibodies] are less common. These autoantibodies have been detected years prior to first symptoms of SLE and are responsible for certain disease manifestations such as photosensitive rashes, cytopenias, thromboses, and glomerulonephritis.

SLE Classification

Clinical presentation and laboratory testing are used together in making a diagnosis. The current criteria for disease classification were developed by the American College of Rheumatology (ACR) in 1982 and revised in 1997, with the addition of antiphospholipid antibody testing (Table 1.1). These criteria aim to

---

J.F. Simard, Sc.D. (✉)
Clinical Epidemiology Unit, T2, Karolinska University Hospital,
171 76 Stockholm, Sweden
e-mail: julia.simard@ki.se

K.H. Costenbader, M.D., M.P.H.
Lupus Center, Brigham and Women's Hospital, Boston, MA, USA

Harvard Medical School, Boston, MA, USA

P.H. Schur and E.M. Massarotti (eds.), *Lupus Erythematosus:*
Clinical Evaluation and Treatment, DOI 10.1007/978-1-4614-1189-5_1,
© Springer Science+Business Media New York 2012

Table 1.1 The evolution of the American College of Rheumatology classification criteria for SLE

Criterion	1971[a]	1982[b]	1997[c]
Malar rash	Malar rash	Malar rash	Malar rash
Discoid rash	Discoid rash	Discoid rash	Discoid rash
Raynaud's phenomenon	Raynaud's phenomenon		
Alopecia	Alopecia		
Photosensitivity	Photosensitivity	Photosensitivity	Photosensitivity
Oral or nasopharyngeal ulcers	Oral or nasopharyngeal ulcers	Oral or nasopharyngeal ulcers	Oral or nasopharyngeal ulcers
Arthritis	Arthritis without deformity	Nonerosive arthritis in at least two peripheral joints	Nonerosive arthritis in at least two peripheral joints
Serositis	Pleurisy Pericarditis	Pleurisy Pericarditis	Pleurisy Pericarditis
Renal disorder	Profuse proteinuria Cellular casts	Profuse proteinuria Cellular casts	Profuse proteinuria Cellular casts
Neurologic disorder	Psychosis Convulsions	Psychosis Seizures	Psychosis Seizures
Hematologic disorder	Hemolytic anemia Leukopenia Thrombocytopenia	Hemolytic anemia Leukopenia Thrombocytopenia Lymphopenia	Hemolytic anemia Leukopenia Thrombocytopenia Lymphopenia
Immunologic disorder	LE cells False-positive serologic test for syphilis (STS)	LE cells False-positive STS Anti-DNA Anti-Sm	False-positive STS Anti-DNA Anti-Sm Antiphospholipid antibodies Lupus anticoagulant
Antinuclear antibody	Positive ANA	Positive ANA	Positive ANA

[a] Cohen AS, Reynolds WE, Franklin EC, et al. Preliminary criteria for the classification of systemic lupus erythematosus. Bull Rheum Dis 1971; 21: 643–8
[b] Tan EM, Cohen AS, Fries JF, et al. The 1982 revised criteria for the classification of systemic lupus erythematosus (SLE). Arthritis Rheum 192; 25: 1271–7
[c] Hochberg MC. Updating the American College of Rheumatology revised criteria for the classification of systemic lupus erythematosus (letter). Arthritis Rheum 1997; 40: 1725

be comprehensive, requiring at least 4 of 11 criteria, but are far from exhaustive given the many clinical manifestations of SLE that are not included. These classification criteria were developed to allow definition of disease populations for research purposes not clinical diagnosis. The shortcomings of the current system have been outlined and modified criteria, including weighting of the different manifestations (more weight for severe organ involvement and less weight for more subjective signs and symptoms such as photosensitivity and oral ulcers) have been proposed and have greater sensitivity, but slightly lower specificity for disease classification.

SLE Heterogeneity and Subtypes

As SLE is a heterogeneous disease, the ACR criteria do not distinguish well among clinically disparate subtypes of SLE. Although it remains unclear whether SLE subtypes are distinct diseases, some non-mutually exclusive clinical subtypes of SLE can be identified.

Anti-Double-Stranded DNA Antibodies/Glomerulonephritis

Anti-dsDNA antibodies are strongly associated with severe SLE and the development and activity of glomerulonephritis.

Anti-Ro Antibodies/Subacute Cutaneous LE and Sjögren's Syndrome (SS)

Anti-Ro antibodies (also called SSA antibodies) target RNA–protein conjugates and can be found in SLE with photosensitive rashes, SS/SLE overlap syndrome, subacute cutaneous LE (SCLE), neonatal lupus, and primary biliary cirrhosis among other autoimmune diseases. In SLE, anti-Ro/SSA antibodies are also associated with cutaneous vasculitis. Although >50% SCLE patients may fulfill the ACR criteria for SLE, they likely represent a distinct but closely related subtype with recognizable annular or psoriasiform photosensitive rashes, less visceral involvement, and the need for immunosuppressive therapy. The related anti-La/SSB antibodies, which also target RNA–protein conjugates, are more strongly associated with Sjögren's syndrome.

Antiphospholipid Antibody Syndrome

Strokes, miscarriage, occlusive vasculopathy (including deep vein thromboses and pulmonary emboli), and livedo reticularis are associated with antiphospholipid antibodies, including lupus anticoagulant, anticardiolipin antibodies, antiprothrombin antibodies, and anti-β2 glycoprotein-1 antibodies.

SLE/Mixed Connective Tissue Disease Overlap

Anti-U1 RNP antibodies, puffy hands, Raynaud's phenomenon, pulmonary hypertension arthritis that is sometimes erosive, and relative protection from renal disease characterize this syndrome.

Additionally, investigators have demonstrated that not only are certain autoantibodies linked with specific SLE phenotypes but also that some autoantibodies may cluster. Three autoantibody clusters were observed in the Hopkins Lupus Cohort: (1) Anti-Sm/anti-RNP, (2) Anti-dsDNA/anti-Ro/anti-La, and (3) Anti-dsDNA/LAC/aCL. The first presented with predominantly dermatologic manifestation and little organ involvement, while the third was associated with neurologic and thrombotic events.

SLE Incidence and Prevalence

Age, Sex, Race, and Ethnicity

SLE can present early or late in life though appears most commonly between 15 and 45 years of age. The female predominance in SLE is present across all ages; there is an approximate 2:1 female-to-male ratio before puberty and after menopause and a peak of 12:1 during childbearing years. Of these, the groups less commonly affected by SLE, including men and children, may have more severe disease, with more organ damage and requiring more intensive treatments. The reasons for these differences are largely unknown. Postmenopausal SLE in women, however, appears similar or slightly less severe than premenopausal disease.

Non-Caucasian populations in the USA, including African, Hispanic, Asian, and Native Americans, have higher incidences of SLE than do Caucasians. They also have younger ages at presentation, more severe disease, more rapid accrual of organ damage, and higher mortality rates.

Worldwide Epidemiology

Although likely underrecognized and underdiagnosed in developing countries, SLE does occur throughout the world. Recent studies examined the worldwide epidemiology of SLE over the past half century using two different approaches (Fig. 1.1). Although direct comparisons are complicated by differing designs, SLE appears to be more common in non-Caucasian racial groups. For instance, in the UK, Asian and African-Caribbean residents had higher incidence rates, while in Australia and New Zealand, Aboriginal populations had higher prevalence and occurrence compared to the Caucasians. In North America, the lowest incidences of SLE were seen among Caucasian Americans, Canadians, and Hispanics with incidences of 1.4, 1.6, and 2.2 cases per 100,000 persons per year, respectively. Similar patterns were observed with the prevalence studies, but no clear North–South or East–West pattern emerged in North America. Racial and genetic differences, as well as more complex social factors related to poverty and healthcare, are likely associated with SLE detection, a factor without which incidence and prevalence cannot be accurately determined.

A "prevalence gradient" between sub-Saharan Africa, where SLE prevalence is reportedly low, and Western countries, such as the USA and Canada, where similar

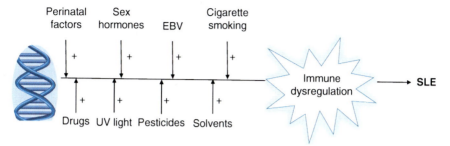

Fig. 1.1 Genes and the environment in the pathogenesis of SLE

populations have more disease, has been reported. Such a gradient could suggest the possibility of genetic admixture or nongenetic/environmental factors in Western countries to increase the risk of SLE. Alternative explanations may also explain the finding of a prevalence gradient, including competing causes of morbidity and mortality in Africa, and the lack of accurate diagnosis and treatment of SLE in Africa. Some studies suggest that SLE is in fact not rarer in Africa.

Risk Factors for SLE

A complex interplay between genetic and environmental factors likely underlies the development of SLE. Genetic factors are thought to predispose to loss of self-tolerance and autoimmunity among individuals after exposure to endogenous or exogenous influences (Fig. 1.2). Epidemiologic studies have sought to identify the factors that might trigger or increase the risk of SLE. Often these investigations compare groups of SLE patients with controls or look at the risk of disease associated with an exposure in a large population. In doing so, much of the published work presents results as relative risk measures. It is important to bear in mind that even a fivefold higher risk can still be a quite small absolute risk as the risk of developing SLE is small.

Hormonal/Reproductive Factors

Endogenous and exogenous hormones have been and continue to be scrutinized in relationship to risk of SLE. Both male and female SLE patients have demonstrated abnormal sex steroid metabolism, but this may be a consequence, rather than a cause, of their disease. Compared to controls, women with SLE have lower androgen (testosterone and DHEA-s) levels and higher estradiol and prolactin levels. Both oral contraceptive and postmenopausal hormone use have been statistically

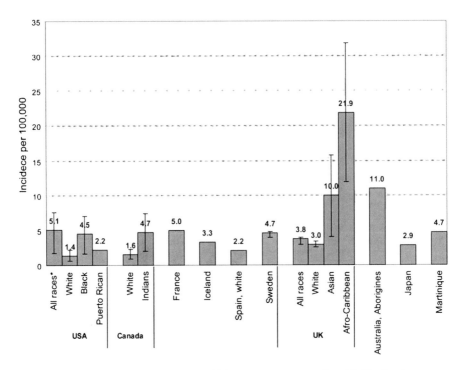

Fig. 1.2 Incidence of SLE around the world from a recent report. *Asterisk*: Total estimates are higher than race specific since former are estimated by more recent studies. *Note*: Median value presented if more than one source is available. The error bars show a range of values reported in different studies and/or in different study years within a single study (Danchenko N, Satia JA, Anthony MS. Epidemiology of systemic lupus erythematosus: a comparison of worldwide disease burden. Lupus 2006;15(5):308–18. Needs copyright release)

significantly associated with increased SLE incidence among women. Moreover, early menarche (≤10 years old) has been identified as increasing SLE risk in some, but not all, studies. It is also unclear from past studies whether either menstrual irregularity or history of breastfeeding is clearly related to risk of developing SLE. Some posit that sex hormones may be modulators of disease expression, but not necessarily causative agents. There may be other important sex-related factors, other than hormones, explaining the predominance of female patients. X-inactivation may play a role in determining disease susceptibility or disease severity.

Early Life Factors

Perinatal exposures may have influences on the developing immune system, thereby influencing the risk of autoimmune disease later in life. Preterm birth and high birth weight have both been associated with small increased risks of SLE among women. These findings have not been yet confirmed. Early exposure to cigarette smoking in utero and in early childhood was not associated with SLE developing in adult females.

Cigarette Smoking

A meta-analysis of past cohort and case–control studies in 2004 suggested that the risk of SLE was significantly 50% increased among current cigarette smokers in comparison to the risk among never smokers. A dose–response relationship has been suggested but not confirmed in all studies. Methodological differences pertaining to who was included in the study, what data were collected, and how exposures were defined may account for some of the discrepant results. A significantly higher rate of anti-dsDNA antibody seropositivity was observed in current smokers compared to nonsmokers in a California lupus cohort, and a statistically significant interaction between cigarette smoking and N-acetyltransferase-2 (NAT-2) slow acetylator genotype has been found in Japanese SLE patients with the odds of SLE increased by over six times. Two recent North American studies have not shown any relationships between cigarette smoking and risk of SLE, however.

Alcohol

Alcohol consumption appears to be inversely associated with risk of SLE. However, it is still not clear whether the early onset of constitutional symptoms could lead to a decrease in alcohol intake prior to disease diagnosis, leading to a spurious association, or whether there is another biologic mechanism underlying this finding.

Environmental Contaminants

Recreational and occupational exposures to petroleum distillates, trichloroethylene and organochlorines, have been associated with increased risk of undifferentiated connective tissue disease and SLE symptoms, although conclusive evidence of an association between trichloroethylene and SLE in humans is still lacking. In the Carolina Lupus Study, occupational exposure to mercury, in particular among dental workers (as dental amalgams contain mercury), was associated with over three times the odds of developing SLE. No epidemiologic research has addressed potential increased risk associated with synthetic chemical exposures such as plasticizers (e.g., phthalates and bisphenol A).

Pesticides

Residential and agricultural exposures to pesticides have been linked to doubling of the risk of developing SLE in the Carolina Lupus Study and the Women's Health Initiative (WHI) Cohort Study. In the WHI Study, a fairly strong dose–response was detected as well. In the highest categories of exposure, the hazard ratio was over twice as high for those who reported a personal application of pesticides/

insecticides in their homes for more than six times a year or for more than 20 years.

Crystalline Silica

The epidemiologic evidence points to a statistically significantly elevated risk of developing SLE associated with crystalline silica from a variety of sources. The Carolina Lupus Study, a case–control study of SLE patients and randomly selected controls from the US South, found an increased odds of SLE associated with silica exposure, mainly through agricultural/soil and dusty trade exposures. Using similar exposure assessment methods, but in an urban environment where exposures to silica included construction work and sandblasting, a similar dose–response relationship was observed in a predominantly African-American community outreach study in Boston. Strong dose effects were observed in both of these case–control studies: high level of exposure of greater than 5 years duration was associated with a greater than fivefold elevated risk. The association between silica and increased relative risk of SLE was further confirmed in a recent Canadian study in which a dose–response was again observed with a greater than double risk of SLE among those in the highest exposure category.

Solvents

Epidemiologic data on the possible role of solvents in the development of SLE have been conflicting. No association between SLE and the use of solvents was seen in the Carolina Lupus Study, and a suggested, but not significant, increased risk was observed in the Roxbury Community Lupus Study. However, in a recent Canadian case–control study, with work applying nail polishes and work with paints, dyes, or film developing, all implying solvent exposures, an increased relative risk of SLE was observed.

Breast Implants, Hair Dyes, and Lipstick

Despite speculations of silicone breast implants as triggers of SLE, the association between silicone breast implants and SLE has not been confirmed. Furthermore, use of permanent hair dyes has also not been consistently associated with SLE. Lipstick use was associated with increased risk of SLE in an Internet-based case–control study and has been hypothesized to explain some of the female preponderance of the disease.

Socioeconomic Position

Low socioeconomic position is associated with increased incidence, severity, and mortality in SLE. Socioeconomic position likely incorporates several different risk factors such as poverty, lack of education, nonadherence to medical care, environmental exposures, and lack of social support. In addition to poverty, low education, and lack of social support, Hispanic and African-American ancestry were significant predictors of poor outcomes and disease progression.

Nutritional Factors

Lower levels of antioxidants and vitamin D have been found among individuals with SLE, but this may be driven by active inflammation, corticosteroid use, decreased intake, frailty, lack of sun exposure, and use of sun screens. Patients with SLE are frequently advised to avoid sun exposure, a common source of vitamin D. No protective effect of increased vitamin D or antioxidant vitamin intake from foods or supplements was found when looking at incident disease in the large prospective Nurses' Health Study cohorts. As far as food chemicals or additives, which are reported as risk factors of autoimmune diseases in the popular press, case reports and animal studies have linked tartrazine and L-canavanine in alfalfa sprouts to the induction of SLE. Bengtsson and colleagues investigated a large number of potential exposures in relation to risk of SLE in a case–control study in Sweden and found no association between ingestion of alfalfa sprouts (which contain L-canavanine) and SLE risk. To date, however, no other epidemiologic studies investigating associations of any food chemicals, dyes, or additives with risk of developing SLE have been performed.

Epstein–Barr Virus

The association between Epstein–Barr virus (EBV) and SLE has been shown repeatedly. Titers of EBV-specific anti-EBNA-1 and anti-VCA antibody titers were significantly higher in patients with SLE than in healthy controls. In one study, titers rose gradually from their first detectable levels years prior to the first symptoms of SLE until the time of diagnosis of SLE, paralleling, and in some cases preceding, the development of SLE-specific antibodies, implicating EBV-specific immune responses in the pathogenesis of SLE.

Immunizations

The association between immunization and incident SLE is not known, although some case reports and series have suggested links with various vaccinations. Much of the published literature has focused on vaccination safety and effectiveness in SLE patients.

Ultraviolet Light

UV light and radiation exist in three forms: UV-A (315–400 nm, long wave), UV-B (280–315 nm, medium wave), and UV-C (<280 nm, short wave). At least one serious sunburn before age 20 and sunburn-susceptible skin type have been associated with increased risk of SLE. Another study using cumulative months of occupational sunlight exposure as a proxy for past UV exposure found no association with the risk of SLE overall but did find an increased risk among the subset who had the glutathione-*S*-transferase (GST)-MI null homozygous genotype, suggesting a gene–environment interaction. Another recent case–control study of SLE risk factors in Canada confirmed an association between outside work, in particular among those with a history of blistering sunburns or rashes, and increased risk of SLE. In the last study, however, 9 years had elapsed between diagnosis and data collection, potentially leading to some recall bias, and cases may have been reporting SLE-related photosensitivity that predated their SLE diagnosis.

SLE Disease Activity/Flare

UV radiation, immunizations, pregnancy, physical and psychological stress, and infections have been associated with increases in SLE disease activity in some studies. UV radiation causes keratinocyte apoptosis that is normally cleared within 2 days of sunburn; in patients with SLE, the abnormal immune response may trigger photosensitive rashes and systemic symptoms. In a large randomized trial, oral contraceptive use was not associated with increased SLE disease activity among patients with stable, low-activity disease and no antiphospholipid antibodies. Because of the heterogeneous and dynamic nature of SLE, these studies are challenging to perform, and we do not have good epidemiologic evidence about the triggers of SLE flares.

Conclusions

SLE is a heterogeneous disease with a large variety of presentations and manifestations, complicating classification and epidemiologic research. Although women of childbearing age are most affected by SLE, SLE may present throughout the lifespan. Disease may be more severe among children and men. Ethnic and socioeconomic factors affect the incidence, prevalence, and severity of SLE with all non-Caucasian groups having higher incidence. Several environmental exposures, including crystalline silica, solvents, pesticides, female hormones, cigarette smoking, ultraviolet light, and EBV infection, have been associated with statistically significant increased relative risks of developing SLE. Identifying the interactions between these environmental risk factors and specific risk genotypes in determining susceptibility to autoimmune disease, to SLE, and to specific disease phenotypes is an important avenue for future research.

Sources

1. Hochberg MC. Updating the American College of Rheumatology revised criteria for the classification of systemic lupus erythematosus. Arthritis Rheum. 1997;40(9):1725.
2. Tan EM, Cohen AS, Fries JF, Masi AT, McShane DJ, Rothfield NF, Schaller JG, Talal N, Winchester RJ. The 1982 revised criteria for the classification of systemic lupus erythematosus. Arthritis Rheum. 1982;25(11):1271–7.
3. Costenbader KH, Karlson EW, Mandl LA. Defining lupus cases for clinical studies: the Boston weighted criteria for the classification of systemic lupus erythematosus. J Rheumatol. 2002;29(12):2545–50.
4. Petri M. Review of classification criteria for systemic lupus erythematosus. Rheum Dis Clin North Am. 2005;31(2):245–54. vi.
5. To CH, Petri M. Is antibody clustering predictive of clinical subsets and damage in systemic lupus erythematosus? Arthritis Rheum. 2005;52(12):4003–10.
6. Brunner HI, Gladman DD, Ibanez D, Urowitz MD, Silverman ED. Difference in disease features between childhood-onset and adult-onset systemic lupus erythematosus. Arthritis Rheum. 2008;58(2):556–62.
7. Tucker LB, Uribe AG, Fernandez M, Vila LM, McGwin G, Apte M, Fessler BJ, Bastian HM, Reveille JD, Alarcon GS. Adolescent onset of lupus results in more aggressive disease and worse outcomes: results of a nested matched case-control study within LUMINA, a multiethnic US cohort (LUMINA LVII). Lupus. 2008;17(4):314–22.
8. Sanchez-Guerrero J, Villegas A, Mendoza-Fuentes A, Romero-Diaz J, Moreno-Coutino G, Cravioto MC. Disease activity during the premenopausal and postmenopausal periods in women with systemic lupus erythematosus. Am J Med. 2001;111(6):464–8.
9. McCarty DJ, Manzi S, Medsger Jr TA, Ramsey-Goldman R, LaPorte RE, Kwoh CK. Incidence of systemic lupus erythematosus. Race and gender differences. Arthritis Rheum. 1995;38(9):1260–70.
10. Alarcon GS, Friedman AW, Straaton KV, Moulds JM, Lisse J, Bastian HM, McGwin G, Jr., Bartolucci AA, Roseman JM, Reveille JD. Systemic lupus erythematosus in three ethnic groups: III. A comparison of characteristics early in the natural history of the LUMINA cohort. LUpus in MInority populations: NAture vs. Nurture. Lupus. 1999;8(3):197–209.
11. Vasudevan A, Krishnamurthy AN. Changing worldwide epidemiology of systemic lupus erythematosus. Rheum Dis Clin North Am. 2010;36(1):1–13. vii.
12. Danchenko N, Satia JA, Anthony MS. Epidemiology of systemic lupus erythematosus: a comparison of worldwide disease burden. Lupus. 2006;15(5):308–18.
13. Bae SC, Fraser P, Liang MH. The epidemiology of systemic lupus erythematosus in populations of African ancestry: a critical review of the "prevalence gradient hypothesis". Arthritis Rheum. 1998;41(12):2091–9.
14. Costenbader KH, Feskanich D, Stampfer MJ, Karlson EW. Reproductive and menopausal factors and risk of systemic lupus erythematosus in women. Arthritis Rheum. 2007;56(4):1251–62.
15. Bernier MO, Mikaeloff Y, Hudson M, Suissa S. Combined oral contraceptive use and the risk of systemic lupus erythematosus. Arthritis Rheum. 2009;61(4):476–81.
16. Costenbader KH, Kim DJ, Peerzada J, Lockman S, Nobles-Knight D, Petri M, Karlson EW. Cigarette smoking and the risk of systemic lupus erythematosus: a meta-analysis. Arthritis Rheum. 2004;50:849–57.
17. Cooper GS, Dooley MA, Treadwell EL, St Clair EW, Gilkeson GS. Smoking and use of hair treatments in relation to risk of developing systemic lupus erythematosus. J Rheumatol. 2001;28(12):2653–6.
18. Cooper GS, Wither J, Bernatsky S, Claudio JO, Clarke A, Rioux JD, Fortin PR. Occupational and environmental exposures and risk of systemic lupus erythematosus: silica, sunlight, solvents. Rheumatology. 2010;49(11):2172–80.

19. Parks CG, Walitt BT, Pettinger M, Chen JC, De Roos AJ, Hunt J, Sarto G, Howard BV. Insecticide use and risk of rheumatoid arthritis and systemic lupus erythematosus in the women's health initiative observational study. Arth Care Res. 2011;63(2):184–94.
20. Parks CG, Cooper GS, Nylander-French LA, Sanderson WT, Dement JM, Cohen PL, Dooley MA, Treadwell EL, St Clair EW, Gilkeson GS, Hoppin JA, Savitz DA. Occupational exposure to crystalline silica and risk of systemic lupus erythematosus: a population-based, case-control study in the southeastern United States. Arthritis Rheum. 2002;46(7):1840–50.
21. Finckh A, Cooper GS, Chibnik LB, Costenbader KH, Fraser PA, Watts J, Pankey H, Karlson EW. Occupational silica and solvent exposures and risk of systemic lupus erythematosus in urban women. Arthritis Rheum. 2006;54(11):3648–54.
22. Sanchez-Guerrero J, Karlson EW, Colditz GA, Hunter DJ, Speizer FE, Liang MH. Hair dye use and the risk of developing systemic lupus erythematosus. Arthritis Rheum. 1996;39(4):657–62.
23. Sutcliffe N, Clarke AE, Gordon C, Farewell V, Isenberg DA. The association of socio-economic status, race, psychosocial factors and outcome in patients with systemic lupus erythematosus. Rheumatology (Oxford). 1999;38(11):1130–7.
24. Duran S, Apte M, Alarcon GS. Poverty, not ethnicity, accounts for the differential mortality rates among lupus patients of various ethnic groups. J Natl Med Assoc. 2007;99(10):1196–8.
25. Costenbader KH, Feskanich D, Holmes M, Karlson EW, Benito-Garcia E. Vitamin D intake and risks of systemic lupus erythematosus and rheumatoid arthritis in women. Ann Rheum Dis. 2008;67(4):530–5.
26. Costenbader KH, Kang JH, Karlson EW. Antioxidant intake and risks of rheumatoid arthritis and systemic lupus erythematosus in women. Am J Epidemiol. 2010;172(2):205–16.
27. Bengtsson AA, Rylander L, Hagmar L, Nived O, Sturfelt G. Risk factors for developing systemic lupus erythematosus: a case-control study in southern Sweden. Rheumatology (Oxford). 2002;41(5):563–71.
28. James JA, Neas BR, Moser KL, Hall T, Bruner GR, Sestak AL, Harley JB. Systemic lupus erythematosus in adults is associated with previous Epstein-Barr virus exposure. Arthritis Rheum. 2001;44(5):1122–6.
29. Peralta-Ramirez MI, Jimenez-Alonso J, Godoy-Garcia JF, Perez-Garcia M. The effects of daily stress and stressful life events on the clinical symptomatology of patients with lupus erythematosus. Psychosom Med. 2004;66(5):788–94.
30. Buyon JP, Petri MA, Kim MY, Kalunian KC, Grossman J, Hahn BH, Merrill JT, Sammaritano L, Lockshin M, Alarcon GS, Manzi S, Belmont HM, Askanase AD, Sigler L, Dooley MA, Von Feldt J, McCune WJ, Friedman A, Wachs J, Cronin M, Hearth-Holmes M, Tan M, Licciardi F. The effect of combined estrogen and progesterone hormone replacement therapy on disease activity in systemic lupus erythematosus: a randomized trial. Ann Intern Med. 2005;142 (12 Pt 1):953–62.

Chapter 2
The Immunopathogenesis and Immunopathology of Systemic Lupus Erythematosus

David S. Pisetsky

Systemic lupus erythematosus (SLE) is a prototypic autoimmune disease characterized by autoantibody production in association with systemic inflammatory manifestations that vary in pattern and severity. This disease occurs primarily in young women, with a peak incidence during the childbearing years suggesting an important influence of sex on disease pathogenesis. Like most autoimmune diseases, lupus results from the interplay of genetic and environmental factors which together promote immune hyperactivity. While the precise environmental triggers for lupus are unknown, these factors likely induce changes in both the innate and adaptive arms of immune system as well as initiate or potentiate the production autoantibodies to components of the cell nucleus. These autoantibodies (antinuclear antibodies or ANAs) are directed to proteins, nucleic acids, and protein–nucleic acid complexes and represent the serological hallmark of SLE.

While the pathogenesis of SLE has elements in common with other autoimmune diseases, studies on human lupus as well as mouse models of this disease have established a strong conceptual and experimental framework to understand the generation of ANAs as well as the mechanisms for tissue inflammation and damage. Key to this framework is the recognition that the nuclear macromolecules that are the target of ANA reactivity have potent immunological activities that can promote both underlying immune disturbances and tissue injury. Indeed, the immunological activities of these target antigens may distinguish SLE from other autoimmune diseases (whose target antigens lack intrinsic immune activity) and account for its characteristic clinical features as well as the response to therapy.

D.S. Pisetsky, M.D., Ph.D. (✉)
Department of Medicine and Immunology, Duke University Medical Center, Durham, NC, USA

Medical Research Service, Durham VA Hospital, 151G Durham VAMC,
508 Fulton Street, Durham, NC 27705, USA
e-mail: dpiset@acpub.duke.edu

For lupus, like other autoimmune diseases, current models of pathogenesis posit that disease arises in a genetically susceptible individual in whom a propensity to autoreactivity is triggered by an environment agent. This event in turn initiates a cascade of B and T cell disturbances that lead to autoantibody production. For SLE, the consequences of autoantibody production are amplified by the formation of immune complexes that have pro-inflammatory properties that reflect the intrinsic immune activity of their component antigens. Thus, understanding the immunopathogenesis of SLE requires consideration of the determinants of susceptibility, the nature of the underlying immune disturbances, the properties of autoantibodies, and the role of immune complexes in pathology.

Determinants of Disease Susceptibility

One of the most notable features of SLE is its striking occurrence in women. Thus, depending on the study, SLE is 5–10 times more common in females compared to males and, furthermore, has a peak incidence during their childbearing years. Since the incidence of disease is more similar between males and females before puberty and after menopause in women, these findings suggest an important role for sex hormones in creating a susceptibility to autoreactivity. This susceptibility extends to many autoimmune diseases, suggesting a general influence of female sex on immune regulation.

While the female preponderance of lupus has long been recognized, little is known about the precise effects of hormones on the immune system. The susceptibility of women to autoimmunity, however, has been linked to aspects of the immune system regulation related to pregnancy. Pregnancy represents an extraordinary immune challenge since a woman bearing a child must accept what is in essence a foreign tissue graft for 9 months. No doubt there are many modifications in the immune system necessary to accommodate the fetus that bears a set of histocompatibility antigens from the father. While these modifications would be expected to lead to immune suppression during pregnancy, they may actually modulate immune cell function to increase, rather than decrease, immune responsiveness.

Estrogen and progesterone have diverse effects on various cells of the innate and adaptive immune systems. In terms of B cells, these actions can affect fundamental events in the establishment of tolerance, skewing the antibody repertoire to increase ANA generation. Hormones can also affect T cells and macrophage function, for example, although hormonal effects may not be the only influence conferred by sex. Thus, differences in the expression of genes on X and Y chromosomes as well as the number of X chromosomes may also determine the tendency to autoreactivity. Since manipulation of sex hormones, including androgens, can modify disease in murine models, direct effects of these mediators appear important.

As shown in both family studies and population-based genome-wide association studies (GWAS), genetic factors have a powerful influence on disease susceptibility. Thus, SLE shows a high concordance among identical twins and occurs at increased frequencies among first-degree relatives; furthermore, in extended family pedigrees, SLE may occur along with other autoimmune diseases such as rheumatoid arthritis or thyroiditis. These findings suggest an inheritable tendency toward autoreactivity that may be shaped by either other inherited factors or environmental exposures to induce a specific pattern of disease.

Building upon studies of family as well as candidate gene approaches, GWAS analyses have now identified over 30 different loci that contribute to disease susceptibility in lupus. These genes include HLA-DRB1, IRF5, STAT4, BLK, and ITGAM among many other. While identifying loci with susceptibility alleles, in general, these studies diseases have not yet defined the actual gene involved or the functional changes conferred by a polymorphism. Even for genes whose link to disease seems compelling, the relationship to pathogenesis is nevertheless speculative and will require extensive deep sequencing as well as functional studies to clarify the effect on immune system.

From these studies, certain conclusions about the genetics of lupus are possible. Thus, lupus appears to be a multigenic disease, with the contribution of each locus to susceptibility limited. Whether the risk to disease is additive or synergistic is not known although abnormalities affecting different arms of the immune systems seem necessary to create a tendency to autoreactivity. Significant heterogeneity in the genetic substrate in disease is therefore likely especially if disease susceptibility involves a threshold effect in which a certain number of susceptibility alleles need to be present. This situation suggests that screening for genetic risk factors will be difficult especially if disease is also influenced by private variants that are not detected by current GWAS technique.

The genetic analysis of lupus suggests possible mechanisms by which inherited factors influence pathogenesis. Thus, gene variants thus far identified appear to influence elements of the immune system related to both the induction of immune responses and inflammation. With respect to B and T cells, the effects of these variants could occur at key steps in immune activation affecting the establishment of central or peripheral tolerance as well as the triggering of cellular responses during disease. Other polymorphisms could influence the function of neutrophils and their role in inflammation. Finally, as suggested by studies on complement genes, variation in copy numbers could affect the overall capacity to clear foreign or self-antigen that could trigger immune responses.

Studies on genetics of lupus in mouse models in general preceded the work on human disease. Murine studies have been of two major types. The first involves detailed dissection of the genetics of an inbred lupus strain such as the (NZB/NZW) hybrid or the NZM2410 inbred strain. The second type is the development and characterization of a knockout or transgenic strain with a lupus phenotype. In general, these genetic models have indicated that a multitude of disturbances of B and/or T cell function can lead to lupus although other genes in the strain background can influence the severity of disease. These studies have also demonstrated a role for genes encoding complement and other proteins (e.g., SAA) involved in the clearance of microorganisms or cellular debris in creating a predisposition to autoimmunity.

The studies on the lupus models have been informative in showing that lupus is multigenic, with the clinical outcome reflecting a summation of positive and negative influences. These genes can regulate the function of B and T cells. While a single locus can lead to serological disturbance, the development of a full-blown lupus syndrome (i.e., nephritis) requires the presence of more than one locus. Interestingly, among loci identified, a gene for interferon response is important in the NZB/NZW hybrid, while, in the BXSB mouse, duplication in the gene encoding TLR7, the toll receptor that recognizes single-stranded RNA, is important for the development of a Y-linked lupus illness. Both interferon and toll-like receptor (TLR) systems appear important in human lupus, suggesting similarity in pathogenetic mechanisms among species.

Serological Disturbances in Lupus

ANA production is a defining immunological disturbance in both human and murine disease. While patients with lupus produce over 100 different autoantibodies, certain specificities have diagnostic and prognostic significance and are associated with particular disease manifestations. Regarding ANA, two specificities represent criteria in the classification of patients with SLE: anti-DNA and anti-Sm. DNA is deoxyribonucleic acid, a polymeric macromolecule that encodes genetic information. Sm (or Smith antigen) is a complex of uridine-rich RNA molecules in association with a series of proteins to which the antibodies are directed. Sm and the related molecular complex called RNP play important roles in RNA processing. While antibodies to RNP occur commonly in SLE, often in association with anti-Sm, they have a wider distribution among other rheumatological disorders and do not have status as classification criteria.

While DNA displays a potentially enormous array of antigenic determinants corresponding to base sequence, antibodies in SLE patient sera predominantly bind conformational determinants on the DNA backbone, either double-stranded (ds) or single-stranded (ss) structure. These backbone structures are highly conserved and occur widely on DNA independent of species origin or basic composition. While, by definition, anti-DNA antibodies are autoantibodies, they are not specific for human (self) DNA since they also react with foreign DNA. These antibodies display high affinity for DNA, likely reflecting the interaction of each Fab binding site with a determinant along an extended polymeric structure. This type of interaction is termed monogamous or bivalent. Anti-dsDNA and anti-ssDNA antibodies commonly coexist in patient sera because many antibodies can bind both ss- and dsDNA. Nevertheless, anti-dsDNA directed to the B conformation of the DNA helix occurs almost exclusively in SLE; anti-ssDNA can occur in other clinical settings.

While anti-DNA can be analyzed by using biochemically and purified DNA, these antibodies are part of a spectrum of specificities that bind to chromatin, the form of DNA in the cell nucleus. In chromatin, DNA is wrapped around a core of histones to form nucleosomes which are the essential building block for chromatin

Table 2.1 Properties of anti-DNA autoantibodies

Subset of antibodies to nucleosomes
Bind conserved sites on single- and double-stranded DNA backbone
Monogamous or bivalent interaction
Can form pathogenic immune complexes
Levels can vary with disease activity

structure and are likely the source of antigenically active DNA. Consistent with a role of DNA as a component or epitope of a larger antigenic structure, anti-DNA antibodies appear commonly in association with antibodies to nucleosomes and histones. These responses are all closely linked, allowing anti-DNA to be studied as a representative of a large antibody family.

The expression of anti-DNA occurs in approximately 30–70 % of patients at some time during the course of their disease but shows marked variability in levels. Anti-DNA levels can rise and fall in association with disease activity, in particular, glomerulonephritis. These fluctuations, which underlie anti-DNA as a measure of disease activity, are a distinctive feature of this response that is not observed commonly with other autoantibody responses. These fluctuations also indicate sensitivity of antibody expression to agents such as glucocorticoids or cyclophosphamide, which, when used to treat flares, can reduce and even eliminate anti-DNA production. Table 2.1 summarizes properties of anti-DNA antibodies.

In contrast to anti-DNA, anti-Sm antibodies bind to proteins even though the Sm antigen has both protein and RNA components. Unlike levels of anti-DNA, levels of anti-Sm (and anti-RNP) tend to be stable during the course of disease, limiting delineation of an association with disease manifestations. Furthermore, in the USA, anti-Sm antibodies have a higher expression in African-Americans than European-Americans; while linked to anti-RNP, anti-Sm is expressed independently of anti-DNA. These features suggest that anti-DNA and anti-Sm antibodies result from different underlying immune disturbances that culminate ultimately in their distribution among B cell subsets, including long-lived plasma cells.

Other autoantibodies found in SLE have diverse antigenic targets and potential roles in disease. Thus, antibodies to the Ro and La antigens bind RNA–protein complexes and occur in SLE as well as Sjogren's syndrome and rheumatoid arthritis; in the context of SLE, anti-Ro and anti-La antibodies are associated with the neonatal lupus syndrome including congenital heart block, as well as subacute cutaneous lupus. Like anti-Sm and anti-RNP, anti-Ro and anti-La are linked.

Another important group of autoantibodies has been identified as lupus anticoagulants and includes antibodies to phospholipids and the lipid-binding protein β2-glycoprotein 1. These antibodies occur prominently in patients with the antiphospholipid syndrome (APS) which is characterized by venous and arterial thrombosis, pregnancy loss, and thrombocytopenia; in this syndrome, antibodies may promote clotting disturbances by their in vivo interaction with clotting factors or endothelial cells. Finally, among antibodies with a potential role in pathogenesis, antibodies to the NMDA receptor, which can cross-react with DNA, have been

Table 2.2 Clinical associations of SLE autoantibodies

Anti-DNA and nephritis
Anti-Ro and neonatal lupus and subacute cutaneous LE and photosensitivity
Anti-ribosomal P and CNS lupus
Anti-RNP and Raynaud's
Antibodies to phospholipids and clotting
?Anti-NMDA antibodies and cognitive dysfunction

implicated in CNS on the basis of studies in mouse models. While the data in the murine models indicate that such antibodies can induce behavioral and cognitive disturbances, the complexity of neuropsychological manifestations of patients has limited determination of the role of these antibodies in human lupus. Table 2.2 summarizes clinical association of selected lupus autoantibodies.

The Induction of ANA

The most striking feature of SLE autoantibody production relates to the targeting of nucleic acids or nucleic acid-containing complexes, which are highly conserved molecules key to essential cell functions such as replication, transcription, and translation. Furthermore, as a group, the nuclear antigens targeted in SLE display features which may be relevant to ANA induction: (1) these molecules can have intrinsic immunological activity; (2) the intracellular location of these molecules is dynamic and can vary depending on the state of the cell, including extracellular translocation; and (3) as conserved molecules, nuclear antigens bear determinants that can displayed by foreign versions of the same molecule or a foreign molecule that is structurally and functionally similar. As such, induction of ANA responses by the mechanism of molecular mimicry may be particularly likely. Of note, intrinsic immune disturbances in patients may predispose to molecular mimicry and the generation of cross-reactive antibodies with autoantibody activity.

The expression of ANA can be divided to three stages: antibody induction, antibody maintenance, and antibody reduction of elimination. Importantly, in current models for pathogenesis, the antigens involved in the first two stages may not be the same. Indeed, there is evidence that bacterial and viral antigens can induce ANA production while self molecules may mediate antibody maintenance. The stage of antibody elimination and reduction usually occurs in response to immunosuppressive therapy; since agents used for this purpose have broad immunomodulatory (and even cytotoxic activity), antibody elimination may be nonspecific and not directly involve a role of antigen in stimulating a regulatory response.

As shown in both patients and animal models, the production of antibodies to RNA-binding proteins (RBPs) (e.g., Sm, RNP, Ro, and La) may differ mechanistically from the production of antibodies to DNA. Thus, antibodies to RBPs may temporally precede those to DNA in humans and may evolve from cross-reactions to foreign responses such as proteins in the Epstein–Barr virus, which can bear sequences similar to those in the RBP. Furthermore, immunization of normal mice with such EBV antigens can lead to generation of autoantibodies as well as the spreading of the response to other self-antigens, including DNA. In contrast, in spontaneous autoimmune mice, the expression of anti-RBP antibodies is much less common than anti-DNA expression, which is essentially universal in murine lupus.

The induction of antibodies to DNA, while a feature of spontaneous autoimmune disease, is much more difficult to replicate by immunization of normal animals. Even if dsDNA is coupled to an immunogenic protein and presented in an adjuvant, immunization of normal mice leads to very limited antibody production. This finding initially suggested that DNA is immunologically weak or inert and that anti-DNA production arises by a mechanism other than direct DNA immunization. Such an alternative mechanism could be either polyclonal activation or molecular mimicry.

While usual models for molecular mimicry for anti-DNA production implicate foreign proteins as the inducing molecule, foreign DNA can serve that function. As shown in studies in vitro and in vivo, DNA is not uniform in its immunological properties, with viral and foreign DNA demonstrating potent immunostimulatory properties. This stimulation arises from interaction of DNA with toll-like receptor 9 (TLR9) as well as other non-TLR internal nucleic acid sensors. These sensors are likely important elements of the innate immune system and serve as pattern recognition receptors (PRR) that respond to foreign molecules termed PAMPs for pathogen-associated molecular patterns.

For bacterial DNA, key determinants of stimulation of TLR9 result from short DNA sequences that center on unmethylated cytosine-guanosine dinucleotide repeats (CpG motifs). These motifs occur much more commonly in bacterial than mammalian DNA because of differences in the pattern of base methylation and a phenomenon known as CpG suppression. Because of CpG suppression, the CpG dinucleotide occurs much less commonly in mammalian DNA than would be predicted on the basis of the base sequence. The combination of base methylation and CpG suppression leads to a PAMP structure that can stimulate TLR9. Stimulation of non-TLR sensors may reflect the intracellular localization of DNA as opposed to a unique structural element, with access to these sensors occurring during infection with viruses or bacteria.

Even though anti-DNA antibodies are considered essentially unique to lupus, anti-DNA production also occurs in normal individuals, with levels approaching those found in patients with lupus. The antibodies in normal individuals, however, differ markedly from those in SLE with respect to specificity and immunochemical properties. Thus, antibodies in normal individuals bind with high selectivity to DNA from particular bacterial species but do not cross-react with either mammalian DNA or other bacterial DNA. These antibodies predominantly bear the IgG2 isotype and κ light chain, whereas anti-DNA antibodies in patients with lupus are predominantly IgG1 and IgG3 and have a more equivalent expression of κ and λ. Table 2.3 describes properties of anti-DNA antibodies in normal human subjects.

The development of antibodies to foreign DNA occurs with DNA from certain bacteria or viruses and does not occur with DNA from *E. coli*, for example; the high

Table 2.3 Properties of anti-DNA in normal subjects

Bind to non-conserved sites on bacterial and DNA
High affinity
IgG2 predominance
κ light chain restriction
Inducible in normal mice by immunization

specificity of these antibodies for DNA from particular species likely accounts for the previous failure to detect this type of anti-DNA antibodies in many studies. The rules for the antigenicity of bacterial and viral DNA are not known although the type of exposure (e.g., infection vs. colonization or location such as skin vs. lung) may influence antibody production. Whatever the basis of this response, the generation of antibodies to foreign DNA may occur because bacterial and viral DNA is immunostimulatory and has sequential determinants not present in mammalian DNA.

In the context of lupus, the immunogenicity of bacterial or viral DNA provides a mechanism for the induction of anti-DNA antibodies that has analogy to the induction of anti-RBP antibodies. Thus, in patients with lupus, bacterial DNA, rather than inducing antibodies to non-conserved sequential determinants, may stimulate a cross-reactive response to conserved backbone determinants shared by bacterial and mammalian DNA; viral DNA may play a similar role. These cross-reactive antibodies would have autoreactivity even if the inducing antigen was foreign nucleic acid. Furthermore, deficient expression in lupus of the normal IgG2 response to bacterial DNA may promote the cross-reactive response because of more prolonged exposure to bacterial DNA and persistent immune stimulation.

Studies in mice support this possibility and demonstrate differences in the immune recognition of DNA in normal and autoimmune animals which likely have a counterpart in patients. Whereas immunization of normal and autoimmune mice with mammalian DNA (as protein complexes in complete Freund's adjuvant) fails to induce an anti-DNA response, immunization with bacterial DNA induces a significant anti-DNA production. In normal mice, the induced antibodies are specific for bacterial DNA, while in autoimmune NZB/NZW mice, the induced antibodies cross-react with both bacterial and mammalian DNA. These findings suggest that an autoimmune background may determine the pattern of antibody recognition of DNA, leading to antibodies to conformational rather than sequential determinants. Since recognition of conformational determinants can confer autoreactivity, an alteration in binding specificity may be key to development of SLE.

An interesting aspect of the immunization model concerns the differences in the response to bacterial and mammalian DNA, in particular, in the autoimmune NZB/NZW mice. These mice are destined to produce anti-DNA spontaneously as they age and can produce anti-DNA in response to immunization with bacterial DNA. Nevertheless, they do not produce anti-DNA in response to immunization with mammalian DNA. These findings suggest that self DNA is poorly immunogenic but that response can occur once tolerance is broken by immunization with a foreign molecule. Coupled with studies on response to protein antigens, these observations highlight the potential role of infection in initiating lupus. While exposure to bacterial and viral antigens may stimulate autoantibody production, self-antigen may underlie ongoing antibody production and affinity maturation.

Cellular Immune Disturbances

Studies on both murine and human SLE demonstrate phenotypic and functional abnormalities of B cells, T cells, macrophages, dendritic cells, and neutrophils among elements of the immune system. While these abnormalities may reflect primary disturbances which are genetically determined, others may be secondary to other events in lupus, in particular, cytokine production. Among these cytokines, type 1 interferon appears to have an important role in pathogenesis. As shown in studies of patients with lupus, peripheral blood cells display patterns of gene expression consistent with stimulation by type 1 interferon. This pattern, which can be demonstrated by either microarray analysis or PCR analysis of selected genes, is termed the interferon signature. An increase in interferon can also be demonstrated by the ability of patient serum to stimulate transcription of interferon responsive genes in cell lines.

The interferon signature may be important in pathogenesis since interferon can induce autoimmunity in patients treated for other diseases. Furthermore, genetic studies point to an etiological role of genes involved in the response to interferon. Interferon has multiple actions that can impact on immune cell function. In addition, interferon can also modulate endothelial cells, an important target tissue in lupus, and lead to vasculopathy. While the interferon signature is present in only some patients, its association with antibodies to RBPs and DNA suggests a mechanism by which these antibodies may promote immunological disturbance in SLE.

In a scenario in which anti-DNA and anti-RBP antibodies drive pathogenesis, a self-reinforcing cycle of autoantibody production leads to the formation of immune complexes which in turn drive interferon production to potentiate inflammation and antibody production. As shown in in vitro systems, antibodies to RBPs and DNA antigen can form immune complexes which stimulate interferon production by plasmacytoid dendritic cells (pDCs). This stimulation involves TLR and non-TLR sensors and occurs most likely because autoantibodies allow internalization of DNA and RNA to access the internal nucleic acid receptors; depending on intracellular location, DNA can become immunoactive and may not need CpG motifs to induce stimulation. Since nucleic acids originating from cells may be attached to nuclear proteins such as the high mobility group box 1 protein (HMGB1), the RAGE receptor (receptor for advanced glycation end products), which binds this protein, may also contribute to immune stimulation; HMGB1 also has immune activity and is a prototype for an alarmin or not of DAMP [a death (or damage)-associated molecular pattern] by analogy with a PAMP (pathogen-associated molecular pattern).

Evidence for the role of stimulatory complexes containing DNA and RNA comes from studies on the inhibitory effects of antagonists of TLR9 and TLR7, receptors for DNA, and single-stranded RNA, respectively, in both in vitro systems as well as lupus mice. Importantly, these mechanisms derive from the intrinsic immunostimulatory activity of DNA and RNA although the presence of these molecules in immune complexes is critical for the stimulation of the pDCs.

In addition to aberrant cytokine production, the pathogenesis of SLE involves intrinsic immune cell abnormalities that may alter, for example, thresholds for activation and signaling. The end result is aberrant tolerance among B and T cells, either peripherally or centrally. These abnormalities perturb the checkpoints for normal deletion or inactivation and can skew the respective repertoires to predispose to autoreactivity. In the B cell compartment, these repertoire disturbances are characterized by an increased number of autoantibody precursors that show broad reactivity among autoantigens including DNA. With an increase in autoantibody precursors in the pre-immune repertoire, stimulation by DNA or a cross-reactive antigen can induce anti-DNA in a way not possible with the ordinary pre-immune repertoire.

Once an autoantibody response is initiated among such precursors, affinity maturation occurs, with related members of clones showing the hallmark of antigen-driven selection in turns of somatic mutations. For anti-DNA antibodies, these mutations can lead to the presence of arginine and other positively charged amino acids to promote the binding of negatively charged DNA. While affinity maturation may occur in lupus, the outcome may differ from that of a conventional antibody response because of the distortion in the pre-immune repertoire, the adjuvant activity of the antigen, the presence of the antigen in a complex with other molecules (e.g., histones), and promiscuous T cell help. These processes could lead to the expression of antibodies that prefer conformational epitopes and display polyreactivity.

Consistent with ongoing immune stimulation, patients with lupus show an increase in the number of plasma cells in the peripheral blood. The level of these cells, which may result from germinal center activity, is dynamic and can correlate with disease activity. The role of plasma cells in autoantibody production is also important in terms of disease pathogenesis since these can be very long-lived cells and difficult to eliminate using current therapy including anti-B cell reagent such as anti-CD20. The presence of cytokines such as B cell activating factor (BAFF) can contribute to the activity of these cells.

The Role of Self-Antigen

For DNA and other nuclear autoantigens to induce responses or form immune complexes, they must exist outside of cells in an immunologically relevant form. The translocation process appears to occur most commonly during cell death, either physiologic or pathologic. During apoptosis, a regulated process called programmed cell death, nuclear molecules undergo extensive cleavage and translocation, appearing on the surface as well as in small subcellular structures called blebs. Furthermore, as apoptosis proceeds, the cell itself can undergo compaction and fragmentation, leading to production of apoptotic bodies. These bodies contain DNA and other nuclear molecules; microparticles which may correspond to blebs also form and detach to cells. While circulating nuclear molecules can be both free and particulate, most of the RNA appears to be in particles. The processes of RNA and DNA release from cells may be distinct, perhaps accounting for the difference in expression of antibodies to RBP and DNA.

Reflecting cell death during ordinary turnover, the blood of even normal subjects has significant amounts of circulating DNA. These levels can increase during a wide variety of conditions, including lupus, that are characterized by inflammation or cell death although these processes can commonly coexist. Thus, levels of circulating DNA can rise because of either an increased cell death or impaired clearance of dead and dying cells. The body has extensive systems for removal of these cells which includes cellular elements such as macrophages as well as humoral elements such as complement, C-reactive protein, and IgM. With impairment of these systems, dead cells may persist and can spill or leak their contents.

A role of impaired clearance in disease pathogenesis can explain the association of SLE with genetic abnormalities in elements of the clearance system, whether cellular or humoral immune. As such, an increase in apoptosis and a decrease in clearance of dead cells in patients may represent fundamental abnormalities that boost the supply of self-antigen to drive autoantigen-specific response or form immune complexes. The consequences of this increase may be particularly important because of the immunostimulatory activity of nuclear molecules as well as subcellular structures such as HMGB1 and microparticles.

Mechanisms of Tissue Inflammation and Damage

Given the array of cellular and humoral disturbances in patients with lupus, tissue inflammation is most likely multifactorial and diverse, differing among organ systems that are commonly affected. For many manifestations, the mechanisms of inflammation are unknown although in general autoantibodies have been implicated as important effectors. These antibodies can cause functional disturbances (e.g., clotting system for antibodies to phospholipid antigens), induce cytotoxicity or promote elimination (e.g., anti-red blood cell antibodies), or form immune complexes with tissue deposition. Abnormal levels of cytokines such as interferon or TNF may either directly induce inflammation or increase inflammation resulting from these other mechanisms. Interferon, for example, can perturb endothelial cell function and promote vasculopathy.

Of organs involved in SLE, the kidney has been studied most intensively to elucidate immunopathogenesis. Compelling data indicate that glomerulonephritis results from the deposition of immune complexes that are comprised of DNA and anti-DNA. This evidence for this mechanism includes the observations as summarized in Table 2.4. While evidence that lupus is an immune complex disease is

Table 2.4 Mechanisms of SLE renal disease

Association with anti-DNA immune complexes
High anti-DNA and low complement with activity
"Full house" immune deposition (IgG, IgA, IgM, and C3)
Immune complexes in sub-epithelial and sub-endothelial location
Impact of antibody and antigen charge on glomerular localization

strong, many aspects of this process remain unknown. Thus, it is not clear whether immune complexes form systemically in the circulation or locally in the kidney. Furthermore, if the complex formation is local, it may occur in a two-step process in which DNA first binds to the glomerular basement membrane to form a nidus to bind anti-DNA. Alternatively, the process may involve the local generation of nucleosomal antigen for assembly of an immune complex within the confines of the kidney. For some anti-DNA antibodies, direct binding to a glomerular antigen may occur by cross-reactivity.

For immune complexes, whether formed in the circulation or in the kidney, the properties of both antibody and antigen can influence renal deposition; DNA is a negatively charged molecule although, when present in nucleosomes, it can display regions of positive and negative charge; charged antigens may have a predilection for glomerular binding. Similarly, anti-DNA antibodies are charged and also may contribute to glomerular interaction. In the kidney, the immune complexes can activate complement, promoting inflammation that can ultimately lead to scarring and fibrosis.

The operation of these mechanism can be assessed by a variety of serological and immunopathological assays. Thus, active nephritis can be associated with high levels of anti-DNA and decreased complement; cytokines can also appear in the urine, indicative of renal inflammation. By histopathology, the immune complexes in the kidney can be detected by immunofluorescent microscopy which shows the presence of IgG, IgM, IgA, and complement in a pattern called "full house." By electron microscopy, the complexes appear as electron-dense material that can localize to either sub-epithelial or sub-endothelial sites. The site of localization can affect the pattern of nephritis and the occurrence of nephritic and nephrotic disease.

Figure 2.1 presents an overall picture of lupus pathogenesis, indicating the role of immune complexes in both cytokine disturbance and nephritis. Although immune complexes may contribute to both facets of pathogenesis, the anti-DNA complexes that drive cytokine production may differ from those that stimulate nephritis, for example. Complexes of other specificities may also contribute to these and other manifestations. While the term "nephritogenic" denotes anti-DNA antibodies that can cause nephritis, a term for antibodies that drive cytokines has not yet been developed. Furthermore, assays to distinguish those specificities with various pathogenic properties (i.e., nephritis and cytokine production) would be very valuable but are not yet available.

Lupus is associated with a dramatically increased frequency of atherosclerosis, an important source of morbidity and mortality. This manifestation is likely multifactorial

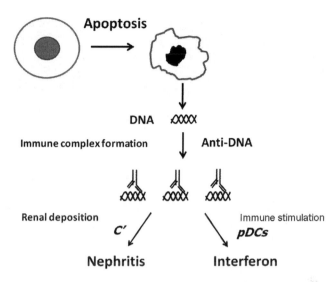

Fig. 2.1 The role of immune complexes in lupus pathogenesis. As illustrated in this figure, the pathogenesis of SLE is critically dependent on the formation of immune complexes whose antigenic components can derive from dead and dying cells. The levels of these components may rise because of impairment of the cellular and humoral immune systems involved in the clearance of dead and dying cells. In the presence of extracellular nuclear antigens, immune complexes can form with antibodies to DNA and other nuclear molecules; this figure depicts the DNA system. These complexes can in turn deposit in the kidney to incite nephritis or stimulate pDCs to produce cytokines such as type 1 interferon. Interferon has broad immunological activities that can impact on other cells to intensify immune disturbances. This schema indicates steps where genetic disturbances can promote susceptibility and, correspondingly, steps where treatment can ameliorate disease

and results from inflammation, vasculopathy, and thrombosis that characterize lupus. Some of these effects may relate to cytokines while others may relate to autoantibodies (e.g., antiphospholipid antibodies) that promote thrombosis in coronary or cerebral arteries. The recognition of this manifestation emphasizes the importance in disease management of agents to reduce cholesterol, lower blood pressure, and prevent clotting (i.e., anticoagulants) as part of the overall therapeutic approach.

Conclusion

SLE is a systemic autoimmune disease that results from interaction of genetic and environmental factors which together promote autoantibody production directed prominently to nuclear macromolecules. Since the nuclear molecules can have intrinsic immunological activity, the resulting immune complexes can cause potent stimulation of the immune system including the production of type 1 interferon.

In addition, these complexes can deposit in the kidney to incite inflammation and damage. The formation of the immune complexes requires an available source of nuclear material. In SLE, this material may arise because of an increase in the amount of cell death as well as impaired clearance dead and dying cells. Thus, pathogenesis of SLE entails important abnormalities that affect both autoantibody and autoantigen production.

Sources

1. Arbuckle MR, McClain MT, Rubertone MV, et al. Development of autoantibodies before the clinical onset of systemic lupus erythematosus. N Engl J Med. 2003;349(16):1526–33.
2. Ardoin SP, Pisetsky DS. Developments in the scientific understanding of lupus. Arthritis Res Ther. 2008;10(5):218.
3. Boulé MW, Broughton C, Mackay F, Akira S, Marshak-Rothstein A, Rifkin IR. Toll-like receptor 9-dependent and -independent dendritic cell activation by chromatin-immunoglobulin G complexes. J Exp Med. 2005;199(12):1631–40.
4. Chaussabel D, Quinn C, Shen J, et al. A modular analysis framework for blood genomics studies: application to systemic lupus erythematosus. Immunity. 2008;29:150–64.
5. Crispin JC, Kyttaris VC, Juang Y-T, Tsokos GC. How signaling and gene transcription aberrations dictate the systemic lupus eruthematosus T cell phenotype. Trends Immunol. 2008;29(3):110–5.
6. Hom G, Graham RR, Modrek B, et al. Association of systemic lupus erythematosus with *C8orf13-BLK* and *ITGAM-ITGAX*. N Engl J Med. 2008;358:1–10.
7. Huerta PT, Kowal C, DeGiorgio LA, Volpe BT, Diamond B. Immunity and behavior: antibodies alter emotion. Proc Natl Acad Sci U S A. 2006;103(3):678–83.
8. Jørgensen TN, Gubbels MR, Kotzin BL. New insights into disease pathogenesis from mouse lupus genetics. Curr Opin Immunol. 2004;16:787–93.
9. Kelly KM, Zhuang H, Nacionales DC, et al. "Endogenous adjuvant" activity of the RNA components of lupus autoantigens Sm/RNP and Ro 60. Arthritis Rheum. 2006;54(5):1557–67.
10. Lafyatis R, Marshak-Rothstein A. Toll-like receptors and innate immune responses in systemic lupus erythematosus. Arthritis Res Ther. 2007;9(6):1–7.
11. Lauwerys BR, Wakeland EK. Genetics of lupus nephritis. Lupus. 2005;14:2–12.
12. Mortensen ES, Fenton KA, Rekvig OP. Lupus nephritis: the central role of nucleosomes revealed. Am J Pathol. 2008;172(2):275–83.
13. Muller S, Dieker J, Tincani A, Meroni PL. Pathogenic anti-nucleosome antibodies. Lupus. 2008;17:431–6.
14. Munoz LE, Lauber K, Schiller M, Manfredi AA, Hermann M. The role of defective clearance of apoptotic cells in systemic autoimmunity. Nat Rev Rheumatol. 2010;6(5):280–9.
15. Odendahl M, Jacobi A, Hansen A, et al. Disturbed peripheral B lymphocyte homeostasis in systemic lupus erythematosus. J Immunol. 2000;165:5970–9.
16. Pisetsky DS. Immune responses to DNA in normal and aberrant immunity. Immunol Res. 2000;22(2–3):119–26.
17. Rahman A, Isenberg DA. Systemic lupus erythematosus. N Engl J Med. 2008;358(9):929–39.
18. Seshan SV, Jennette JC. Renal disease in systemic lupus erythematosus with emphasis on classification of lupus glomerulonephritis. Arch Pathol Lab Med. 2009;133:233–48.
19. Shlomchik MJ. Activating systemic autoimmunity: B's, T's and tolls. Curr Opin Immunol. 2009;21(6):626–33.
20. Yurasov S, Wardemann H, Hammersen J, et al. Defective B cell tolerance checkpoints in systemic lupus erythematosus. J Exp Med. 2005;201(5):703–11.

Chapter 3
Diagnosing and Monitoring Lupus

Elena M. Massarotti and Peter H. Schur

Introduction

Making the diagnosis of lupus can be challenging. Patients with SLE are subject to a myriad of symptoms, complaints, as well as inflammation that can affect virtually every organ. The most common pattern is a mixture of constitutional complaints with skin, musculoskeletal, hematologic, and serologic involvement. However, some patients have predominately hematologic, renal, cardiopulmonary, or central nervous system manifestations. The pattern that dominates during the first few years of illness tends to prevail subsequently.

The approach to the diagnosis and differential diagnosis of SLE will be reviewed here. An overview of the symptoms and signs that can occur in SLE, discussions of particular sites of involvement (e.g., skin, kidneys, and central nervous system), and the treatment and prognosis of SLE are presented separately in other chapters.

E.M. Massarotti, M.D. (✉)
Division of Rheumatology, Center for Clinical Therapeutics,
Brigham and Women's Hospital, 75 Francis Street,
Boston, MA 02115, USA

Harvard Medical School, Boston, MA, USA
e-mail: emassarotti@partners.org

P.H. Schur, M.D., F.A.C.P.
Division of Rheumatology, Brigham and Women's Hospital, Boston, MA 02115, USA

Harvard Medical School, Boston, MA, USA
e-mail: pschur@partners.org

Table 3.1 Questionnaire for the diagnosis of systemic lupus erythematosus

Have you ever had arthritis or rheumatism for more than 3 months?
Do your fingers become pale, numb, or uncomfortable in the cold?
Have you had any sores in your mouth for more than 2 weeks?
Have you been told that you have low blood counts (anemia, low WBC count, or low platelet count)?
Have you ever had a prominent rash on your cheeks for more than 1 month?
Does your skin break out after you have been in the sun (not sunburn)?
Has it ever been painful to take a deep breath for more than a few days (pleurisy)?
Have you ever been told that you have protein in your urine?
Have you ever had rapid loss of lots of hair?
Have you ever had a seizure, convulsion, or fit?

Diagnosis

The diagnosis of SLE is straightforward in a patient who presents with several characteristic clinical features and has supportive laboratory abnormalities. A typical example is a young woman who presents with complaints of fatigue, painful swollen joints, and a photosensitive malar rash with a CBC test that reveals leukopenia. This scenario should trigger testing for the presence of antinuclear antibodies (ANAs).

However, SLE can also present as

- Raynaud's phenomenon
- Serositis (pleuritis, pericarditis, and peritonitis)
- Nephritis or nephrotic syndrome
- Neurologic symptoms such as seizures or psychosis
- Alopecia
- Phlebitis
- Recurrent miscarriage
- Anemia
- Leukopenia
- Thrombocytopenia

SLE should also be suspected in young women presenting with fatigue, low-grade fever, rashes, myalgia, nausea, headaches, cognitive disturbances, loss of appetite, weight gain or loss, purpura, easy bruising, diffuse adenopathy, hepatosplenomegaly, peripheral neuropathy, endocarditis, myocarditis, interstitial pneumonitis, hypertension, or aseptic meningitis—or any combination thereof. The symptoms may be mild, severe, fleeting, or persistent.

Diagnostic Criteria

The diagnosis of lupus is especially challenging because the presenting symptoms can be indicative of many different entities. A useful approach to the detection of

Table 3.2 ACR criteria for diagnosis of systemic lupus erythematosus

Criterion	Definition
Malar rash	Fixed erythema, flat or raised, over the malar eminences, tending to spare the nasolabial folds
Discoid rash	Erythematosus raised patches with adherent keratotic scaling and follicular plugging; atrophic scarring may occur in older lesions
Photosensitivity	Skin rash as a result of unusual reaction to sunlight, by patient history or physician observation
Oral ulcers	Oral or nasopharyngeal ulceration, usually painless, observed by a physician
Arthritis	Nonerosive arthritis involving two or more peripheral joints, characterized by tenderness, swelling, or effusion
Serositis	Pleuritis—convincing history of pleuritic pain or rub heard by a physician or evidence of pleural effusion OR
	Pericarditis—documented by EKG, rub, or evidence of pericardial effusion
Renal disorder	Persistent proteinuria greater than 0.5 g/day or greater than 3+ if quantitation not performed OR
	Cellular casts—may be red cell, hemoglobin, granular, tubular, or mixed
Neurologic disorder	Seizures or psychosis—in the absence of offending drugs or known metabolic derangements (uremia, ketoacidosis, or electrolyte imbalance)
Hematologic disorder	Hemolytic anemia—with reticulocytosis OR
	Leukopenia—less than 4,000/mm^3 total on two or more occasions OR
	Lymphopenia—less than 1,500/mm^3 on two or more occasions OR
	Thrombocytopenia—less than 100,000/mm^3 in the absence of offending drugs
Immunologic disorders	Positive antiphospholipid antibody OR
	Anti-DNA—antibody to native DNA in abnormal titer OR
	Anti-Sm—presence of antibody to Sm nuclear antigen OR
	False-positive serologic test for syphilis known to be positive for at least 6 months and confirmed by Treponema pallidum immobilization or fluorescent treponemal antibody absorption test
Antinuclear antibody	An abnormal titer of antinuclear antibody by immunofluorescence or an equivalent assay at any point in time and in the absence of drugs known to be associated with "drug-induced lupus" syndrome

SLE and in differentiating it from other systemic disorders has been the use of a validated questionnaire (Table 3.1). If three or more questions are answered positively, SLE is a possibility and an ANA test is indicated.

Most physicians rely on diagnostic criteria for lupus that were developed by the American Rheumatism Association (ARA, now the American College of Rheumatology or ACR) (Table 3.2). These criteria were developed for the *classification* of SLE patients when SLE was compared to other rheumatic diseases *for study purposes*. The criteria were established by cluster analyses, primarily in academic centers and primarily in Caucasian patients.

Whether these criteria apply to other populations has not been established, although they have been used to demonstrate that the frequency of SLE is higher among Afro-Americans, Afro-Caribbeans, Anglo-Asians, and American-Hispanics than in Caucasians.

The diagnosis of SLE is made if four or more of the manifestations are present, either serially or simultaneously, during any interval of observations. When tested against other rheumatic diseases, these criteria have a sensitivity and specificity of approximately 96 %.

These criteria have some inherent weaknesses. As an example, one can have a renal biopsy demonstrating lupus nephritis, but the patient still fails to fulfill four criteria.

Using the analogy of the 1987 ACR criteria for the diagnosis of rheumatoid arthritis, we suggest that patients be classified as follows:

- Classical SLE—many criteria
- Definite SLE—four or more criteria
- Undifferentiated connective tissue disease (UCTD)

UCTD is defined as a patient with ANAs and evidence of inflammation on examination who does not meet the ACR criteria for SLE or any other autoimmune/rheumatic/connective tissue disorder. Up to one-third of patients with UCTD have all their symptoms and signs disappear over a 10-year follow-up period; anywhere from 40 % to 60 % continue with their initial clinical features, while 5–30 % evolve and meet classification criteria for a definite disease, such as rheumatoid arthritis, SLE, scleroderma, or an inflammatory myositis. Thus, patients with UCTD need to be followed carefully and encouraged to report new symptoms and to have periodic laboratory testing to assess for the emergence of new clinical features or laboratory findings.

Laboratory Testing

Laboratory tests that may provide diagnostically useful information when SLE is suspected include

- Complete blood count and differential
- Comprehensive chemistry profile
- Creatine kinase
- Erythrocyte sedimentation rate and/or C-reactive protein
- Urinalysis
- 24-h urine collection for calculation of creatinine clearance and quantitation of proteinuria or protein/creatinine ratios using spot urine protein and spot urine creatinine

Autoantibody testing is also indicated (see Section "Autoantibodies"). The autoantibodies that are routinely assayed are

- ANAs
- Antiphospholipid antibodies (see Chap. 15)
- Antibodies to double-stranded DNA (dsDNA)
- Anti-Smith (anti-Sm) antibodies

Autoantibodies

The ANA test, as performed using an immunofluorescent method, is the best diagnostic test for SLE and should be performed whenever SLE is suspected. Two features of the immunofluorescent test are important to evaluate: the titer and the pattern of immunofluorescence.

The ANA is positive in significant titer (usually 1:160 or higher) in virtually all patients with SLE. Depending upon the titer of the ANA, the false-positive rate in healthy controls varies from approximately 30 % with ANA titers of 1:40 (high sensitivity, low specificity) to as little as 3 % with ANA titers of 1:320 (low sensitivity, high specificity). The probability of having SLE in a population at variable risk for lupus is less than 0.14 % if the ANA test is negative.

Immunofluorescent "patterns" are reported as homogenous or diffuse, speckled, nucleolar, and centromere. SLE can be associated with all the patterns, though the homogeneous/diffuse pattern is most commonly seen. Speckled and nucleolar patterns are seen in scleroderma and mixed connective tissue disease, and the centromere pattern is highly suggestive of what was commonly known as CREST or limited scleroderma.

Since diseases other than SLE are associated with a positive ANA, the predictive value of a positive test depends upon the population being studied. In a review of 276 patients referred to a rheumatologist for a positive ANA (titer ≥1:40) without a diagnosis, 52 (19 %) were diagnosed with SLE.

One of the most challenging scenarios confronted by primary care physicians and rheumatologists is the evaluation of a group of patients with fibromyalgia-like manifestations and a positive ANA. These patients differ clinically and serologically from patients with definite SLE and generally do not merit the diagnosis of SLE.

ANAs are also present, often in lower titer and depending on the assay system used, in a variety of other disorders as well:

- Sjögren's syndrome—68 %
- Scleroderma—40–75 % (especially with a speckled or anticentromere pattern of ANAs)
- Juvenile rheumatoid arthritis—16 %
- Rheumatoid arthritis—25–50 % (especially with a diffuse pattern of ANAs)

dsDNA and Sm Antibodies

There are two autoantibodies that are highly specific for SLE: anti-dsDNA and anti-Sm antibodies. For antibodies to dsDNA, the sensitivity is 66–95 %, specificity is

75–100 %, and the positive predictive value is 89–100 %. For antibodies to Sm, the sensitivity is up to 55 % and the specificity is 58–100 %.

Some autoantibodies produced in patients with SLE or other rheumatic diseases tend to be associated with certain clinical settings with a variable degree of sensitivity and specificity:

- Antibodies to ribonucleoprotein (RNP) are associated with SLE, mixed connective tissue disease, rheumatoid arthritis, and scleroderma.
- Antibodies to Ro (SS-A) and La (SS-B) are associated with both SLE and Sjögren's syndrome.

The following associations have been noted between specific antibodies and manifestations of SLE:

- Anti-dsDNA with nephritis and active systemic disease
- Anti-RNP (U1 RNP) with myositis, Raynaud's phenomenon, and less severe lupus
- Anti-Ro/SSA with lymphopenia, photosensitivity, neonatal lupus, C2 deficiency, subacute cutaneous lupus erythematosus, and secondary Sjögren's syndrome; and anti-La/SSB with neonatal lupus and secondary Sjögren's syndrome
- Anti-ribosomal P protein and neuropsychiatric manifestations

Measurement of serum complement levels C3 and C4 may also be helpful, since hypocomplementemia is a frequent finding in active SLE.

Imaging

Diagnostic imaging may be valuable but is not routinely obtained unless indicated by the presence of symptoms, clinical findings, or laboratory abnormalities. Examples include

- Plain radiographs of involved joints.
- Renal ultrasonography to assess kidney size and rule out urinary tract obstruction when there is evidence of renal impairment.
- Chest radiography.
- Echocardiography (e.g., for suspected pericardial involvement, to assess for a source of emboli, or noninvasive estimation of pulmonary artery pressure).
- Computed tomography (CT) (e.g., for abdominal pain, suspected pancreatitis).
- Magnetic resonance imaging (e.g., for focal neurologic deficits or cognitive dysfunction).
- Contrast angiography may be valuable if vasculitis affecting medium-sized arteries is suspected (e.g., mesenteric or limb-threatening ischemia).

Biopsy

Biopsy of an involved organ (e.g., skin or kidney) is necessary in some cases.

Other Tests

Other tests that may be necessary are typically dictated by the clinical presentation and associated differential diagnostic possibilities. Examples include

- Electrocardiography in the assessment of chest pain that may be due to pericarditis
- Tests to assess for pulmonary embolism in a patient with pleuritic chest pain and dyspnea
- Diffusing capacity for carbon monoxide (DLCO) to assess for suspected pulmonary hemorrhage and estimate the severity of interstitial pneumonitis

Differential Diagnosis

Given the protean manifestations of SLE, the differential diagnosis is correspondingly broad. In a particular patient in whom the diagnosis of SLE is being considered, a combination of a focused history, physical examination, certain laboratory tests, and imaging will usually facilitate making a correct diagnosis.

Systemic Symptoms

Fatigue occurs in most patients. It can be due to SLE, a sleep disorder, psychosocial issues, deconditioning, anemia, renal disease, endocrine disorders, infections, cardiopulmonary disorders, other rheumatic disorders, medications, etc. A low-grade fever is common; when associated with chills and leukocytosis, infection should be considered, while no chills and leukopenia may represent SLE. Weight gain can be due to renal disease or fluid retention from cardiac disease; weight loss can be due to any chronic illness, including endocrine, GI, malignancy, infection, renal, cardiopulmonary, neurological, psychiatric, or another rheumatic disorder.

Cutaneous Lesions

Lupus skin lesions are typically photosensitive and are observed in sun-exposed areas, especially the face, forearms, neck, and chest. However, "polymorphous light eruption" can be present in the same area, and rosacea can present as a malar rash. Furthermore, patients with any rash may develop chronic changes including hyper- and hypopigmentation and telangiectasias. Patchy alopecia may be seen in lupus. Other skin disorders can be confused with lupus including vasculitis, hypertrophic lichen planus, actinic keratosis, and various macular eruptions, and medication-induced rashes. Patients may have bruising due to thrombocytopenia or the use of corticosteroids. A skin biopsy that includes H&E and immunofluorescence staining may help to differentiate lupus from other disorders.

Raynaud's Phenomenon

Raynaud's phenomenon may be primary but is also associated with scleroderma, MCTD, PM/DM, and a number of other diseases.

Mucosal Lesions

SLE typically causes painless ulcers and should not be confused with painful chancre sores/blisters (herpes simplex) or aphthous stomatitis.

Polyarthritis/Polyarthralgia

Widespread joint pain and/or periarticular pain is common. In patients with SLE, morning stiffness is in minutes, while in RA, it is measured in hours. Arthritis in patients with SLE is usually migratory and may last for a few days—while in rheumatoid arthritis, it is symmetrical, persistent, and may last for months. In SLE, it tends to affect the hands, fingers, and less often other joints; this contrasts with the propensity to affect the MCPs and MTPs in RA. Arthritis has many other etiologies including OA, crystal induced, spondyloarthropathy, infectious, postinfectious, and other rheumatic diseases. If there is uncertainty about the presence or absence of inflammation in a patient with polyarthralgia, imaging of symptomatic joints may be informative. Joint fluid analysis and serologic tests facilitate making the differential. Avascular necrosis and osteoporosis should always be considered in patients on chronic corticosteroids.

Lymphadenopathy

Enlarged lymph nodes palpable in the neck and axilla are a common finding in patients with active SLE, not on corticosteroids—which tend to quickly make palpable nodes disappear. Lymphadenopathy is also often appreciated in patients with active SLE on radiographic evaluation of the chest and abdomen. On the other hand, enlarged nodes in patients already taking corticosteroids should make one concerned about a malignant lymphoproliferative disorder or an infection warranting a biopsy.

Hepatomegaly is not unusual in patients with SLE, but other causes including liver disease, CHF, and malignancy should also be considered.

Splenomegaly is uncommon in SLE and is usually associated with thrombocytopenia. One should also consider liver disease, malignancy (especially lymphoma), and infections.

GI System

More than one-third of patients develop symptoms related to the GI system including dyspepsia, reflux, nausea, vomiting, or abdominal pain. The differential is long and includes peptic ulcer disease, GERD, liver disease (including biliary tract disease), pancreatitis, peritonitis, motility disorders, mesenteric vasculitis, and the use of medications, especially NSAIDs and corticosteroids. Appropriate workup may include endoscopy and CT scans to differentiate the various causes.

Renal Disease

Clinical kidney involvement develops in approximately 50 % of patients with SLE. Most patients develop kidney disease during the first 2 years of illness. Renal disease is typically asymptomatic. The first clue may be hypertension in a young person, but more typically it is detected when a urinalysis shows protein and/or an excess number of red blood and/or white blood cells. When these abnormalities are observed, one must consider whether to perform a renal biopsy to determine whether the pathology represents focal or diffuse proliferative glomerulonephritis, membranous nephropathy, due to SLE—or something else [e.g., postinfectious, IgA nephropathy, Henoch-Schönlein, diabetes, RPGN, and vasculitis (including ANCA associated)]. Immunofluorescent staining of the biopsy, EM, and serologic testing often facilitates differentiation between the different forms of nephritis.

Patients with SLE nephritis may develop chronic renal diseases. One form is nephritic syndrome, with peripheral edema and marked proteinemia. The other is glomerulonephritis with active urinary sediment, proteinuria, hypertension, and the development of uremia (with its associated nausea and fatigue and anemia).

Other causes of impaired renal function can be seen that are not directly caused by SLE, including superimposed problems such as hypovolemia, urinary tract obstruction, infection, and drug toxicity.

Cardiovascular Disease

The heart is uncommonly affected in SLE. However, pericarditis is not uncommon but should also make one think of infections (especially viral), malignancy, postirradiation, CHF, renal failure, and other rheumatic diseases (RA, MCTD, scleroderma, sarcoidosis, and ARF). In recent years, there has been a greater appreciation of accelerated atherosclerosis in lupus patients, resulting in coronary artery disease at a much earlier age, especially in young women.

Asymptomatic valvular disease has been observed in up to 25 % of patients with SLE. It may be associated with the presence of antiphospholipid antibodies, but rarely becomes symptomatic (e.g., cause emboli as in verrucous, Libman–Sacks, and culture-negative endocarditis).

Lung Disease

The lung is involved in about 50 % of patients with SLE. Chest pain can be seen in lupus, and it is important to differentiate chest wall pain (characterized by pain to touch and movement) from symptomatic coronary artery disease (e.g., angina, MI with its associated diaphoresis, EKG, and enzyme changes) from pleurisy (true inflammation of the pleura) with its associated pain with breathing, pleural rub, and abnormal chest X-ray. Pleuritis and/or pleural effusion may also be caused by infections, PE, malignancy, pneumothorax, uremia, liver failure, CHF, and other rheumatic diseases (RA, MCTD, and drug-induced LE). Radiographic evaluation as well as an examination of pleural fluid will usually facilitate making the correct diagnosis.

Pneumonitis

Acute infectious pneumonia with fever, productive cough, physical findings, and lung infiltrate present on chest radiograph will generally be initially approached as a community-acquired pneumonia. In a patient with SLE taking corticosteroids and/or immunosuppressive drugs, opportunistic or nosocomial infections must also be considered. One should suspect interstitial lung disease, cryptogenic pneumonia, or malignancy if the process does not respond to empiric antibiotic therapy.

Pulmonary Hypertension

Symptomatic severe pulmonary hypertension is rare in SLE. Rather, one should consider recurrent pulmonary thromboembolism or scleroderma.

Alveolar Hemorrhage

Alveolar hemorrhage is a rare manifestation of SLE and has a variety of other causes [e.g., vasculitis, infection, Goodpasture's syndrome, Wegener's (proper term now granulomatosis with polyangiitis), Henoch-Schönlein purpura, bleeding disorders, or other rheumatic disorders (MCTD<RA, PM)].

Shrinking Lung Syndrome

This rare entity is related to diaphragmatic muscle weakness and characterized by low lung volumes evident on chest X-ray and by pulmonary function testing.

Neuropsychiatric Symptoms

Virtually all patients with SLE have some form of NP symptoms including headaches, anxiety, depression (not uncommon in any patient with a chronic disease), cognitive defects, and behavioral disturbances. Only two NP symptoms are part of the ACR criteria for the classification of SLE: psychosis and seizures. Psychosis is actually uncommon and has a broad differential including psychiatric causes as well as metabolic disorders and caused by many medications, especially corticosteroids. Seizures also have a broad differential including infections, strokes, hypertension, and the use of some medications. Strokes are not infrequent in patients with SLE; one should consider the antiphospholipid antibody syndrome, as well as the more common causes of stroke such as emboli, hemorrhage, and atherosclerotic thrombosis. Vasculitis is exceedingly rare. Appropriate workup with lab work (especially a metabolic panel), MRI/MRA, EEG, and CSF analysis facilitates making an appropriate diagnosis.

Eye Disease

The most common manifestation of eye disease is associated Sjögren's, although Sjögren's is more commonly either primary or associated with RA. Retinal vasculitis, scleritis, and episcleritis are rare, and one should consider its other causes (infection, Behcet's, Wegner's, sarcoidosis, systemic vasculitis, RA, polychondritis, and IBD).

Hematologic Abnormalities

A variety of hematologic abnormalities can occur in SLE, each of which can be caused by other diseases.

The abnormalities include

- Anemia can be associated with comorbid chronic disease, renal failure, malignancy, diet, or medication, as well as hemolytic anemia.
- Leukopenia is common in SLE, more so in patients with active disease. The association of leukopenia with a positive ANA test usually reflects SLE. Other causes of leukopenia include infection (especially viral), hypersplenism, and malignancy.
- Thrombocytopenia is common in SLE but may also be associated with infections, hypersplenism, thrombotic thrombocytopenic purpura (TTP), malignancy, the use of heparin, and the antiphospholipid syndrome (APS).
- Hypercoagulable state (thrombophilia)—patients with SLE have a marked increased frequency of antiphospholipid antibodies which predispose to venous

and/or arterial thromboemboli as well as recurrent miscarriage. Other causes of hypercoagulable states should be considered including inherited forms, malignancy, trauma, surgery, pregnancy, use of oral contraceptives (and HRT), immobilization, and nephritic syndrome.

Sources

1. Von Feldt JM. Systemic lupus erythematosus. Recognizing its various presentations. Postgrad Med. 1995;97:79.
2. Cervera R, Khamashia MA, Font J, et al. SLE: clinical and immunologic patterns of disease expression in a cohort of 1000 patients. Medicine. 1993;72:113.
3. Estes D, Christian CL. The natural history of systemic lupus erythematosus by prospective analysis. Medicine (Baltimore). 1971;50:85–95.
4. Fessler BJ, Boumpas DT. Severe organ involvement in SLE. Diagnosis and management. Rheum Dis Clin North Am. 1995;21:81.
5. Rothfield N. Clinical features of systemic lupus erythematosus. In: Kelley WN, Harris ED, Ruddy S, Sledge CB, editors. Textbook of rheumatology. Philadelphia: Saunders; 1981.
6. Nakamura RM, Bylund DJ. Contemporary concepts for the clinical and laboratory evaluation of SLE and "lupus-like" syndromes. J Clin Lab Anal. 1994;8:347.
7. Heinlen LD, McClain MT, Merrill J, et al. Clinical criteria for systemic lupus erythematosus precede diagnosis, and associated autoantibodies are present before clinical symptoms. Arthritis Rheum. 2007;56:2344.
8. Liang MH, Meenan RF, Cathcart ES, Schur PH. A screening strategy for population studies in systemic lupus erythematosus: series design. Arthritis Rheum. 1980;23:152.
9. Hochberg MC. Updating the American College of Rheumatology revised criteria for the classification of systemic lupus erythematosus. Arthritis Rheum. 1997;40:1725.
10. Tan EM, Cohen AS, Fries JF, et al. The 1982 revised criteria for the classification of systemic lupus erythematosus. Arthritis Rheum. 1982;25:1271.
11. Citera G, Wilson WA. Ethnic and geographic perspectives in SLE. Lupus. 1993;2:351.
12. Johnson AE, Gordon C, Palmer RG, Bacon PA. The prevalence and incidence of s systemic lupus erythematosus in Birmingham, England. Arthritis Rheum. 1995;38:551.
13. Meyer O. A critical appraisal of the classification criteria for systemic lupus erythematosus. Clin Exp Rheumatol. 1994;12 Suppl 11:S41.
14. Symmons DPM. Lupus around the world. Frequency of lupus in people of African origin. Lupus. 1995;4:176.
15. Petri M. SLICC revision of the ACR classification criteria for SLE (abstract). Arthritis Rheum. 2009;60:S336.
16. Greer JM, Panush RS. Incomplete lupus erythematosus. Arch Intern Med. 1989;149:2473.
17. Lom-Orta H, Alarcon-Segovia D, Diaz-Jouanen E. Systemic lupus erythematosus. Differences between patients who do, and who do not, fulfill classification criteria at the time of diagnosis. J Rheumatol. 1980;7:831.
18. Bodolay E, Csiki Z, Szekanecz Z, et al. Five-year follow-up of 665 Hungarian patients with undifferentiated connective tissue disease (UCTD). Clin Exp Rheumatol. 2003;21:313.
19. Stahl Hallengren C, Nived O, Sturfelt G. Outcome of incomplete systemic lupus erythematosus after 10 years. Lupus. 2004;13:85–8.
20. Mosca M, Tani C, Bombardieri S. A case of undifferentiated connective tissue disease: is it a distinct clinical entity? Nat Clin Pract Rheumatol. 2008;4:328.
21. von Muhlen CA, Tan EM. Autoantibodies in the diagnosis of systemic rheumatic diseases. Semin Arthritis Rheum. 1995;24:323.
22. Tan EM, Feltkamp TE, Smolen JS, et al. Range of antinuclear antibodies in "healthy" individuals. Arthritis Rheum. 1997;40:1601.

23. Shiel Jr WC, Jason M. The diagnostic associations of patients with antinuclear antibodies referred to a community rheumatologist. J Rheumatol. 1989;16:782.
24. Griner PF, Mayewski RJ, Mushlin AI, Greenland P. Selection and interpretation of diagnostic tests and procedures. Principles and applications. Ann Intern Med. 1981;94:557.
25. Calvo-Alen J, Bastian HM, Straaton KV, et al. Identification of patient subsets among those presumptively diagnosed with, referred, and/or followed up for SLE at a large tertiary care center. Arthritis Rheum. 1995;38:1475.
26. Smeenk R, Brinkman K, van den Brink H, et al. Antibodies to DNA in patients with SLE. Their role in the diagnosis, the follow-up and the pathogenesis of the disease. Clin Rheumatol. 1990;9:100.
27. Eaton RB, Schneider G, Schur PH. Enzyme immunoassay for antibodies to nDNA. Specificity and quality of antibodies. Arthritis Rheum. 1983;26:52.
28. Munves EF, Schur PH. Antibodies to Sm and RNP: prognosticators of disease involvement. Arthritis Rheum. 1983;26:848.
29. Avina-Zubieta JA, Galindo-Rodriquez G, Kwan-Yeung L, et al. Clinical evaluation of various selected ELISA kits for the detection of anti-DNA antibodies. Lupus. 1995;4:370.
30. Harley JB. Autoantibodies are central to the diagnosis and clinical manifestations of lupus. J Rheumatol. 1994;21:1183.

Chapter 4
Recommendations on How to Monitor the Patient with Systemic Lupus Erythematosus in the Clinic or at the Bedside

Vivian P. Bykerk

Introduction

Systemic lupus erythematosus (SLE) is a heterogeneous disease with each patient having a unique expression of his or her disease. Clinicians will follow patients with SLE in the clinic when the disease is mild to moderate and or well controlled. At times patients with SLE are hospitalized and are monitored much more intensively according to extent of their disease activity. In clinical studies investigators frequently use complex outcome measures to determine disease activity although these are not yet routinely used in all clinics or at the bedside. Patients with SLE need to be assessed regularly for clinical symptoms, physical findings, and laboratory parameters to determine the extent of disease activity, damage from the disease, quality of life, comorbidities, and drug toxicity. Immunosuppressive therapy is frequently used to control the manifestations of SLE, and potential adverse effects of the medications must be monitored for on a regular basis during regular clinical evaluations and laboratory parameters should be performed when monitoring the patient with SLE.

This chapter provides an overview as to how to best monitor the patient with lupus in the clinic and bedside for clinical and laboratory manifestations of SLE and effects of medications.

V.P. Bykerk, M.D. (✉)
Hospital for Special Surgery,
535 East 70th St, New York, NY 07030, USA
e-mail: bykerkv@hss.edu

General Principles

Frequency of Monitoring the Patient

When determining the type and frequency of monitoring of the patient with SLE, the physician needs to take into account the history of the patient's prior symptoms, flare frequency, current disease activity status, and severity of current or prior flares. Some patients with higher risk having very active disease with consequences of potential serious organ system damage will need to be followed more frequently and intensively, as often as every 1–2 weeks. Those patients with controlled disease with a history of mild–moderate disease manifestations may require follow-up only every few months as outlined in Table 4.1. A thorough physical exam evaluating signs and symptoms in each organ system should be performed according to the schedule noted in the table. The physical examination needs to be extensive and includes examination of the skin (including scalp and mucous membranes), lymph nodes as well as respiratory, cardiovascular, abdominal, musculoskeletal, and neurologic systems. Corresponding laboratory monitoring is also recommended.

Baseline and Repeat Laboratory Monitoring of the Patient with SLE

It is helpful to have a baseline assessment of most laboratory parameters routinely used in SLE assessment including the following autoantibodies and complement: ANA, anti-dsDNA, anti-Ro, anti-La, anti-RNP, anti-Sm, antiphospholipid antibodies (anticardiolipin, anti-beta 2 glycoprotein 1, lupus anticoagulant), and complement (CH50, C3, C4). If attempting to determine if the patient is serologically active or quiescent or in remission, an anti-dsDNA, C3, and C4 would need to be repeated to support evidence of disease activity/remission. Regardless of the level of disease activity or risk of disease severity some parameters should be routinely monitored for all patients with SLE. These include baseline and routine monitoring of a complete blood count (CBC), serum creatinine, urea, liver function tests, urinalysis at each visit and periodically an assessment of GFR (24-h urine creatinine clearance), and a urine protein/creatinine at least annually. For some patients, the erythrocyte sedimentation rate (ESR), C-reactive protein (CRP), complement (C3, C4), and anti-dsDNA are informative, especially in those with renal disease. Patients with inactive disease should have laboratory monitoring at 6–12 months intervals including CBC, ESR, CRP, serum albumin, serum creatinine (or eGFR), urinalysis, and urine protein/creatinine ratio. If a patient is on a specific drug treatment, monitoring for toxicity and therapeutic effects associated with that drug is required as well.

Table 4.1 Clinical symptoms and signs and corresponding laboratory tests which require regular monitoring for patients with lupus in the clinic

Organ system involvement	Symptoms and signs	Monitoring of specific physical findings and laboratory tests	Special considerations
Constitutional	Chills, sweats, weight loss, malaise, loss of appetite, fatigue	Fevers, weight loss Lab tests: ESR or CRP; may have low C3, C4, high anti-dsDNA	Nonspecific manifestations of active disease, monitor at every visit; fatigue rarely resolves completely
Mucocutaneous	Hair thinning, bald spots, photosensitive rashes (sun-exposed distribution), painful nasal or oral mucosal ulcers	Hair pull test, patchy alopecia, malar or discoid rashes, diffuse rashes, mucosal ulcers of the nasopharynx, oral mucosa, upper palate Lab tests: not required	Evaluated at every visit
Musculoskeletal	Joint pain, swelling and/or stiffness, proximal weakness	Complete joint exam for joint tenderness, swelling, ROM, deformity; tests of muscle strength Lab tests: ESR, CRP, SF analysis, X-ray, bone density, MRI	Synovitis nonerosive but potentially deforming; myositis pathogenesis similar to dermatomyositis
Renal	Usually asymptomatic[a]—may have hypertension-related headaches and nephritic-related edema	Pedal edema, hypertension Lab tests: [a]urinalysis for sediment, cells, casts; 24 h protein and creatinine clearance, urine protein/creatinine, serum creatinine and albumen, anti-DNA, complement, renal biopsy	Nephritis (consider any of 5 types of (WHO classification) renal involvement)
Hematologic	Usually asymptomatic, possibly bruising, unusual bleeding[b]	Bruising, petechiae Lab tests: complete blood counts, PT, PTT, bone marrow	Thrombocytopenia, leukopenia, hemolytic anemia
Gastrointestinal	Pain, bloating, nausea, vomiting	Abdominal tenderness, distension, guarding Radiology: abdominal CT, US, angiography Labs: stool guaiac, amylase, lipase, *H. pylori*	GI symptoms are rare but may be due to vasculitis of the bowels, intestinal pseudo-obstruction, abdominal serositis
Pulmonary	Pleuritic pain, dyspnea, cough, hemoptysis	Air entry, rales, rhonchi, rubs, diaphragmatic excursion Labs: PFT with DLCO Radiology: CT	Monitoring for pleuritis, pneumonitis, shrinking lung syndrome, alveolar hemorrhage

(continued)

Table 4.1 (continued)

Organ system involvement	Symptoms and signs	Monitoring of specific physical findings and laboratory tests	Special considerations
Cardiovascular	Positional or inspiratory chest pain, chest pressure, palpitations	Evaluate for coronary insufficiency (pain/pressure/palpitations), rubs, murmurs, pulsus paradoxus Labs: baseline EKG; 2D echo as indicated, lipids, ESR, CRP, stress test, carotid US[c]	Can include pericarditis, Libman-Sacks endocarditis; (premature) coronary atherosclerosis—as angina, MI, consequences of MI, TIA, CVA
Neuropsychiatric	Headaches, loss of coordination, movement disorders, numbness, trouble thinking, loss of consciousness, seizures, cognitive abnormalities	Cranial nerve exam, fundoscopic exam, mini-mental status, tests of coordination Labs: consider neuropsychiatric testing, EEG, MRI, LP	Seizures, CVAs, psychosis, aseptic meningitis, cranial or peripheral neuropathies

ROM range of motion

[a] As lupus nephritis is usually asymptomatic, monitoring for this manifestation requires regular analysis of the urinary sediment to assess for active inflammation. A second morning urine looking for pyuria, proteinuria, hematuria and casts can often identify renal disease in SLE. In the case of pyuria in the absence of other findings, a urinary tract infection should be excluded. If hematuria is the only finding, this could also indicate recent menses, or if the patient is receiving cyclophosphamide, it might indicate cyclophosphamide-induced cystitis

[b] A complete blood count looking for thrombocytopenia; anemia, considering hemolytic anemia and anemia of chronic disease; and leukopenia can indicate active SLE

[c] Physical examination and simple tests may not always detect cardiopulmonary findings. If there are clinical suspicion for these, consider stress testing, transesophageal echocardiography, and angiography

Monitoring for Clinical Manifestations in the Patient with SLE in the Clinic

Caveats on Monitoring the SLE Patient with Blood Tests

Generally patients with SLE will require frequent monitoring of laboratory tests, usually at each patient encounter. Many of these will be to look at specific manifestations of lupus activity. These should typically include a CBC looking for leukopenia, anemia, and thrombocytopenia, and creatinine and urinalysis looking for signs of nephritis. These laboratory tests will also look for signs of disease activity that may not correspond to specific organ system involvement. Such tests would include complement levels (CH50, C3, and C4) and anti-dsDNA that tend to track with level of disease activity and can even be harbingers of disease flare. As well, tests of acute phase reactants, usually an ESR and CRP, can be useful and important measures that allow the clinician to confirm or refute the presence of active disease. These and more specific laboratory measures to be evaluated in the patient with lupus are also described in Table 4.1. In general there is no utility in monitoring ANA or antibodies to extractable nuclear antibodies (e.g., anti-Ro, La, Sm, RNP) in SLE as they are unlikely to change over time and even less likely to be convergent with disease activity. Monitoring anti-dsDNA levels may have some clinical utility as there is evidence that anti-dsDNA levels will increase with disease activity and will even be a harbinger of a flare of disease going up prior to clinical manifestations of disease, especially lupus nephritis.

Monitoring the Patient at the Clinic or Bedside Using Validated Outcome Measure for SLE

Several composite outcome measures have been developed over time for the assessment of SLE. At this point in time these are not routinely used in clinical practice to monitor patients' disease activity or to document damage. Only the SLEDAI has been found to be responsive to change in SLE patients followed over time in clinics. More recently only two measures, the SELENA-SLEDAI and the SLEDAI-2K, have been shown to be more responsive to change and treatment. Further study of composite indices to monitor patients with SLE in routine practice may be needed before most clinicians will perform these routinely, even though the use of one of these tools in its current state has the potential to be the basis of a comprehensive responsive monitoring tool in the clinic or at the bedside.

Monitoring the In-Hospital Patient with SLE at the Bedside

In the case of a patient with SLE having a severe flare who is hospitalized monitoring for disease activity needs to be much more intensive to determine response to

Table 4.2 Clinical signs and symptoms and laboratory tests which require regular moniutary for medications used to treat lupus

Medication	Potential adverse effects requiring regular monitoring	Monitor for	Frequency
NSAIDs, ASA	GI bleeding, hypertension, renal dysfunction, edema	Hemoglobin/hematocrit, blood pressure, unexplained weight gain Lab: creatinine	Q2–4 weeks initially, then twice annually if on a stable dose
Prednisone (short term)	Weight gain, hypertension, hyperglycemia, increased infection, poor wound healing	Weight, BP Lab: periodic fasting glucose or HgbA1C	
Prednisone (long term)	Bone loss, cataracts, long term glucose tolerance, atherogenic potential	Height (ophthalmologic exam looking for cataracts) Lab: bone mineral density, HgA1C; lipids	At treatment initiation, consider repeating at 3–6 months if high dose and then annually
Hydroxychloroquine (HCQ) or chloroquine (CQ)	GI toxicity, rashes, visual disturbances, rarely retinopathy, myopathy, cardiomyopathy	Ophthalmologic exam (keep maintenance dose based on lean body weight for HCQ at <6.5 mg/kg/day and for CQ at <3 mg/kg/day)	Baseline exam within first year and annual eye exam with Amsler grid or visual field testing after 5 years or annually if comorbid ocular conditions
Methotrexate[a]	Mucosal ulcers, alopecia, diarrhea, suppressed appetite, malaise, elevated LFTs (rarely hepatic fibrosis, cirrhosis, pulmonary toxicity, myelosuppression)	Monitor weight, oral mucosa, scalp (toxicity can increase if renal dysfunction) Cutaneous exam and strength testing at each visit	CBC, creatinine, AST, ALT, ALP, Albumen Q month × 3 and then Q3 months
Azathioprine	Mucosal ulcers, alopecia, diarrhea, suppressed appetite, malaise, elevated LFTs	Myelosuppression [risk higher if thiopurine methyltransferase (TMPT) gene deficient (risk 6/1,000)	CBC, creatinine, AST, ALT, Q month × 3 and then Q3 months, consider initial genetic testing for TMPT
Mycophenolate mofetil (MMF)	Nausea, vomiting, diarrhea, alopecia, increased risk of infection and serious infections	Myelosuppression	CBC monthly × 3 and then Q3–6 months
Cyclophosphamide	Nausea, alopecia, hemorrhagic cystitis, increased risk of infection	Myelosuppression	CBC, urinalysis, monthly
Rituximab[a]	Infusion reactions, increased risk of infection, very rarely PML, long term vaccination status unknown if used >5 years	CBC, IgG, IgM, IgA levels prior to treatment	Repeat immunoglobulin levels prior to each infusion if using longer than 2 years

[a]Medications that are known to be used in SLE may but not have indications for this in all countries (This table has been modified from [Mandl and Liang 2004])

intensive therapy(ies). These patients can have life-threatening multisystem organ involvement and require daily monitoring of disease activity. Clinicians also need ways to determine if their patients are responding quickly to therapeutic measure being taken in these circumstances (pulse steroid, cyclophosphamide, IVIg, plasmaphoresis). Clinical monitoring of these patients will center on the organ system(s), which flared causing hospitalization in the first place. In these circumstances disease activity can be particularly monitored with the use of a CBC, acute phase reactants, complement (C3, C4), and urinary sediment, all of which will change quickly as the patient's condition worsens or as the patient responds to therapy.

Monitoring for the Effects of Treatment in Patients with SLE

Many potentially toxic and immunosuppressive therapies are needed to treat SLE. Table 4.2 includes the majority of therapies used in the treatment of SLE and provides a schema as to how to monitor potential adverse effects of the treatments used in SLE.

Monitoring for Disease and Treatment-Related Comorbidities and Special Situations in SLE

Renal Disease

Fifty percent of SLE patients will develop lupus nephritis (LN). A protein/creatinine ratio or 24-h urine for protein, a urine microscopy, and if abnormal a renal ultrasound with consideration for biopsy should be considered at baseline and in followup as indicated. The best parameter to monitor in LN is urine protein. A recent American College of Rheumatology position paper recommended that using the spot urine protein to creatinine ratio is important to monitor lupus nephritis in addition to a urinalysis. Of note however, spot urine is inadequate for clinical care as a diurnal rhythm in proteinuria, and changes in posture, diet, and exercise can affect the spot urine protein to creatinine ratio during the day. The most reliable way to quantitate urine protein is by using the 24-h urine protein to creatinine ratio rather than a 24-h urine protein collection as collection samples may not be complete. A recent prospective 6-year follow-up of over 600 patients with SLE showed that renal exacerbations were not present if C3, C4, anti-dsDNA, and anti-C1q values were normal. In this study none of these tests were completely reliable in confirming the clinical diagnosis of renal relapses although the anti-C1q was slightly better than the other tests to confirm the clinical activity of LN particularly in patients with focal and diffuse proliferative LN. However the anti-C1q is not routinely available in clinical practice, and most rheumatologists and nephrologists monitor complement (C3, C4) and anti-DNA routinely when monitoring renal disease in SLE. Thus, patients with established nephropathy should be monitored with a protein/creatinine ratio (or 24 h proteinuria), as well as immunological tests (C3, C4, anti-dsDNA), urine microscopy, serum creatinine (including an eGFR), serum albumin, and blood pressure at least every 3 months for the first 2–3 years. Patients with established chronic renal disease (eGFR <60 ml or stable proteinuria >0.5 mg/24 h) should be followed according to the National Kidney Foundation guidelines for chronic kidney disease including urinalysis, serum creatinine, serum albumin, and urine protein.

Neuropsychiatric SLE

How to monitor for neuropsychiatric manifestations of SLE remains one of the most difficult challenges in managing patients with SLE. Patients with SLE should be monitored for the presence of neuropsychological symptoms (seizures, paresthesia, numbness, weakness, headache, epilepsy, depression, etc.) by focused history.

Cognitive impairment may be assessed by evaluating attention, concentration, word finding, and memory difficulties (i.e., by asking the patient about problems with multitasking, with household tasks, or memory). If there is evidence to suggest significant cognitive impairment, then the patient should be assessed in using neuropsychiatric testing by psychologists knowledgeable in the disease. In the event that significant neuropsychiatric SLE (NPSLE) is present, further imaging needs to be considered.

Magnetic resonance imaging (MRI) is the technique of choice to define anatomy in NPSLE. MRI is more likely to show abnormalities if there are focal neurologic defects, seizures, chronic cognitive dysfunction, or manifestations of antiphospholipid syndrome (APS), and less likely to show abnormalities in patients with affective disorders, confusional states, or headache. However, in a note of caution, a cranial MR study should be obtained within 24 h of the initial neurologic event since the typical reversible, high-intensity lesions associated with diffuse presentations resolve rapidly with corticosteroid therapy.

Electroencephalography (EEG) findings are often nonspecific for identifying or monitoring the status of NPSLE as it is unable to determine active from inactive and new versus old disease. EEG measures regional, mostly cortical brain electrical activity and is often abnormal in NPSLE. EEG cannot always distinguish abnormalities associated with active NPSLE from unrelated confounding disorders common to SLE patients such as idiopathic epilepsy, cognitive disorders, drug effects, primary affective disorders, or metabolic encephalopathy. Thus findings from this test must take all these potential manifestations into account when monitoring the patient with SLE. It will be most useful when a SLE-related seizure disorder is suspected.

PET scanning is a very sensitive and expensive, but nonspecific tool for the monitoring of NPSLE, and although not usually recommended because of high cost, limited availability, and high radiation dose, its utility is hampered by the fact that it is often unable to differentiate old from new NPSLE lesions and from confounding lesions. At this point PET is still for the most part a research tool and not recommended for use in routine clinical monitoring of the patient.

Angiography should only be reserved for cases where medium-to-large vessel disease is suspected and then MR angiography should be used initially because of greater safety and lesser expense.

Monitoring the SLE Patient During Pregnancy

Pregnancy still constitutes a major challenge for women with SLE. A coordinated medical/obstetric care is essential to maximize the chance of success. Close surveillance, with monitoring of blood pressure, proteinuria, and placental blood flow by Doppler studies, helps the early diagnosis and treatment of complications such as preeclampsia and fetal distress. Postpartum follow-up is also essential as this is a time when SLE can flare. Other special monitoring is required during pregnancy. At the first pregnancy visit, anti-Ro and anti-La are measured. If positive, weekly fetal four-chamber cardiac ultrasounds should be scheduled from week 16 to week 32 of the pregnancy to detect congenital heart block. Monitoring of complement and dsDNA can be helpful in the last trimester as very low complement or high anti-dsDNA, in the setting of lupus activity, are highly predictive of preterm birth. See Chap. 14 for more details.

The Antiphospholipid Syndrome (APS)

The APS manifests with venous and arteriolar macro- and microthromboses and recurrent miscarriage. Its diagnosis is supported by the presence of antiphospholipid antibodies measured twice at least 12 weeks apart. As noted, these should be assessed at baseline, and in previously negative patients, these antiphospholipid antibodies should be reassessed prior to pregnancy, surgery, and transplant and prior to the use of estrogen-containing treatments, or in the presence of a new neurological or vascular event. See Chap. 15 for more details.

Cardiovascular Disease

Patients with SLE are at higher than expected risk for cardiovascular disease (CVD); however, increased incidence of CVD and of premature atherosclerosis in SLE cannot be fully explained by traditional CVD risk factors. Premature CVD is much more common in young premenopausal women with lupus as they are over 50 times more likely to have a myocardial infarction. Older age at lupus diagnosis, longer lupus disease duration, longer duration of corticosteroid use, hypercholesterolemia, and postmenopausal status are factors that have been noted to be more common in the women with lupus who had a cardiovascular event as compared to those who did not have cardiovascular event. Thus it becomes important to monitor for risk of CVD in patients with SLE by monitoring traditional CVD risk factors and managing modifiable risk factors according to the existing guidelines at baseline and during follow-up at least once a year. This would include the assessments of smoking, vascular events (cerebral/cardiovascular), blood pressure, physical activity, oral contraceptives, and family history of CVD and performing blood cholesterol, glucose, and body mass index (and/or waist circumference) calculations. Patients such as those on glucocorticoids may require more frequent follow-up. See Chap. 8 for more details.

Diabetes

Lupus patients should have a fasting glucose checked yearly. The American Diabetic Association (ADA) defines diabetes with either a fasting plasma glucose of >126 mg dl or a glucose tolerance test of >200 mg dl. Goals of therapy should be near-normal glucose levels and a hemoglobin A1C level of <7 %.

Summary

This chapter has provided an overview on how to monitor the patient with SLE in the clinic and at the bedside to best identify active disease and monitor its treatment. Other sections of this text will provide more in depth information as to how to best manage different aspects of this difficult disease and provide further context for the suggestions noted here. Although this has not been a comprehensive review of the literature, it highlights the key elements the clinician and associated health-care professionals need to take into consideration while looking after their patients with SLE. Key references that address various aspects of monitoring these patients have been included and warrant reading to better understand the complexities of monitoring and managing this disease.

Sources

1. Mosca M, Tani C, Aringer M, Bombardieri S, Boumpas D, Brey R, et al. European League Against Rheumatism recommendations for monitoring patients with systemic lupus erythematosus in clinical practice and in observational studies. Ann Rheum Dis. 2010;69(7):1269–74.
2. Petri M. Monitoring systemic lupus erythematosus in standard clinical care. Best Pract Res Clin Rheumatol. 2007;21(4):687–97.
3. Mandl L, Liang M. Monitoring patients with SLE. In: Lahita RG, editor. Systemic lupus erythematosus. 4th ed. Philadelphia: Elsevier Science (USA); 2004. p. 619–31.

4. Bruce IN, Clark-Soloninka CA, Spitzer KA, Gladman DD, Urowitz MB, Laskin CA. Prevalence of antibodies to beta2-glycoprotein I in systemic lupus erythematosus and their association with antiphospholipid antibody syndrome criteria: a single center study and literature review. J Rheumatol. 2000;27(12):2833–7.
5. LeBlanc BA, Urowitz MB, Gladman OD. Serologically active, clinically quiescent systemic lupus erythematosus—longterm followup. J Rheumatol. 1994;21(1):174–5.
6. Gladman DD, Goldsmith CH, Urowitz MB, Bacon P, Bombardier C, Isenberg D, et al. Sensitivity to change of 3 Systemic Lupus Erythematosus Disease Activity Indices: international validation. J Rheumatol. 1994;21(8):1468–71.
7. Fortin PR, Abrahamowicz M, Clarke AE, Neville C, Du Berger R, Fraenkel L, et al. Do lupus disease activity measures detect clinically important change? J Rheumatol. 2000;27(6):1421–8.
8. Petri M, Kim MY, Kalunian KC, Grossman J, Hahn BH, Sammaritano LR, et al. Combined oral contraceptives in women with systemic lupus erythematosus. N Engl J Med. 2005;353(24):2550–8.
9. Furie RA, Petri MA, Wallace DJ, Ginzler EM, Merrill JT, Stohl W, et al. Novel evidence-based systemic lupus erythematosus responder index. Arthritis Rheum. 2009;61(9):1143–51.
10. Ibanez D, Gladman D, Urowitz M. Summarizing disease features over time: II. Variability measures of SLEDAI-2K. J Rheumatol. 2007;34(2):336–40.
11. Marmor MF, Carr RE, Easterbrook M, Farjo AA, Mieler WF, American Academy of Ophthalmology. Recommendations on screening for chloroquine and hydroxychloroquine retinopathy: a report by the American Academy of Ophthalmology. Opthalmology. 2002;109:1377–82.
12. Marmor M. New American Academy of Ophthalmology recommendations on screening for hydroxychloroquine retinopathy. Arthritis Rheum. 2003;48(6):1764.
13. Anon. TPMT testing before azathioprine therapy. Drug Ther Bull. 2009;47(1):9–12.
14. Marra CA, Esdaile JM, Anis AH. Practical pharmacogenetics: the cost effectiveness of screening for thiopurine s-methyltransferase polymorphisms in patients with rheumatological conditions treated with azathioprine. J Rheumatol. 2002;29(12):2507–12.
15. Appel A, Appel G. An update on the use of mycophenolate mofetil in lupus nephritis and other primary glomerular diseases. Nat Clin Pract Nephrol. 2009;5:132–42.
16. Sinclair A, Appel G, Dooley MA, Ginzler E, Isenberg D, Jayne D, et al. Mycophenolate mofetil as induction and maintenance therapy for lupus nephritis: rationale and protocol for the randomized, controlled Aspreva Lupus Management Study (ALMS). Lupus. 2007;16(12):972–80.
17. Criteria RDSotACoRAHCoSLER. The American College of Rheumatology response criteria for proliferative and membranous renal disease in systemic lupus erythematosus clinical trials. Arthritis Rheum. 2006;54(2):421–32.
18. Christopher-Stine L, Petri M, Astor B, Fine D. Urine protein-to-creatinine ratio is a reliable measure of proteinuria in lupus nephritis. J Rheumatol. 2004;31(8):1557–9.
19. Moroni G, Radice A, Giammarresi G, Quaglini S, Gallelli B, Leoni A, et al. Are laboratory tests useful for monitoring the activity of lupus nephritis? A 6-year prospective study in a cohort of 228 patients with lupus nephritis. Ann Rheum Dis. 2009;68:234–7.
20. Sibbitt Jr WL, Sibbitt RR, Brooks WM. Neuroimaging in neuropsychiatric systemic lupus erythematosus. Arthritis Rheum. 1999;42(10):2026–38.
21. Lampropoulos CE, Koutroumanidis M, Reynolds PP, Manidakis I, Hughes GR, D'Cruz DP. Electroencephalography in the assessment of neuropsychiatric manifestations in antiphospholipid syndrome and systemic lupus erythematosus. Arthritis Rheum. 2005;52(3):841–6.
22. Ruiz-Irastorza G, Khamashta MA. Managing lupus patients during pregnancy. Best Pract Res Clin Rheumatol. 2009;23(4):575–82.
23. Buyon J, Clancy R. Neonatal lupus: basic research and clinical perspectives. Rheum Dis Clin North Am. 2005;31(2):299–313. vii.
24. Clowse ME, Magder LS, Witter F, Petri M. The impact of increased lupus activity on obstetric outcomes. Arthritis Rheum. 2005;52(2):514–21.

25. Abu-Shakra M, Urowitz MB, Gladman DD, Gough J. Mortality studies in systemic lupus erythematosus. Results from a single center. II. Predictor variables for mortality. J Rheumatol. 1995;22(7):1265–70.
26. Esdaile JM, Abrahamowicz M, Grodzicky T, Li Y, Panaritis C, du Berger R, et al. Traditional Framingham risk factors fail to fully account for accelerated atherosclerosis in systemic lupus erythematosus. Arthritis Rheum. 2001;44(10):2331–7.
27. Manzi S, Meilahn EN, Rairie JE, Conte CG, Medsger Jr TA, Jansen-McWilliams L, et al. Age-specific incidence rates of myocardial infarction and angina in women with systemic lupus erythematosus: comparison with the Framingham Study. Am J Epidemiol. 1997;145(5): 408–15.
28. Genuth S, Alberti K, Benett P, et al. Follow-up report on the diagnosis of diabetes mellitus. Diabetes Care. 2003;26:3160–7.
29. Elliott JR, Manzi S. Cardiovascular risk assessment and treatment in systemic lupus erythematosus. Best Pract Res Clin Rheumatol. 2009;23(4):481–94.

Chapter 5
The Treatment of Lupus: General Principles

Elena M. Massarotti and Peter H. Schur

Effective patient care entails the development of a trusting relationship and workable treatment plan between patient and physician. Clear mutual goals should be set whose basic aims are to alleviate symptoms, prevent exacerbations, treat relapses, prevent permanent organ dysfunction, and prevent damage from treatment.

The Patient–Doctor Relationship

Probably the most important part of a successful long-term treatment program for the lupus patient is the development of open communication and a sense of trust between patient and physician. To the physician, this means not only regular office visits with time for discussion, answering questions, and offering explanations but also availability for emergencies (e.g., by telephone and e-mail).

Patients with lupus are confronted with the unknown, a potentially disabling chronic disease and at times the fear of dying. The patient may have seen a definition of lupus on line as a "fatal disease of young women." Patients with lupus need reassurance, sympathy, support, and frank discussions, not just initially but on subsequent visits, regarding their disease as well as the stress the disease puts on them.

E.M. Massarotti, M.D. (✉)
Division of Rheumatology, Center for Clinical Therapeutics,
Brigham and Women's Hospital, 75 Francis Street,
Boston, MA 02115, USA

Harvard Medical School, Boston, MA, USA
e-mail: emassarotti@partners.org

P.H. Schur, M.D., F.A.C.P.
Division of Rheumatology, Brigham and Women's Hospital, Boston, MA 02115, USA

Harvard Medical School, Boston, MA, USA
e-mail: pschur@partners.org

Patients often have to deal with the fact that they "look well" but may be suffering from significant organic disease.

Often it is helpful to discuss the nature of the illness with other members of a patient's family and to enlist their support. The Lupus Foundation of America (LFA) sponsors many local support groups in which patients and family members gather under the guidance of a skilled professional and discuss ways of managing disease-related stress. In addition a large number of books, booklets, pamphlets, newsletters, articles, videos, internet articles have been published by the LFA, Arthritis Foundation, NIH, and UpToDate to assist patients and their families.

The physician should educate the patient with regard to signs suggesting that the disease is becoming more severe. These signs include malaise, poor appetite, weight loss, weight gain, fatigue, pallor, irregular and heavy menses, fever, arthritis, seizures, cognitive abnormalities, mood changes, difficulty coping, chest pain, edema, excessive hair loss, oliguria, rashes, and mouth sores. The physician should routinely ask about these signs at each visit and encourage patients to bring in problem/question lists. In some instances these symptoms have causes other than lupus and should be investigated and treated. Patients often become anxious regarding the interpretation of laboratory tests. Explanations of test rationale and results are helpful.

Often patients are more concerned with the side effects of medication than with their benefits. The physician should monitor for drug allergies; drug interactions, whether medications should be taken prior to, with, or after meals; and medication cost.

The physician needs to focus not just on prolonging life but also on improving the quality of life.

Determination of Disease Activity and Severity

Patients with lupus may present and follow up with a variety of symptoms and concerns. Determining whether these symptoms are due to lupus activity, other processes related to another cause, or the effects of injury from previously active disease is critical in the rheumatologist's clinical assessment. Disease activity usually refers to the degree of inflammation from ongoing, uncontrolled disease; severity implies that organ function and perhaps its underlying structure is quantitatively impaired. The degree of organ dysfunction has been referred to as the "damage index."

The presence of severe organ dysfunction does not necessarily imply ongoing inflammation. As an example, marked proteinuria and a decreasing glomerular filtration rate may result from either active inflammation or from scarred glomeruli in the absence of active inflammatory disease. The ability to differentiate between these two possibilities is extremely important since immunosuppressive therapy is not indicated in the latter setting. Similarly, joint pain may be related to active synovitis, for which anti-inflammatory agents or corticosteroids may be indicated, while avascular necrosis—another cause of musculoskeletal pain in lupus patients—is not due to active inflammation and is treated with analgesics and possibly surgery.

Table 5.1 SLE activity indices

- Over 60 systems to gauge disease activity have been assessed, but agreement on a definition of disease activity has not been reached
- *BILAG* (British Isles Lupus Assessment Group)
- Systemic lupus erythematosus disease activity index (*SLEDAI with SELENA* modification)
- Systemic lupus activity measure (*SLAM*)
- Lupus activity index (*LAI*)
- These indices are reliable, valid, and correlate with each other
- Rarely used in the clinical setting—may not practical for busy clinicians
- Were not designed for clinical trials but for be cohort or cross-sectional studies
- None is perfect
- Validated in English

Clinically Useful Markers of Activity

Validated disease activity measures have been developed to assess lupus-related disease in clinical research but have not gained widespread use in busy clinical practices (Table 5.1). In clinical practice, disease activity is assessed using a combination of the clinical history, physical examination, selected laboratory tests, and serologic studies, examples of which include

- Active SLE (particularly lupus nephritis) is often preceded by a rise in IgG anti-double-stranded DNA titers, a fall in complement levels (especially CH50, C3, and C4), and an elevation in complement split and activation products.
- Persistently low serum levels of complement C1q are associated with continued activity of proliferative glomerulonephritis.
- Increases in the erythrocyte sedimentation rate (ESR) and serum C-reactive protein (CRP) concentration are also commonly seen in the context of inflammation. There are conflicting data on the diagnostic value of a marked elevation of CRP in distinguishing active lupus from infection. Infection should be considered in the differential diagnosis of an elevated CRP.

However, not all patients with these serologic markers have active disease, and these markers do not necessarily predict disease exacerbation. In one study, for example, 12 % of patients with hypocomplementemia and elevated anti-DNA antibody titers had no clinical evidence of active disease.

In general, we do not use laboratory tests alone to primarily guide treatment and favor an approach in which patients are closely monitored; therapy is adjusted if there are signs of *clinical* worsening of the disease. For example, a patient presenting in follow-up with quiescent symptoms and laboratory testing showing hypocomplementemia and an elevated dsDNA would not necessarily require any change in pharmacotherapy but would be reassessed within weeks for any evolving symptoms suggestive of disease activity.

Frequency of Laboratory Testing

The frequency with which monitoring laboratory tests are performed should be tailored to each patient. In general, patients with more active disease are monitored more frequently, while those with inactive disease require less frequent monitoring. In general, for stable patients without active disease, a complete blood count, chemistry profile, and urinalysis done every 6 months or so is probably adequate. Following specific serological markers like C3, C4, CH50, and dsDNA can be tailored to the individual patient; if a patient's known disease activity correlates with CH50 and dsDNA, testing for these serological studies may give insight into the particular symptom at hand. Routinely testing these laboratory parameters in the absence of specific symptoms is probably not cost effective or clinically useful.

Investigational Markers

Numerous investigations of other immunologic tests as indicators of disease activity have been reported, including antibodies to C1q and nucleosomes, complement activation products, soluble T-cell activation markers, serum levels of various cytokines and cytokine receptors, angiogenic factors, adhesion molecules, chemokines, and cell surface markers of immunologic activation (e.g., erythrocyte/reticulocyte-bound C4d).

Gene expression profiling and proteomic approaches may eventually provide additional indices of disease activity. As examples

- An increased expression of genes activated by interferon in peripheral blood mononuclear cells has been noted.
- Active disease may be associated with a constellation of autoantibodies that can be detected using proteomic arrays.
- A proteomic approach identified a pattern of proteins that was both sensitive and specific for active nephritis.
- Increased amounts of erythrocyte-bound C4d were correlated with increased disease activity in one but not another study.

The putative usefulness of the investigational markers of disease activity noted above has either been unconfirmed or has generally not yet been proven to be as useful as monitoring complement and anti-double-stranded DNA antibodies.

General Treatment Considerations

Although organ involvement requires specific drug therapy, a number of general issues are applicable to every patient with SLE. More details regarding the treatment of specific manifestations can be found in other chapters in this text.

Sun Protection

Emotional and physical adjustment to avoiding the sun is a difficult battle that lupus patients face in our sun-loving society. Some patients are more photo-sensitive than others, but generally all direct sun exposure should be avoided for most SLE patients. This includes sun bathing, tanning parlors, sitting on the beach, areas with lots of reflection off concrete surfaces, or snow! In general, we recommend that lupus patients avoid exposure to direct or reflected sunlight and other sources of ultraviolet light (e.g., fluorescent and halogen lights, sunlamps, welding arcs) and use sunscreens, preferably those that block both UV-A and UV-B, with a high skin protection factor (SPF). A sunscreen with a SPF of 55 or greater is suggested. Sunscreen should be applied 1 h before exposure and reapplied for those very sensitive, and exposed, every 2–4 h. Protective clothing helps including broad-brimmed hats and sun-protective clothing. Photosensitizing medications like phenothiazines should be avoided—patients who complain of being light-headed or dizzy after sun exposure do not qualify as being "photosensitive" by the classification criteria.

Diet and Nutrition

Limited data exist concerning the effect of dietary modification in SLE. A conservative approach is to recommend a balanced diet consisting of carbohydrates, proteins, and fats. However, the diet should be modified based upon disease activity and the response to therapy:

- Patients with active inflammatory disease and fever may require more calories.
- Glucocorticoids enhance appetite, resulting in potentially significant weight gain. Hunger can be somewhat lessened by the ingestion of water, antacids, proton pump inhibitors, and/or histamine H2 blockers. A low-salt and low-calorie diet should be instituted if there is significant weight gain.

For those patients who are overweight, moderate increases in physical activity and calorie reduction should be encouraged. Inactivity produced by acute illness causes a rapid loss of muscle mass and stamina resulting in a sense of fatigue, so that patients tend to rest more. Too much rest will result in more loss of muscle mass, and more fatigue, which may then result in a reactive depression, thus resulting in even less activity. This vicious cycle needs to be broken and there needs to be a balance between rest and exercise. In fact there are no diseases that have been shown to be benefited by rest. The patient should be encouraged once they are feeling better to begin graded exercise. Exercise can be walking, swimming, and biking—anything a patient enjoys. Jogging may be too strenuous for an already weakened musculoskeletal structure. Physical and occupational therapy and a formal exercise program can be of help. Antimalarial drugs (e.g., hydroxychloroquine) can help fatigue.

- Hyperlipidemia may be induced by the nephrotic syndrome or the administration of glucocorticoids. Patients with hyperlipidemia should be encouraged to eat a low-fat diet. A lipid-lowering agent (usually a statin) should be considered if serum cholesterol remains above the recommended values despite a change in diet.
- Vitamins are rarely needed when patients eat a balanced diet. However, a daily multivitamin should be taken by patients who are not able to obtain an adequate diet or who are dieting to lose weight, or are pregnant. Vitamins or other alternatives will rarely help fatigue.
- The majority of patients with SLE have low serum levels of 25-hydroxyvitamin D (calcidiol), probably due at least in part to avoidance of sun exposure. Patients with low vitamin D levels should be treated with supplemental vitamin D. Patients taking long-term glucocorticoids and postmenopausal women should ingest 1,000 units of vitamin D plus 1,500 mg of calcium per day.
- Herbs are of unproven benefit and may cause harm.

A low-salt diet, to prevent fluid retention and hypertension, is recommended if the patient is receiving glucocorticosteroids.

Cosmetics and Hair Products

Many patients with SLE develop skin lesions, especially on the face, that they, and others, consider unsightly and disturbing. One should therefore educate patients about preventing skin lesions by avoiding UV exposure (especially sunlight) and the regular use of sunscreens. If skin lesions do develop, prompt treatment with topical and injectable corticosteroids and antimalarials should be considered. If scars or blemishes develop, we recommend that patients seek the advice of a cosmetologist (often found through large department stores) who can prescribe appropriate makeup to "hide" areas of hyper- or hypopigmentation or telangiectasias.

Smoking Cessation

Cigarette smoking may increase the risk of developing SLE, and smokers in general have more active disease. Smoking may affect the efficacy of some medications (e.g., hydroxychloroquine). Patients should be counseled not to smoke or to quit smoking and provided with help to do so.

Immunizations

It had been previously thought that immunization could exacerbate SLE. However, influenza vaccine and pneumococcal vaccines are safe, but resultant antibody titers are somewhat less in patients with SLE than in controls. Use of glucocorticoids, such as prednisone, or other immunosuppressive agents may contribute to the blunted antibody response.

In contrast, it is inadvisable to immunize lupus patients, especially those receiving corticosteroids or immunosuppressives with live vaccines [e.g., measles, mumps, rubella, polio, varicella, and vaccinia (smallpox)].

While the issue of efficacy of vaccination with hepatitis B vaccine has not been completely resolved, the risks posed by hepatitis B vaccine to patients with SLE must at most be very small.

Radiation Therapy

Anecdotal reports of increased toxicity following therapeutic ionizing radiation have made radiation oncologists wary of treating patients with SLE and other connective tissue disorders. However, if needed, radiation therapy may be used in patients with SLE to treat malignant disease, and all agree that the potential benefits outweigh any risks.

Contraception and Pregnancy (Also see Chap. 14)

The physician may be asked to provide counsel regarding contraception and family planning. Barrier methods and spermicides are the safest form of contraception. Oral contraceptives, especially those low in estrogen, are generally safe but should be avoided in those SLE patients prone to thromboembolic disease (e.g., those with antiphospholipid antibodies), patients with migraine headaches, and/or a history of phlebitis. Hormone replacement therapy in postmenopausal women may be associated with a modest increase in the rate of flares, and decisions about use of estrogen for postmenopausal symptoms must be carefully considered weighing the potential benefits against risks of thrombotic events, breast cancer, and uterine cancer.

Family planning generally revolves around timing, when a patient has not had active disease for a number of months (to avoid the risk of lupus exacerbation), does not have significant organ impairment (e.g., renal insufficiency, CNS, or cardiopulmonary impairment), and is not taking medications that may put a fetus at risk. Patients should be tested for antibodies to Ro (SSA) and La (SSB) to determine if their child is at risk for neonatal lupus (including heart block) but told if positive that the risk is only about 3 %. Nevertheless the fetus should be monitored with fetal ECHO starting at about 15 weeks to determine if heart block has developed, and persists, so that a pacemaker can be put in at birth. In addition the patient should be tested for antiphospholipid antibodies to determine if they are at (increased) risk for miscarriage. Most patients should be monitored by an obstetrician used to be dealing with high-risk pregnancies.

Another issue of concern for all is what medications are safe during pregnancy. Again, one always has to balance benefit and risk. Some medications are clearly not safe such as the immunosuppressives methotrexate, leflunomide, mycophenolate, and cyclosporine; some should be used with caution, if the clinical situation warrants it and nothing else is available, such as azathioprine and cyclophosphamide. Prednisone is the drug of choice for most flares of lupus and has some well-recognized risks for the mother and rare for the fetus. During pregnancy hydroxychloroquine appears to be safe. Aspirin and nonsteroidal anti-inflammatory drugs (NSAIDs) appear to be safe but are generally discontinued in the third trimester.

Nevertheless, patients should be reassured that most pregnancies have good outcomes, both for mother and child.

A frequent question asked by prospective parents is as follows: what is the risk that their child will develop lupus when they grow up? Current epidemiological studies suggest that the risk is approximately 5 %.

Breast-feeding is generally recommended and is not a problem for many patients, unless they are too ill to do so. During that time the medication list should be carefully reviewed to avoid medication getting into breast milk. Generally one uses the minimum dose to be given right after breast-feeding. Prednisone 10–15 mg/day appears safe as are short-acting NSAIDs and 200 mg hydroxychloroquine. Immunosuppressive medications should be avoided.

Treating Comorbid Conditions

Accelerated atherosclerosis, pulmonary hypertension, antiphospholipid antibodies, and osteopenia or osteoporosis are among the comorbid conditions that can be treated and for which screening tests are appropriately used. These comorbid disorders, for which patients with SLE have an increased risk, include

- Accelerated atherosclerosis.
- Pulmonary hypertension.
- Antiphospholipid antibodies—the presence of antiphospholipid antibodies is assessed by assays for antibodies to cardiolipin (aCL), beta 2 glycoprotein-1 (anti-β2 glycoprotein-1), and for the presence of lupus anticoagulant (LA) activity.
- Osteopenia or osteoporosis—bone mineral density determination may detect the presence of osteopenia or osteoporosis and allow dietary or medical interventions to prevent or reverse bone demineralization. Patients taking high-dose and/or long-term therapy with corticosteroids are at increased risk.

Avoidance of Specific Medications

Some data suggest that sulfonamide-containing antibiotics (e.g., sulfadiazine, trimethoprim–sulfamethoxazole, sulfisoxazole) may cause exacerbations and should therefore be avoided.

In contrast, medications that cause drug-induced lupus, such as procainamide and hydralazine, do not cause exacerbations of idiopathic SLE. On the other hand we tend to avoid prescribing minocycline to patients with SLE.

Treatment of Specific Organ Involvement (Also see Chap. 17)

A number of medications are commonly used in the treatment of SLE, including NSAIDs, antimalarials (primarily hydroxychloroquine), glucocorticoids, and immunosuppressive agents (including cyclophosphamide, methotrexate, azathioprine, and mycophenolate). Patient compliance with recommended treatment is, as expected, associated with better outcomes than noncompliance.

What follows is a general overview of which drugs are preferred in selected clinical settings.

- Topical therapies for rashes are often useful and reduce the risk of side effects that are associated with systemic use of NSAIDs, glucocorticoids, or immunosuppressants.
- NSAIDs are generally effective for musculoskeletal complaints, fever, headaches, and mild serositis. Cyclooxygenase (COX)-2 selective inhibitors may also be effective and safe in such patients.
- Antimalarials are most useful for skin manifestations and for musculoskeletal complaints. Their use may also reduce the risk of disease flares, though this is less clear for renal and central nervous system manifestations.
- Systemic glucocorticoids (e.g., high doses of 1–2 mg/kg/day of prednisone or equivalent or as intermittent intravenous "pulses" of methylprednisolone) used alone or in combination with immunosuppressive agents are generally reserved for patients with significant organ involvement, particularly renal and central nervous system disease. There are a paucity of data to support the use of intravenous "pulse" versus daily oral glucocorticoids. Patients with organ-threatening disease (e.g., cardiopulmonary, hepatic, renal, hemolytic anemia, immune thrombocytopenia) usually are given the above-mentioned oral doses, whereas non-organ-threatening disease (e.g., cutaneous, musculoskeletal, constitutional) patients usually respond to 5–15 mg of prednisone equivalent a day until a steroid-sparing agent or antimalarial can take effect.

Treatment with immunosuppressive medications other than glucocorticoids (e.g., methotrexate, cyclophosphamide, azathioprine, or mycophenolate) is generally reserved for patients with significant organ involvement and/or patients who have had an inadequate response to glucocorticoids.

Immunosuppressive agents such as mycophenolate, azathioprine, or cyclophosphamide are given with glucocorticoids to patients with more than mild lupus nephritis and cyclophosphamide to those with alveolar hemorrhage, systemic vasculitis, and to most patients with significant central nervous system involvement.

Lower doses of glucocorticoids (e.g., ≤10 mg/day of prednisone) may be used for symptomatic relief of severe arthralgia, arthritis, or serositis while awaiting a therapeutic effect from other medications.

Prognosis

SLE can run a varied clinical course, ranging from a relatively benign illness to a rapidly progressive disease with fulminant organ failure and death. Most patients have a relapsing and remitting course, which may be associated with the use of high-dose steroids during the treatment of severe flares. In general, patients tend to flare with the same manifestations with which they presented, but the clinician must remain hyperalert to the very real possibility of disease occurrence in previously unaffected organ systems.

Patient Survival

The 5-year survival rate in SLE has dramatically increased over the last several decades from approximately 40 % in the 1950s to more than 90 % in studies beginning after 1980, a trend that has continued into the early twenty-first century.

The likelihood of survival can be ranked on the basis of organ involvement (skin and musculoskeletal best, central nervous system and kidney worst) and on the number of American College of Rheumatology criteria for SLE. Older age, male sex, poverty, and a low complement may also be poor prognostic factors, as was noted in a cohort of North American patients. However, increasing age was not a predictor of an increased mortality rate in one Chinese cohort of 442 patients when compared to an age-adjusted population mortality rate. Measures of disease activity and accumulated organ damage may also be predictive of increased mortality while use of antimalarial drugs may reduce mortality rates.

The improvement in patient survival is probably due to multiple factors. These include increased disease recognition with more sensitive diagnostic tests, earlier diagnosis or treatment, inclusion of milder cases, and increasingly judicious therapy and prompt treatment of complications.

Deaths due to lupus differ with respect to gender and race as reported by the CDC in 2002. As examples, the proportion of deaths due to SLE was more than five times higher in women than men and more than three times higher in black compared to white women. More than one-third of deaths due to lupus occurred in people aged 15–44 years.

Causes of Death

The major cause of death in the first few years of illness is active disease (e.g., CNS, renal, or cardiovascular disease) or infection due to immunosuppression, while late deaths are either caused by the illness (e.g., end-stage renal disease), treatment complications (including infection and coronary disease), non-Hodgkin lymphoma, and lung.

Serious infection is most often due to immunosuppressive therapy. Patients at particular risk are those treated with both glucocorticoids and cyclophosphamide, especially if the white blood cell count is less than 3,000/μL and/or high-dose steroids are given. Lymphopenia (<1,000/μL) at presentation may be an independent risk factor.

Premature coronary artery disease is being increasingly recognized as a cause of late mortality.

Is Cancer Risk Increased?

Although the relation of SLE to malignancy was previously unclear because of conflicting data, there appears to be a clear increase of certain malignancies in patients with SLE.

A 2005 meta-analysis concluded that there is an increased risk in patients with SLE, predominantly for that of non-Hodgkin-type lymphoma. Non-Hodgkin lymphoma in patients with SLE is often an aggressive histologic subtype, especially diffuse large B cell lymphoma. Other studies have demonstrated increased frequencies of Hodgkin lymphoma, breast cancer, squamous skin cancer, abnormal cervical Papanicolaou (Pap) smears, cervical cancer, and vaginal/vulvar cancer. Antimalarial drug use may be associated with a reduced risk of cancer in one but not other studies. Although some data suggest that the use of immunosuppressive drugs may be associated with the later development of hematologic malignancies, there is at present insufficient information to conclude whether or not the use of immunosuppressive medications in patients with SLE increases their risk for malignancies.

Prognostic Factors

Poor prognostic factors for survival in SLE include

- Renal disease (especially diffuse proliferative glomerulonephritis)
- Hypertension
- Male sex
- Young age
- Older age at presentation

- Poor socioeconomic status
- Black race, which may primarily reflect low socioeconomic status
- Presence of antiphospholipid antibodies
- Antiphospholipid syndrome
- High overall disease activity (e.g., hemolytic anemia, TTP, alveolar hemorrhage, pulmonary hypertension, mesenteric vasculitis)

Morbidity

Despite a reduction in the risk of premature death, patients with SLE are still at risk for significant morbidity due to both active disease and the side effects of drugs such as glucocorticoids and cytotoxic agents. Steroid-induced avascular necrosis of the hips and knees, osteoporosis, fatigue, and cognitive dysfunction have become particularly important problems as patients live longer with their illness with a concomitant increase in total steroid exposure.

Factors that may be associated with a shorter delay between disease onset and organ damage include

- Hispanic ethnicity
- Greater disease activity
- A history of thrombotic events
- Glucocorticoid use of less than 10 mg/day

Glucocorticoid use at doses equivalent to prednisone ≥10 mg/day was associated with a longer time from SLE onset to organ damage, but, as noted above, long-term use of higher doses of glucocorticoids has significant risks that must be considered.

Clinical Remission

After appropriate therapy, some patients go into a clinical remission lasting 1–5 years requiring no treatment. However, relapses are common.

Summary

Successful treatment of lupus includes a systematic and methodical approach to diagnosis and assessment of which organ systems are affected. While certain treatments can be generally recommended (sun protection, for example), other modalities may be more appropriate for specific aspects. For example, antimalarials are especially useful for cutaneous disease but ineffective for the treatment of active kidney disease. Lupus patients, then, may be treated with different agents in combination. In addition, it is likely that different mechanisms are responsible for the different clinical aspects of lupus, accounting for the use of medications with different mechanisms of action. The FDA approval of belimumab for the treatment of lupus introduces the realm of biological therapy to this prototypic autoimmune illness and will likely help scientists and clinicians better understand the pathogenesis of this disease.

Sources

1. Wallace DJ. Improving the prognosis of SLE without prescribing lupus drugs and the primary care paradox. Lupus. 2008;17:91.
2. Liu CC, Manzi S, Ahearn JM. Biomarkers for systemic lupus erythematosus: a review and perspective. Curr Opin Rheumatol. 2005;17:543.
3. Lloyd W, Schur PH. Immune complexes, complement, and anti-DNA in exacerbations of SLE. Medicine. 1981;60:208.
4. Kao AH, Navratil JS, Ruffing MJ, et al. Erythrocyte C3d and C4d for monitoring disease activity in systemic lupus erythematosus. Arthritis Rheum. 2010;62:837.
5. Gunnarsson I, Sundelin B, Heimburger M, et al. Repeated renal biopsy in proliferative lupus nephritis—predictive role of serum C1q and albuminuria. J Rheumatol. 2002;29:693.
6. Gaitonde S, Samols D, Kushner I. C-reactive protein and systemic lupus erythematosus. Arthritis Rheum. 2008;59:1814.
7. Walz LeBlanc BA, Gladman DD, Urowitz MB. Serologically active clinically quiescent systemic lupus erythematosus—predictors of clinical flares. J Rheumatol. 1994;21:2239.
8. Ronnblom L, Eloranta M-L, Alm GV. The type I interferon system in systemic lupus erythematosus. Arthritis Rheum. 2006;54:408.
9. Ettinger WH, Goldberg AP, Applebaum-Bowden D, Hazzard WR. Dyslipoproteinemia in SLE. Effect of corticosteroids. Am J Med. 1987;83:503.
10. Tench CM, McCarthy J, McCurdie I, et al. Fatigue in systemic lupus erythematosus: a randomized controlled trial of exercise. Rheumatology (Oxford). 2003;42:1050.
11. Wallace DJ. Antimalarial agents and lupus. Rheum Dis Clin North Am. 1994;20:243.
12. O'Neill SG, Isenberg DA. Immunizing patients with systemic lupus erythematosus: a review of effectiveness and safety. Lupus. 2006;15:778.
13. Lin A, Abu Isa E, Griffith KA, Ben-Josef E. Toxicity of radiotherapy in patients with collagen vascular disease. Cancer. 2008;113:648.
14. Pope J, Jerome D, Fenlon D, et al. Frequency of adverse drug reactions in patients with systemic lupus erythematosus. J Rheumatol. 2003;30:480.
15. Buyon JP, Petri MA, Kim MY, et al. The effect of combined estrogen and progesterone hormone replacement therapy on disease activity in SLE: a randomized trial. Ann Intern Med. 2005;142:953.
16. A randomized study of the effect of withdrawing hydroxychloroquine sulfate in systemic lupus erythematosus. The Canadian Hydroxychloroquine Study Group. N Engl J Med. 1991;324:150.
17. Parker BJ, Bruce IN. High dose methylprednisolone therapy for the treatment of severe systemic lupus erythematosus. Lupus. 2007;16:387.
18. Fortin PR, Abrahamowicz M, Ferland D, et al. Steroid-sparing effects of methotrexate in systemic lupus erythematosus: a double-blind, randomized, placebo-controlled trial. Arthritis Rheum. 2008;59:1796.
19. Tyndall A. Cellular therapy of systemic lupus erythematosus. Lupus. 2009;18:387.
20. Merrill JT, Neuwelt CM, Wallace DJ, et al. Efficacy and safety of rituximab in moderately-to-severely active systemic lupus erythematosus: the randomized, double-blind, phase II/III systemic lupus erythematosus evaluation of rituximab trial. Arthritis Rheum. 2010;62:222.

21. Wallace DJ, Stohl W, Furie RA, et al. A phase II, randomized, double-blind, placebo-controlled, dose-ranging study of belimumab in patients with active systemic lupus erythematosus. Arthritis Rheum. 2009;61:1168.
22. Urowitz MB, Gladman DD, Tom BD, et al. Changing patterns in mortality and disease outcomes for patients with systemic lupus erythematosus. J Rheumatol. 2008;35:2152.
23. Bernatsky S, Joseph L, Boivin JF, et al. The relationship between cancer and medication exposures in systemic lupus erythaematosus: a case-cohort study. Ann Rheum Dis. 2008;67:74.
24. Navarra SV, Guzmán RM, Gallacher AE, Hall S, Levy RA, Jimenez RE, Li EK, Thomas M, Kim HY, León MG, Tanasescu C, Nasonov E, Lan JL, Pineda L, Zhong ZJ, Freimuth W, Petri MA, BLISS-52 Study Group. Efficacy and safety of belimumab in patients with active systemic lupus erythematosus: a randomised, placebo-controlled, phase 3 trial. Lancet. 2011;377(9767):721–31.
25. Merrill JT, Burgos-Vargas R, Westhovens R, Chalmers A, D'Cruz D, Wallace DJ, Bae SC, Sigal L, Becker JC, Kelly S, Raghupathi K, Li T, Peng Y, Kinaszczuk M, Nash P. The efficacy and safety of abatacept in patients with non-life-threatening manifestations of systemic lupus erythematosus: results of a twelve-month, multicenter, exploratory, phase IIb, randomized, double-blind, placebo-controlled trial. Arthritis Rheum. 2010;62(10):3077–87.
26. Up to Date: Many articles in UpToDate in rheumatology and UpToDate in nephrology table

Chapter 6
Cutaneous Manifestations of Lupus Erythematosus

Henry Townsend and Ruth Ann Vleugels

Introduction

Lupus erythematosus (LE) is a chronic inflammatory autoimmune disease characterized by diverse clinical features and autoantibodies. LE includes both systemic disease (SLE), which may affect multiple organ systems, and cutaneous disease (CLE) involving the skin and mucous membranes. Cutaneous disease has been estimated to occur as the initial manifestation in 25 % of patients diagnosed with systemic lupus erythematosus and in 70–80 % of patients at some point during their disease course. The skin manifestations of LE are generally classified as either LE specific (clinically and histologically diagnostic of LE) or LE nonspecific (cutaneous eruptions that are not histopathologically specific for LE). LE-specific skin disease has three recognized subtypes: acute cutaneous LE (ACLE), subacute cutaneous LE (SCLE), and chronic cutaneous LE (CCLE). In addition, CCLE may occur in several forms including discoid LE (DLE), hypertrophic LE, lupus panniculitis/profundus, tumid LE, and chilblains LE. LE-nonspecific cutaneous disorders include photosensitivity, alopecia, mucosal lesions, Raynaud's phenomenon, livedo reticularis, cutaneous vasculitis, and urticarial vasculitis. The types of cutaneous LE vary significantly in both their clinical presentations and in their associations with systemic disease.

H. Townsend, M.D.
Division of Clinical Immunology and Rheumatology,
Department of Medicine, University of Alabama at Birmingham,
Birmingham, AL, USA

R.A. Vleugels, M.D., M.P.H. (✉)
Connective Tissue Disease Clinic, Brigham and Women's Dermatology,
221 Longwood Ave, Boston, MA 02115, USA

Harvard Medical School, Boston, MA, USA
e-mail: rvleugels@partners.org

Lupus Erythematosus-Specific Skin Disease

Acute Cutaneous Lupus Erythematosus

ACLE may occur as a localized or diffuse eruption. The most common and well-known form is the malar (butterfly) rash characterized by erythema of the cheeks and nasal bridge with sparing of the nasolabial folds (see Fig. 6.1). The eruption may also involve the forehead, anterior neck, arms, and hands. Other presentations of ACLE include a generalized morbilliform eruption (often referred to as maculopapular), a bullous eruption, and a diffuse toxic epidermal necrolysis (TEN)-like exfoliative process. Overall, ACLE is estimated to occur in approximately 15 % of patients with cutaneous lupus. In addition, ACLE is strongly associated with active SLE or future development of SLE.

Antinuclear antibodies (ANA) are positive in 95 %, and anti-double-stranded DNA antibodies are present in approximately 50 % of patients with ACLE. All forms of ACLE appear to be at least moderately photosensitive. ACLE usually resolves without scarring; however, post-inflammatory pigmentation changes may occur, most commonly in darker skinned patients. Conditions which can mimic the malar rash of ACLE include sunburn, rosacea, seborrheic dermatitis, atopic dermatitis, and dermatomyositis. Of note, a helpful feature to assist in distinguishing the midfacial erythema associated with dermatomyositis versus that of ACLE is that it tends to involve the nasolabial folds with dermatomyositis rather than sparing these areas. The differential diagnosis for generalized ACLE includes viral exanthems and hypersensitivity reactions to medications. Evaluation of TEN-like exfoliative

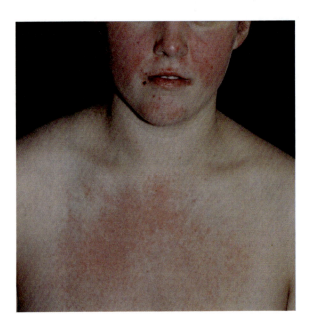

Fig. 6.1 Acute LE

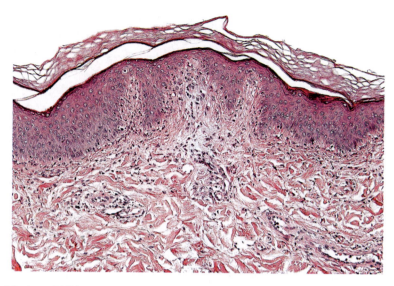

Fig. 6.2 Acute LE histology: karyorrhectic debris and lymphocytic infiltrate along the dermoepidermal junction and focal rare apoptosis of keratinocytes (Picture courtesy of Dr. Alireza Sepehr)

dermatitis should always include a thorough medication review. The drugs most closely associated with TEN are nonsteroidal anti-inflammatory drugs, sulfonamide antibiotics, anticonvulsants, and allopurinol. In patients already diagnosed with LE who present with TEN or a generalized morbilliform eruption, antimalarials should also be added to the list of potential triggering medications. In patients in whom no causal medication can be found, a diagnosis of generalized ACLE should be considered and histopathology can confirm this diagnosis.

The appearance of bullous ACLE can be challenging to distinguish clinically from other blistering disorders. Thus, in addition to serologic studies, a skin biopsy with immunofluorescence should be performed in all bullous dermatoses. Although bullous LE tends to present in patients with active systemic disease, the cutaneous eruption itself should be considered LE nonspecific, given that the histopathology demonstrates a split at the dermoepidermal junction and a predominantly neutrophilic infiltrate, while other classic histopathologic features of cutaneous LE are typically lacking. In bullous LE, direct immunofluorescence (DIF) demonstrates C3 and IgG in a linear or granular pattern at the dermoepidermal junction.

Histologically, the malar rash of ACLE shows a classic interface dermatitis characterized by a lymphocytic infiltrate at the dermoepidermal junction (see Fig. 6.2). Vacuolar degeneration of the epidermal basal cell layer and perivascular and periadnexal inflammation are other common findings. DIF examination in ACLE commonly shows linear or granular deposition of immunoglobulins and complement at the basement membrane zone. This finding, historically known as the lupus band test, occurs in >90 % of lesional skin, 75 % of sun-exposed normal-appearing skin, and 50 % of non-sun-exposed, normal skin in patients with ACLE. The lupus band

Fig. 6.3 Annular SCLE

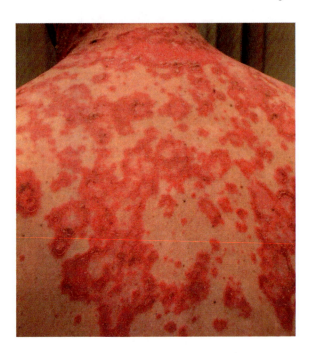

test is most specific when performed on normal, sun-protected skin, as positive band tests have been noted in 20 % of healthy young adults when performed on sun-exposed skin. When performed on normal, sun-protected skin, a positive lupus band test is considered reliable for diagnosis and can also have prognostic utility based on the number of positive immunoreactants.

Subacute Cutaneous Lupus Erythematosus

SCLE traditionally presents with one of two characteristic types of lesions: annular or polycyclic plaques with central clearing, often termed annular SCLE (see Fig. 6.3), or scaly papules and plaques, frequently called papulosquamous or psoriasiform SCLE (see Fig. 6.4). SCLE lesions occur most commonly on the neck, shoulders, upper back, chest, and arms. The face may also be involved; however, this is less common. SCLE is a highly photosensitive condition, and a recent history of sun exposure can often be elicited in patients initially presenting with SCLE. Overall, SCLE is estimated to occur in 8–16 % of patients with cutaneous lupus. Approximately 50 % of patients with SCLE have a sufficient number of the American College of Rheumatology (ACR) criteria to fulfill the diagnosis of SLE. Arthralgias and inflammatory arthritis are the most common noncutaneous manifestations accompanying SCLE. Major organ system involvement such as renal or neurologic disease is uncommon in SCLE. Serologic studies of patients with SCLE indicate

Fig. 6.4 Psoriasiform SCLE

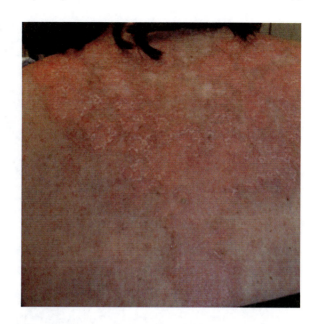

that 50–70 % of patients are ANA positive, 70–95 % are anti-SSA/Ro antibody positive, 30–50 % are anti-SSB/La antibody positive, and 30 % are rheumatoid factor positive. SCLE lesions frequently heal without scarring; however, long-standing and even permanent post-inflammatory pigmentation changes, atrophy, and telangiectasias may occur.

When considering the diagnosis of SCLE, the differential diagnosis typically includes erythema multiforme and other figurate erythemas, psoriasis, lichen planus, dermatomyositis, tinea corporis, pityriasis rosea, pityriasis rubra pilaris, and mycosis fungoides.

Medications are increasingly being recognized as triggers of SCLE and may, in fact, cause up to 20 % of cases. One potential hypothesis of the pathogenesis of drug-induced SCLE is that the medications unmask SCLE in a genetically susceptible individual via a photosensitizing effect. Hydrochlorothiazide is the most common cause of drug-induced SCLE; however, any patient diagnosed with SCLE should have a careful review of their drug history for possible causative medications. A list of medications which have been identified as causes of SCLE include:

Antifungals (e.g., terbinafine)
Antibiotics (e.g., tetracycline)
Anticonvulsants (e.g., phenytoin)
Antimalarials (e.g., hydroxychloroquine)
ACE inhibitors (e.g., captopril)
Beta-blockers (e.g., acebutolol)
Calcium channel blockers (e.g., diltiazem, nifedipine)
Thiazide diuretics (e.g., hydrochlorothiazide)
Sulfonylureas (e.g., glyburide)
NSAIDs (e.g., naproxen)

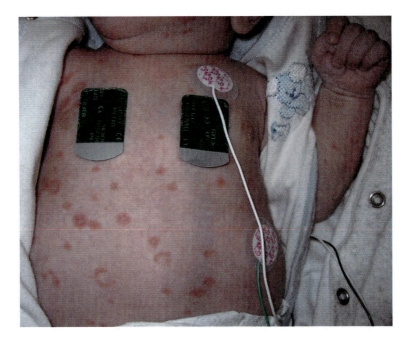

Fig. 6.5 Neonatal LE (Photo courtesy of Dr. Heather Brandling-Bennett)

Proton pump inhibitors (e.g., omeprazole)
Chemotherapeutic agents (e.g., tamoxifen, docetaxel)
Others (e.g., leflunomide, bupropion, interferon-alpha, tumor necrosis factor-alpha inhibitors)

Neonatal Lupus Erythematosus

Neonatal LE (NLE) presents as erythematous macules, papules, and annular plaques on the scalp, face, arms, and trunk (see Fig. 6.5). The skin lesions may be present at birth but more commonly develop during the first several weeks after birth. NLE is caused by transplacental transfer of maternal anti-Ro/SSA and/or anti-La/SSB antibodies from mother to fetus. The eruption generally clears by 6 months of age as the maternal antibodies disappear and usually does not cause residual scarring.

A major concern for infants born with NLE or for those born to mothers with a history of previous children with NLE is possible congenital heart disease. Anti-Ro/SSA antibodies have an affinity for the conduction system of the fetal heart and can directly damage this system, resulting in atrioventricular block (AV) or cardiomyopathy. Congenital AV block has been noted as early as the second trimester of pregnancy and is a life-threatening condition which may require the implantation of a pacemaker. The risk of fetal cardiac disease in pregnancies in which the mother has anti-Ro/SSA antibodies is estimated to be 2 %. In pregnancies in which there is

Fig. 6.6 Discoid LE

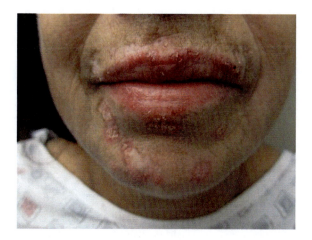

a history of cutaneous NLE, the recurrence rate for cutaneous disease has been found to be 49.4 % and the incidence of cardiac disease to be 18.2 % according to data from the Research Registry for Neonatal Lupus (RRNL). It is recommended that all women with any type of lupus be tested for anti-Ro/SSA and anti-La/SSB antibodies with each pregnancy and that those with positive results be carefully monitored by a high-risk obstetrician.

Chronic Cutaneous Lupus Erythematosus

Discoid Lupus Erythematosus

DLE is the most common form of cutaneous lupus, estimated to comprise 70 % of all cases of cutaneous lupus. In addition, DLE represents 95 % of all cases of chronic cutaneous lupus. DLE usually begins as well-defined erythematous papules or plaques, often with a firmly adherent scale (see Fig. 6.6). Follicular plugging is often an associated feature. Unless treated early and aggressively, DLE lesions progress to cause dyspigmentation, atrophy, and scarring (see Fig. 6.7). Scalp lesions that progress to scarring result in permanent alopecia due to a loss of hair follicles (see Fig. 6.8).

DLE most commonly occurs on the scalp, ears, face, and neck, referred to as localized DLE. When DLE is localized to these sites, the risk of progression to SLE is estimated to be 5–10 %. Less often, a more widespread variant called generalized DLE occurs with lesions also occurring on the trunk and extremities. In the generalized form, there is a corresponding increased association with SLE of approximately 10–20 %. These generalized cases also have a lower likelihood of entering remission when compared to localized cases. ANA is positive in approximately 35 % of patients with DLE, whereas anti-double-stranded DNA and SSA/Ro

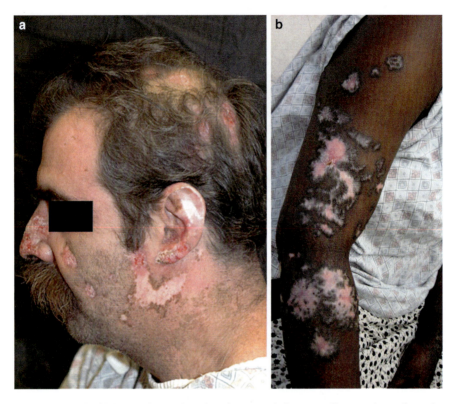

Fig. 6.7 (a)DLE with both active, scaly and erythematous lesions as well as scarring and atrophy on the ear and lateral cheek. (b) DLE lesions demonstrating atrophy and scarring

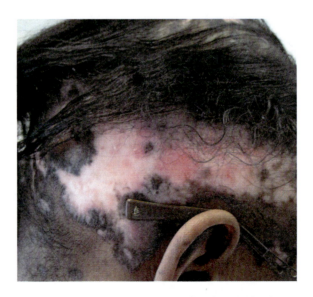

Fig. 6.8 Scarring alopecia from DLE (Photo courtesy of Dr. Joseph Merola)

Fig. 6.9 Lupus panniculitis/profundus. Note the active discoid LE lesions also present on the left cheek

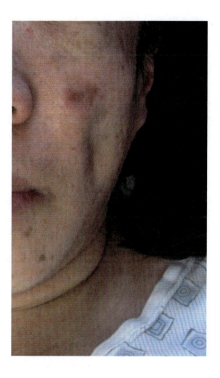

antibodies are found in 5–10 % of DLE patients. The differential diagnosis of suspected DLE should include sarcoidosis, psoriasis, tinea faciei, and actinic keratoses.

Lupus Panniculitis/Profundus

Lupus panniculitis/profundus is a form of chronic cutaneous lupus which manifests as tender subcutaneous nodules and plaques, most commonly involving the face, buttocks, thighs, upper arms, trunk, and breasts. Lupus panniculitis frequently develops at the site of preexisting or concomitant discoid lesions. This disease process tends to have a chronic course, resulting in significant lipoatrophy and depressed scars (see Fig. 6.9). Associated calcification sometimes occurs see Fig. 6.10. Histologically, these lesions demonstrate a lobular panniculitis containing a dense inflammatory infiltrate of lymphocytes and plasma cells as well as mucin deposition between adipocytes. Subcutaneous panniculitis-like T-cell lymphoma, along with other lobular panniculitides, should always be included in the differential diagnosis in these patients.

Tumid Lupus Erythematosus

Tumid LE is characterized by erythematous, urticarial plaques and papules on sun-exposed areas such as the face, upper trunk, and arms (see Figs. 6.11 and 6.12).

Fig. 6.10 Lupus panniculitis/profundus. The hip lesion has associated calcification

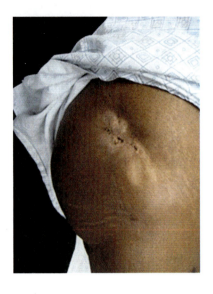

Fig. 6.11 Tumid LE on the face

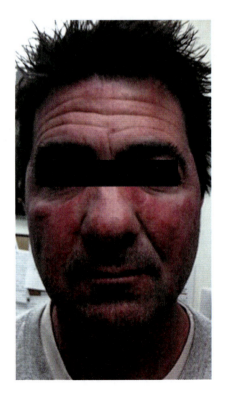

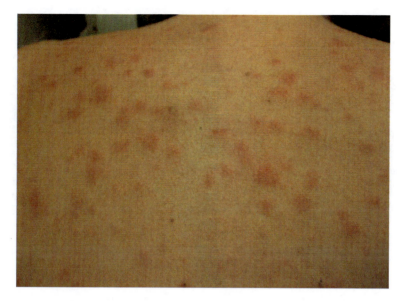

Fig. 6.12 Tumid LE on the upper back

In contrast to DLE and SCLE, the lesions of tumid LE heal without scarring or pigmentary changes. Along with SCLE, tumid LE is one of the most photosensitive types of cutaneous lupus.

The histopathology of tumid LE lesions shows abundant dermal mucin and a dense perivascular and periadnexal lymphocytic infiltrate. Given the fact that there is little to no change at the dermoepidermal junction in tumid LE, some have questioned whether tumid LE should be categorized as a form of LE. Despite this controversy, tumid LE is traditionally categorized as one of the forms of chronic CLE. Tumid LE generally responds very well to treatment with antimalarials, with lesions usually resolving without scarring or atrophy. ANA serologies are typically normal in patients with tumid LE, and the development of SLE is very rare.

Chilblain Lupus Erythematosus

Chilblain lupus erythematosus is a rare form of chronic cutaneous lupus characterized by tender, violaceous to erythematous papules or plaques on acral skin, particularly the fingers, toes, ears, and nose (see Fig. 6.13). Occasionally, these lesions go on to fissure and ulcerate resulting in significant discomfort. Chilblain LE is commonly exacerbated by cold, damp conditions.

Chilblain LE may be accompanied by DLE and is estimated to be associated with SLE in approximately 20 % of cases. In the absence of other clinical features of lupus erythematosus, chilblain LE can be challenging to distinguish from pernio,

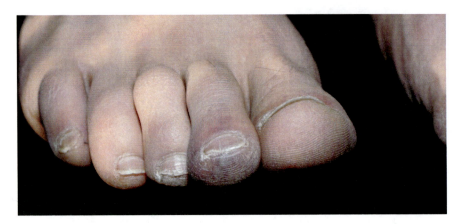

Fig. 6.13 Chilblain LE

which also manifests as tender, inflammatory macules and papules on the fingers and toes that are exacerbated by cold exposure. Some argue that chilblain LE should have the classic histopathologic changes of LE including vacuolar interface change at the dermoepidermal junction; however, these are not always detected, making the distinction from pernio even more challenging. Of note, chilblain LE should never be referred to as "lupus pernio," as this term actually refers to cutaneous sarcoidosis of the face.

Patients with chilblain LE should be followed for signs of systemic disease. Useful tests for aiding in the diagnosis of chilblain LE include ANA, anti-Ro/SSA, antiphospholipid antibodies, rheumatoid factor, and serum immunoglobulins. An autosomal dominant familial form of chilblain LE has also been reported and is characterized by mutations in the *TREX1* (endonuclease repair) gene.

Treatment of chilblain LE includes avoidance of triggering factors, such as cold and damp environments. Class I topical corticosteroids may help minimize inflammation and pain. Unfortunately, chilblain LE is often refractory to antimalarials.

Hypertrophic/Verrucous Lupus Erythematosus

Hypertrophic or verrucous LE is a variant of CCLE in which thick, prominent hyperkeratosis is seen in place of the usual adherent scale of DLE lesions. Hypertrophic LE typically occurs in patients with concomitant, more classic DLE lesions. Given the abundant hyperkeratosis, hypertrophic LE lesions have a clinical appearance resembling warts, hypertrophic lichen planus, keratoacanthomas, or squamous cell carcinomas. Hypertrophic LE tends to be a chronic, refractory disorder; however, systemic retinoids may be beneficial.

Lupus Erythematosus-Nonspecific Skin Disease

Photosensitivity

Photosensitivity is one of the four cutaneous findings included in the ACR criteria for the diagnosis of SLE. In clinical medicine, the term "photosensitive" denotes a cutaneous reaction which is deemed to be outside the normal range of responses to ultraviolet radiation (UVR). Photosensitivity is estimated to occur in 69 % of patients with SLE and is likely more common in patients with cutaneous LE and in those with lighter skin.

In cutaneous lupus erythematosus, the incidence of photosensitivity varies with the subtype of CLE. A study by Kuhn et al. published in 2001 utilized phototesting to estimate the incidence of photosensitivity in the various types of cutaneous lupus. Patients with tumid LE were found to be the most photosensitive, with 72 % developing characteristic skin lesions with phototesting. Photosensitive skin reactions were induced by UVR in 63 % of patients with SCLE, 60 % of patients with ACLE, and 45 % of patients with DLE. Based on the controlled UVR dose and duration utilized in the study protocol, this study likely underestimates the true incidence of photosensitivity in patients with CLE.

The exact mechanisms by which UVR induces and exacerbates CLE and SLE are still unclear; however, prevailing theories involve abnormalities in the processing of apoptotic cells. UVR is a potent inducer of cellular apoptosis, and it has been demonstrated that SLE and CLE patients accumulate apoptotic cells in the epidermis. This occurs via both an increased susceptibility to induction of apoptosis and decreased clearance of apoptotic cells. UVR also induces the production of inflammatory cytokines such as tumor necrosis factor alpha (TNF-α), IL-1, IL-6, TGF-β-1, and type 1 interferons and upregulates expression of the endothelial adhesion molecules E-selectin and ICAM-1. These processes lead to the recruitment of dendritic cells, macrophages, and lymphocytes for removal of apoptotic cellular debris.

In CLE, this culminates in the production of the various types of inflammatory skin lesions.

Alopecia

As mentioned above, scarring alopecia frequently occurs in DLE, and the scalp is often an initial presenting site of this form of CCLE. In fact, a study of 89 patients with DLE noted scarring alopecia in 34 % of patients. The scarring alopecia seen with DLE is, however, considered to be LE-specific skin disease given that the classic histopathologic features of LE are detected on biopsy and is therefore discussed above.

Patients with systemic LE frequently experience non-scarring, diffuse alopecia in association with disease exacerbations. This diffuse hair loss is traditionally considered to be due to telogen effluvium. Other forms of non-scarring alopecia in

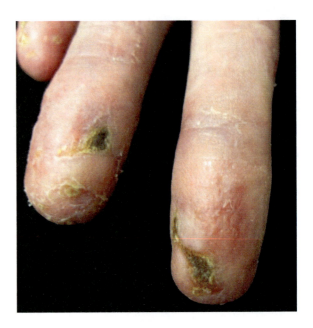

Fig. 6.14 Raynaud's with digital ulcerations

patients with SLE are peripheral or frontal alopecia due to thin weakened hairs at the scalp line ("lupus hairs") and patchy, partial hair loss. Non-scarring alopecia may also be caused by medications used to treat CLE or SLE, including methotrexate, azathioprine, cyclophosphamide, hydroxychloroquine, corticosteroids, acitretin, and isotretinoin. The main differential diagnosis for non-scarring hair loss includes both telogen effluvium, which can occur postpartum or after other significant stressors such as anesthesia, and androgenetic alopecia.

Raynaud's Phenomenon

Raynaud's phenomenon is a vasospastic disorder that causes discoloration of the fingers, toes, and occasionally the nose and ears. Episodes of Raynaud's are most commonly triggered by cold and stress. Raynaud's typically begins with affected areas first turning white secondary to vasoconstriction. This is usually followed by a bluish discoloration secondary to cyanosis with associated numbness, paresthesias, and pain. After removal of the initiating factor, the affected areas may turn red, throb, or swell, which is traditionally thought to result from reactive hyperemia. An affected individual may not experience all of these color changes or associated symptoms. In severe cases, Raynaud's can result in digital infarctions and ulcerations (see Fig. 6.14). Other disorders to consider in patients with Raynaud's include systemic sclerosis, mixed connective tissue disease, Buerger's disease, vasculitis, peripheral vascular disease, infection, or atherosclerotic embolic disease.

Treatment of Raynaud's includes avoidance of triggering and exacerbating factors such as cold, smoking, caffeine, beta-blockers, and vasoconstrictors (e.g., decongestants, amphetamines, ergots, cocaine). If these measures are insufficient, beneficial medications include calcium channel blockers, alpha-blockers, selective serotonin reuptake inhibitors (SSRIs), sildenafil, and losartan.

Livedo Reticularis and Racemosa

Livedo reticularis is a vascular condition characterized by a blue-purple, mottled, reticulated pattern of the skin. It most commonly occurs on the extremities, with the legs usually more affected than the arms. Livedo reticularis is frequently exacerbated by cold exposure. It is a common, usually benign, condition occurring more often in women than men. However, when occurring in the setting of lupus erythematosus, testing for antiphospholipid antibodies should be considered. When associated with lupus erythematosus or antiphospholipid antibody syndrome, cutaneous necrosis or ulcerations can occur with livedo reticularis.

Livedo racemosa is characterized by a violaceous, irregular, often annular or polycyclic netlike pattern on the skin. The distribution of livedo racemosa is more widespread than livedo reticularis, typically involving the extremities, buttocks, and trunk. In addition, livedo racemosa classically remains present on warming of the skin unlike livedo reticularis. Livedo racemosa is frequently associated with antiphospholipid antibody syndrome, SLE, and polycythemia vera, among other disorders, and is the characteristic cutaneous manifestation seen in Sneddon's syndrome, in which it occurs in conjunction with cerebrovascular accidents. Notably, there are also reports linking livedo reticularis and racemosa to cerebrovascular accidents in patients with SLE.

Cutaneous Vasculitis

Cutaneous vasculitis in lupus erythematosus is usually due to small-vessel leukocytoclastic vasculitis. In a series of 670 patients with SLE, vasculitis was diagnosed in 76 (11 %), with cutaneous small-vessel vasculitis being the formal diagnosis in 68 of these 76 (89 %). The classic and most common clinical feature of small-vessel leukocytoclastic vasculitis is palpable purpura, most commonly occurring on the lower. Cutaneous vasculitis in lupus patients may be a predictor of the development of lupus nephritis.

The differential diagnosis for cutaneous vasculitis in lupus patients includes drug-induced hypersensitivity reaction, thrombocytopenic purpura, disseminated intravascular coagulation, viral exanthem, and bacteremia/septic vasculitis. Treatment is based on the underlying cause and disease severity. In immune-mediated, limited cutaneous disease, colchicine and dapsone are reasonable therapeutic options.

Extensive cutaneous disease or end-organ disease is usually treated with a combination of prednisone 0.5–1 mg/kg and a systemic immunosuppressive agent such as methotrexate, mycophenolate mofetil (MMF), azathioprine, or cyclophosphamide.

Urticarial Vasculitis

Urticarial vasculitis may also occur in patients with lupus and presents as urticarial plaques that persist beyond 24 h and often resolve with hyperpigmentation. These features can help distinguish urticarial vasculitis from classic urticaria. Histologically, a neutrophilic infiltrate is frequently seen in urticarial vasculitis. Thus, therapeutic agents such as colchicine and dapsone are often more beneficial than antimalarials. Urticarial vasculitis is frequently associated with hypocomplementemia, particularly in patients with SLE. Other diagnoses to consider in cases of suspected urticarial vasculitis include urticaria, drug eruptions, viral exanthems, chronic bacterial infections, contact dermatitis, hereditary angioedema, lymphoma, and leukemia.

Other LE-Nonspecific Manifestations: Mucosal Ulcerations, Periungual Telangiectasias, Palmar Erythema, and Urticaria

Mucosal disease may occur in cutaneous and systemic LE and usually involves the oral cavity (lips, palate, tongue, and buccal mucosa). Nasal, conjunctival, and anogenital lesions have also been described. Mucosal lesions can be LE specific or LE nonspecific depending upon the pathology of the lesions. Often, LE-nonspecific ulcerations are seen in SLE patients with active disease. In fact, these lesions are one of the formal ACR criteria for diagnosing SLE. LE-specific lesions are most commonly seen in patients with DLE. Oral discoid lesions typically occur as well-demarcated, atrophic, or ulcerated plaques and as cheilitis. Pain is variable. Oral cavity lesions are most commonly asymmetric. This asymmetry is an important distinguishing feature from lichen planus, which should always be included in the differential diagnosis of oral DLE. Squamous cell carcinoma can arise in long-standing oral lesions of all types and should always be considered. Treatment of LE-specific mucosal lesions includes topical corticosteroids, often best delivered in a gel vehicle for mucosal disease (examples include clobetasol gel and fluocinonide gel), intralesional corticosteroids, and hydroxychloroquine.

Hand-specific manifestations of LE include Raynaud's phenomenon (discussed above), periungual telangiectasias, and palmar erythema. Periungual telangiectasias are more frequently seen in dermatomyositis and systemic sclerosis, however, can also occur in LE and tend to accompany systemic disease. Palmar erythema occurs in a small percentage of patients with SLE. Erythromelalgia is a clinical syndrome of erythema, pain, and burning sensation of the hands, feet, face, and/or ears, which has been noted to occur in some patients with SLE.

Urticaria without vasculitis has been described as an initial manifestation of SLE and also occurs in patients with established SLE. Recurrent or chronic urticaria, angioedema, arthralgias, and fevers should prompt consideration of a possible diagnosis of SLE and be followed by testing for ANA and complement levels. Solar-induced urticaria is more common in lupus patients and should also result in consideration of potential underlying SLE.

Treatment of Cutaneous Lupus

An algorithm for the treatment options for cutaneous LE are outlined in Fig. 6.16.

Photoprotection

Cutaneous LE is a highly photosensitive disease, and evidence also exists that UVR can trigger flares of systemic lupus erythematosus as well. All patients with CLE should be counseled on photoprotection strategies including avoidance of outdoor sun exposure during peak periods of the day, wearing of sun protective clothing and broad-brimmed hats, and topical sunscreen use. Ideally, sunscreens should contain both a chemical (e.g., avobenzone or ecamsule) and physical (e.g., titanium dioxide or zinc oxide) blocking agent and protect against both UVA and UVB. The daily use of sunscreens with sun protection factor (SPF) 50 or higher and reapplication every 2–3 h should also be encouraged in patients with SLE and CLE. Patients should be reminded that ordinary glass blocks UVB but not UVA, so tinted glass to block UVA may be useful for those who are very photosensitive. Patients can get enough exposure through ordinary windows in their homes or automobiles to induce disease flares, mandating protection even in these locations. The strict photoprotection regimen required by patients with CLE is a risk factor for vitamin D deficiency and its associated adverse health effects. Thus, daily vitamin D supplementation with approximately 2,000 IU of cholecalciferol and periodic measurement of serum 25-OH vitamin D levels with a target range of 30–60 ng/dl should also be recommended.

Smoking Cessation

Cigarette smoking has been found to reduce the efficacy of chloroquine and hydroxychloroquine in the treatment of cutaneous lupus. The negative effect of smoking on antimalarial efficacy has also been shown to be both dose-related and reversible upon smoking cessation. Postulated mechanisms for smoking interference with antimalarial efficacy include competitive inhibition of antimalarial accumulation within lysosomes by nicotine and enhanced antimalarial metabolism by cytochrome p-450 enzyme activation via aromatic hydrocarbons present in tobacco smoke. Some studies also suggest that smoking itself worsens the cutaneous lesions of LE. In addition, it has been shown that patients with SLE who smoke have a higher level of disease activity and organ damage. For these reasons, all patients with cutaneous lupus who are smokers should be regularly counseled and assisted with smoking cessation.

Corticosteroids

Topical corticosteroids are a mainstay for the treatment of cutaneous lupus. Medium-potency (e.g., triamcinolone acetonide 0.1 %) to high-potency (e.g., clobetasol propionate 0.05 %) topical corticosteroids are most commonly used; however, their use must be closely monitored to reduce the risk of side effects. Most commonly, topical corticosteroids are applied twice daily for up to 1 week on the face and up to 2 weeks on the trunk and/or extremities, followed by a 1- to 2-week rest period. Several topical corticosteroid vehicles are available, and selection of an appropriate vehicle is important for both patient compliance and optimal clinical efficacy. Ointments are the most hydrating and are believed to be the most effective; however, patients may dislike the greasy nature of these topical medications. In this case, a cream or lotion may be an acceptable alternative. Corticosteroid foams, solutions, and occasionally gels or oils are effective, well-tolerated options for scalp CLE. Potential adverse effects of topical corticosteroids include cutaneous atrophy, telangiectasias, dyspigmentation, and striae. Extra precautions to avoid side effects must be observed when treating the face and intertriginous areas.

Intralesional corticosteroid therapy may be an effective treatment strategy for localized, active inflammatory lesions and is most commonly used for DLE to assist with refractory lesions and to avoid permanent scarring. This modality is most frequently employed for active DLE lesions on the scalp. Triamcinolone 2.5–5 mg/ml is typically used for intralesional therapy, and treatment is often repeated every 4–6 weeks, while monitoring closely for side effects. Subcutaneous atrophy is the most common and potentially limiting side effect with intralesional corticosteroid therapy; however, telangiectasias and dyspigmentation also can occur.

Systemic corticosteroids are generally not used as a mainstay of therapy specifically for the cutaneous disease of LE for several reasons. Not only are systemic corticosteroids less effective for cutaneous LE than for the systemic components of LE, but they also tend not to be a remittive agent, with flares in cutaneous disease noted upon tapering. In addition, the doses of systemic corticosteroids required to maintain adequate control of CLE often lead to significant steroid-related morbidity.

Topical Calcineurin Inhibitors

Both tacrolimus ointment and pimecrolimus cream have shown efficacy in the treatment of cutaneous LE lesions. Tacrolimus 0.1 % ointment applied twice a day for 12 weeks showed significant benefit in comparison to placebo in a double-blind, randomized, vehicle-controlled study of 30 patients with various types of CLE. In this study, the greatest degree of improvement was noted in patients with tumid LE, SCLE, and ACLE, whereas patients with DLE showed the least improvement. Pimecrolimus 1 % cream has also shown efficacy in treating various types of CLE. In a randomized, double-blind pilot study comparing pimecrolimus 1 % cream to betamethasone 0.1 % cream in ten patients with moderate to severe DLE, pimecrolimus 1 % cream resulted in similar efficacy as the betamethasone 0.1 % cream.

Topical calcineurin inhibitors are usually well-tolerated and have an excellent safety profile. They are a reasonable complement to topical corticosteroids and are especially useful for treating high-risk areas such as the face, eyelids, and intertriginous skin. Tacrolimus ointment and pimecrolimus cream are usually applied twice a day, either during alternating cycles with topical corticosteroids or concurrently.

Antimalarials

Antimalarial medications are the oldest systemic therapy for the treatment of cutaneous lupus. Reports of their efficacy in CLE specifically date from as early as 1894, when Payne published a report on the efficacy of quinine in patients with DLE. Antimalarials currently used for CLE include hydroxychloroquine, chloroquine, and quinacrine. Antimalarials are potentially effective in all types of CLE and should be considered as first-line agents whenever systemic therapy is warranted, such as with widespread lesions, rapidly progressive or highly inflammatory disease, to halt the development of scarring, or for a lack of an adequate response to topical therapy.

Antimalarials have been found to have several immunomodulatory effects including lysosomal stabilization, inhibition of toll-like receptor signaling, suppression of antigen presentation, and inhibition of prostaglandin and proinflammatory cytokine synthesis. Additional potential benefits of antimalarials include photoprotection, antithrombotic/antiplatelet effects, reduction of LDL cholesterol and triglycerides, improved glucose tolerance, and antiviral effects.

Antimalarials are generally slow-acting medications, requiring at least a 3-month trial period prior to making any determinations of efficacy. Hydroxychloroquine is the most commonly utilized antimalarial for initial treatment of CLE in the USA given its lower ocular toxicity when compared to chloroquine. If satisfactory results have not been achieved after several months of therapy, one should consider either switching to chloroquine (which is used more often in Europe given potential higher efficacy than hydroxychloroquine) or combination therapy with quinacrine, which is only available via compounding pharmacies. Of note, hydroxychloroquine and chloroquine should not be given in combination given potential additive ocular toxicity. In patients with CLE, smoking has been shown to inhibit the efficacy of antimalarials in a dose-dependent manner. Thus, patients with CLE who smoke may need additional or alternative therapies than antimalarials.

Antimalarials accumulate to different degrees in human body tissues and organs. The highest concentrations occur in melanin-containing tissues such as the retina and skin. Accumulation in these tissues results in many of the beneficial as well as the adverse effects of antimalarials. Excretion of antimalarials occurs via the kidneys (~50 %), liver (~40 %), and gastrointestinal system (~10 %).

Antimalarial dosing guidelines are straightforward and, when followed, will minimize the occurrence of potential adverse effects. Dosages should be calculated based on ideal body weight and should always be adjusted accordingly for older patients and those with impaired renal or hepatic function. Hydroxychloroquine is traditionally dosed at 200–400 mg/day (6.5 mg/kg max), chloroquine 250–500 mg/day (4 mg/kg max), and quinacrine 25–100 mg/day.

The most common adverse effect from antimalarial therapy is gastrointestinal upset (nausea, dyspepsia, diarrhea, etc.), which is estimated to occur in 20 % of patients. Dose reduction is usually effective in alleviating gastrointestinal issues. Ocular toxicity is the most well-known potential side effect of antimalarials and occurs as corneal deposits or retinopathy. Corneal deposits are more common with chloroquine and are rare with hydroxychloroquine at a dose of 400 mg/day or less. Symptoms of corneal deposits include transient halos or increased light sensitivity. These symptoms are reversible upon discontinuation of the medication. Irreversible retinopathy is the most serious potential ophthalmologic complication of antimalarial therapy. The exact incidence of retinopathy is unknown but has been estimated to occur in 3–4 % of patients taking hydroxychloroquine and in up to 10 % of patients taking chloroquine after 10 years of therapy. Given that chloroquine is more oculotoxic, its use therefore requires more frequent eye examinations. In addition, the retinal toxicity may progress even after the medication has been discontinued. Quinacrine does not cause retinopathy. In general, ophthalmologic examination should be performed at baseline (ideally prior to starting therapy, but practically within with first 1–2 months after initiating therapy) and every 6–12 months thereafter in patients being treated with hydroxychloroquine or chloroquine. Cutaneous side effects also occur with antimalarials. Blue-gray pigmentation can occur with long-term hydroxychloroquine and chloroquine use, particularly of the shins, palate, and nails (see Fig. 6.15). Quinacrine often causes a reversible yellow discoloration of the skin and sclerae and can also rarely lead to bone marrow suppression. Other less common adverse effects of antimalarial therapy include cutaneous drug eruptions including erythema multiforme, transaminitis, hemolysis/anemia, headaches, and neuromyopathy.

Methotrexate

Methotrexate is a folic acid analog which inactivates dihydrofolate reductase, thus blocking purine and pyrimidine synthesis and resulting in reduced lymphocyte proliferation. In addition, methotrexate inhibits the enzyme AICAR transformylase, leading to increased adenosine concentrations. Adenosine has potent anti-inflammatory effects including inhibition of neutrophil, monocyte, and macrophage inflammatory cytokine release. In 2001, a review of 14 clinical trials involving 207 patients with CLE and SLE found methotrexate, 10–20 mg/week, to be generally

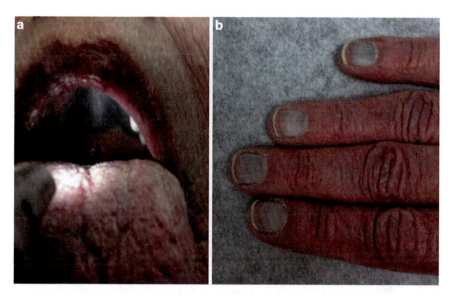

Fig. 6.15 (**a**) Blue-gray palate and (**b**) nail pigmentation due to hydroxychloroquine

effective and well tolerated for the treatment of cutaneous disease and arthritis. Patients in this review had continued significant disease activity despite treatment with antimalarials and oral prednisone prior to treatment with methotrexate. Another study of methotrexate in 43 patients with various subtypes of CLE reported efficacy for skin disease in 98 % of patients. In general, after antimalarials, many consider methotrexate to be the next best option for systemic therapy for cutaneous lupus. In fact, it is often used as add-on therapy to antimalarials when they are not fully effective, or in place of antimalarials when these medications are contraindicated or result in side effects.

Methotrexate is usually dosed at 10–25 mg/week for cutaneous LE and can be administered orally, subcutaneously, or intramuscularly. Potential adverse effects of methotrexate include alopecia, stomatitis, gastrointestinal upset, hepatitis, cytopenias, pneumonitis, pulmonary fibrosis, and teratogenicity. Folic acid, 1–5 mg/day, or folinic acid, 5 mg once a week 12–24 h after taking methotrexate, can reduce the incidence and severity of methotrexate side effects.

Mycophenolate Mofetil

MMF is a lymphocyte-specific immunosuppressive agent which blocks de novo purine synthesis via inhibition of the enzyme inosine monophosphate dehydrogenase. MMF was reported as an effective treatment in a 2007 open-label, pilot study of ten patients with SCLE resistant to standard therapy. MMF has also been shown to be an effective treatment of lupus nephritis, thus increasing its appeal as a therapeutic option in patients with both cutaneous and systemic lupus. On the other hand, many patients on MMF for their lupus nephritis see little to no improvement in their cutaneous disease, requiring other agents to specifically control their skin lesions. MMF is usually dosed at 500–1,000 mg twice a day when treating CLE. The most common side effects of MMF include gastrointestinal upset, cytopenias, and opportunistic infections.

Azathioprine

Azathioprine is a purine analog that affects both cellular and humoral immune function via inhibition of lymphocyte proliferation. In a series of six patients with recalcitrant cutaneous lupus (four with SCLE and two with DLE), four patients responded to treatment with azathioprine. Azathioprine has long been used as a treatment for lupus nephritis and thus should also be considered in patients with overlapping cutaneous and systemic disease with the same caveat as mentioned for MMF that many patients on azathioprine for their lupus nephritis do not have significant improvement in cutaneous disease. Prior to initiation of azathioprine, thiopurine methyltransferase (TPMT) enzyme activity should be considered as this is the safest means to guide dosing and thereby achieve efficacy while reducing the risk of bone marrow toxicity. Given the expense of this laboratory study, some physicians instead titrate the dose of azathioprine slowly up while monitoring closely for leucopenia. The usual dose of azathioprine is 1–2.5 mg/kg/day.

Cyclophosphamide

Cyclophosphamide is an alkylating agent that causes DNA cross-links resulting in cell death. It has long been the gold standard treatment for severe organ-threatening SLE, particularly that with renal or CNS involvement. A small study of cyclophosphamide in DLE and SCLE reported moderate to excellent efficacy in eight of nine patients. Due to the significant risk of serious toxicities (including ovarian failure, bladder cancer, and myeloproliferative disorders), cyclophosphamide is typically not used for the treatment of CLE.

Thalidomide

Thalidomide is an immunomodulatory agent with anti-inflammatory activity. The mechanisms by which thalidomide causes immunomodulatory and anti-inflammatory effects are not fully understood; however, thalidomide appears to reduce TNF-α production, modulate interleukin production, modulate adhesion molecule expression, and inhibit angiogenesis. In vivo, thalidomide has been shown to inhibit UVB-induced keratinocyte apoptosis in patients with CLE and SLE. Clinically, thalidomide has demonstrated considerable efficacy in the treatment of cutaneous LE. In a retrospective study of 48 patients, including 18 with DLE, 6 with SCLE, and 24 with SLE with cutaneous disease, the overall response rate to thalidomide was 81 % with remission achieved in 60 %. A Brazilian study of 65 patients with refractory cutaneous LE treated with thalidomide reported complete or partial remission in 97 % of patients. A major issue limiting the use of thalidomide is the adverse effect profile, most notably peripheral neuropathy and teratogenicity. Strict contraception and monthly monitoring visits following the System for Thalidomide Education and Prescribing Safety (STEPS) program are absolute requirements of thalidomide users. Other potential side effects include sedation, constipation, and hypercoagulability. Typical dosages of thalidomide for cutaneous LE are 50–200 mg/day.

Dapsone

Dapsone, a sulfone compound with anti-inflammatory, immunomodulatory, and antibacterial properties, has been reported to be effective in several subtypes of CLE particularly bullous SLE, lupus profundus/panniculitis, and inflammatory DLE. In addition, dapsone has shown efficacy in urticarial vasculitis and oral ulcerations in lupus patients. The largest study of dapsone in cutaneous LE was published in 1986, in which 15 of 33 patients (48 %) with DLE showed a moderate to excellent response to dapsone. A retrospective review from Japan published in 2006 reported remission of lupus profundus within 8 weeks in eight of ten patients treated with dapsone. Hematologic, hepatic, renal, and gastrointestinal side effects can occur with oral dapsone therapy. Prior to treatment, exclusion of glucose-6-phosphate dehydrogenase (G6PD) deficiency is mandatory. During treatment, patients need to be monitored for hemolysis, methemoglobinemias, and neuropathy. The traditional dose of dapsone is between 25 and 150 mg/day.

Retinoids

Oral retinoids, including acitretin and isotretinoin, are vitamin A (retinol) analogs which act therapeutically to induce keratinocyte differentiation and reduce epidermal hyperplasia. Both compounds have shown efficacy in treating cutaneous LE, particularly the hyperkeratotic and verrucous LE variants. A study conducted in the USA in 1986 reported good results in eight of ten patients with CCLE or

SCLE treated with isotretinoin 80 mg/day for 16 weeks. In a German study from 1988, 15 of 20 patients with cutaneous LE showed a good clinical response to acitretin. The only randomized controlled trial in CLE using two systemic drugs was conducted in 1992 and compared the efficacy of acitretin 50 mg/day with hydroxychloroquine 400 mg/day in 28 and 30 patients, respectively. Improvement of CLE was reported in 46 % of patients treated with acitretin and in 50 % of patients treated with hydroxychloroquine.

Common side effects of retinoids include dry skin and mucous membranes, reversible alopecia, gastrointestinal upset, arthralgias, and myalgias. Oral retinoids may also cause hyperlipidemia, particularly hypertriglyceridemia, elevated liver function tests, and cytopenias; thus, these laboratories must be tested before and during treatment. Acitretin and isotretinoin are both teratogenic, mandating effective contraception during and after treatment (pregnancy avoidance is required for 3 years following acitretin and for 1 month following isotretinoin). Lastly, mood disturbances and inflammatory bowel disease have also been reported to potentially be associated with isotretinoin therapy. Typical dosing of retinoids is 0.5–1 mg/kg/day.

Intravenous Immunoglobulin

IVIG is complex immunomodulatory agent which has shown clinical efficacy in the treatment of several subtypes of CLE. In 2004, a case series was published that included 12 patients with cutaneous LE treated with IVIG. An excellent response was seen in five patients, and a good response was noted in two additional patients. More recently, a report was published demonstrating a good response to IVIG in four cases of refractory SCLE. IVIG is typically administered monthly, as a 2-day course, at a dose of 1 g/kg/day.

Biologics

Rituximab is a chimeric antibody that binds to CD20 on the surface of B cells, leading to B-cell depletion. Case reports have been published describing excellent clinical responses to rituximab for severe, refractory ACLE, SCLE, and lupus profundus.

Belimumab is a humanized monoclonal antibody targeted against the B-lymphocyte stimulator (BLyS). BLyS is a cytokine produced by activated monocytes and macrophages which stimulates the maturation of B cells into antibody-secreting plasma cells. Belimumab was recently approved by the FDA for the treatment of SLE; however, it has not been studies for the treatment of CLE.

Epratuzumab is a humanized monoclonal antibody that binds to CD22 on the surface of B cells, leading to B-cell depletion. Epratuzumab has shown promising results for the treatment of SLE and is currently in phase III clinical trials. Improvement in cutaneous disease has been noted during treatment with epratuzumab as a component of the Systemic Lupus Erythematosus Disease Activity Index (SLEDAI) score, although cutaneous disease has not been individually assessed.

TNF-α is a key mediator of inflammation in many cutaneous and systemic inflammatory diseases. Infliximab, etanercept, and adalimumab all inhibit the biologic effects of TNF-α. There are a few case reports demonstrating the efficacy of etanercept for SCLE in patients with rheumatoid arthritis. On the other hand, each of these medications has been reported to cause the formation of ANA and drug-induced systemic LE as well as ACLE, SCLE, and DLE. Thus, at this time, TNF-α antagonists are not often recommended as treatments for cutaneous LE.

Efalizumab is a recombinant, humanized monoclonal antibody against CD11a, a protein involved in T-cell activation and trafficking. Efalizumab has been reported to be efficacious in CLE; however, this medication has been withdrawn from the market due to an association with several cases of progressive multifocal leukoencephalopathy.

The Cutaneous Lupus Erythematosus Disease Area and Severity Index

In 2005, the cutaneous lupus erythematosus disease area and severity index (CLASI) was developed for the purpose of tracking cutaneous disease activity and damage in patients with cutaneous lupus erythematosus. The CLASI provides a quantitative measure of the skin-specific burden of disease that enables standardized assessments of disease progression. Such a standardized approach to assessing cutaneous disease facilitates the organization of clinical trials, analysis of results, and comparisons among studies, which ideally will ultimately result in additional knowledge regarding the efficacy of various therapeutic options for cutaneous lupus.

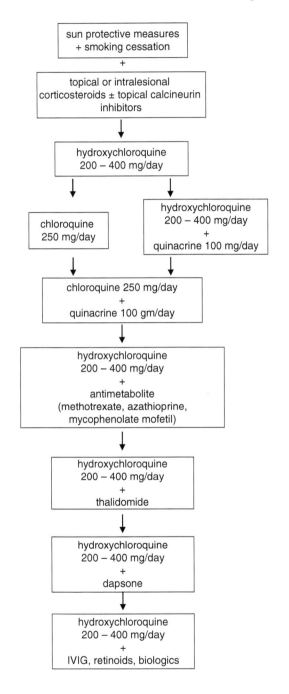

Fig. 6.16 Outline of treatment of cutaneous lupus

Sources

1. Obermoser G, Sontheimer RD, Zelger B. Overview of common, rare, and atypical manifestations of cutaneous lupus erythematosus and histopathological correlates. Lupus. 2010; 19:1050–70.
2. Kuhn A, Ochsendorf F, Bonsmann G. Treatment of cutaneous lupus erythematosus. Lupus. 2010;19:1125–36.
3. Walling HW, Sontheimer RD. Cutaneous lupus erythematosus: issues in diagnosis and treatment. Am J Clin Dermatol. 2009;10:365–81.
4. Kuhn A, Sticherling M, Bonsmann G. Clinical manifestations of cutaneous lupus erythematosus. J Dtsch Dermatol Ges. 2007;5:1124–40.
5. Alireza S, Wenson S, Tahan SR. Histopathological manifestations of systemic diseases: the example of cutaneous lupus erythematosus. J Cutan Pathol. 2010;37:112–24.
6. Izmirly PM, Llanos C, Lee LA, Askanase A, Kim MY, Buyon JP. Cutaneous manifestations of neonatal lupus and risk of subsequent congenital heart block. Arthritis Rheum. 2010; 62:1153–7.
7. Kreuter A, Gaifullina R, Tigges C, et al. Lupus erythematosus tumidus: response to antimalarial treatment in 36 patients with emphasis on smoking. Arch Dermatol. 2009;145:244–8.
8. Hedrich CM, Fiebig B, Hauck FH, Sallmann S, et al. Chilblain lupus erythematosus—a review of the literature. Clin Rheumatol. 2008;27:949–54.
9. Bijl M, Kallenberg CGM. Ultraviolet light and cutaneous lupus. Lupus. 2006;15:724–7.
10. Trueb RM. Involvement of scalp and nails in lupus erythematosus. Lupus. 2010;19:1078–86.
11. Ramos-Casals M, Nardi N, Lagrutta M, et al. Vasculitis in systemic lupus. Erythematosus: prevalence and clinical characteristics in 670 patients. Medicine. 2006;85:95–104.
12. Nico MM, Viela MA, Rivitti EA, Lourenco SV. Oral lesions in lupus erythematosus: correlation with cutaneous lesions. Eur J Dermatol. 2008;18:376–81.
13. Wozniacka A, McCauliffe DP. Optimal use of antimalarials in treating cutaneous lupus erythematosus. Am J Clin Dermatol. 2005;6:1–11.
14. Lampropoulos CE, D'Cruz DP. Topical calcineurin inhibitors in systemic lupus erythematosus. Ther Clin Risk Manag. 2010;6:95–101.
15. Wenzel J, Brahler S, Bauer R, et al. Efficacy and safety of methotrexate in recalcitrant cutaneous lupus erythematosus: results of a retrospective study in 43 patients. Br J Dermatol. 2005; 153:157–62.
16. Kreuter A, Tomi NS, Weiner SM, Huger M, Altmeyer P, Gaimbichler T. Mycophenolate sodium for subacute cutaneous lupus erythematosus resistant to standard therapy. Br J Dermatol. 2007;156:1321–7.
17. Waddington Cruz M, de Souza Papi JA. Long-term thalidomide use in refractory cutaneous lesions of lupus erythematosus: a series of 65 Brazilian patients. Lupus. 2005;14(6):434–9.
18. Lampropoulos CE, Hughes GR, D'Cruz DP. Intravenous immunoglobulin in the treatment of resistant subacute cutaneous lupus erythematosus: a possible alternative. Clin Rheumatol. 2007;26(6):981–3.
19. Wallace DJ. Advances in drug therapy for systemic lupus erythematosus. BMC Med. 2010;8:77.
20. Klein RS, Morganroth PA, Werth VP. Cutaneous lupus and the cutaneous lupus erythematosus disease area and severity index instrument. Rheum Dis Clin North Am. 2010;36:33–51.

Chapter 7
Musculoskeletal Manifestations of SLE

Simon M. Helfgott

Introduction

Musculoskeletal involvement constitutes the most frequent problem seen in patients with SLE. The majority of patients will describe joint pain and achiness either at the onset of the disease or later during its course. Yet the frequency of arthralgia or arthritis in lupus populations is quiet variable; for example, in one series described by Fries, it was observed in 53 % of 193 patients, and in the Dubois series, it was described at some time during the course of the illness in 92 % of 520 patients. Although the traditional teaching considers lupus arthritis to be nondeforming and nonerosive, there are many exceptions to this rule.

In addition, musculoskeletal pain may be due to soft tissue injuries, inflammatory muscle injury (myositis), or noninflammatory pain syndromes such as fibromyalgia. Fibromyalgia symptoms may be observed in a large number of patients. In one lupus cohort of 173 lupus patients, approximately 30 % met criteria for the diagnosis of fibromyalgia. Conversely, approximately 10 % of patients with fibromyalgia have a positive antinuclear antibody test (ANA). Though this test result does not confirm a diagnosis of lupus, it may confuse the clinical picture further, especially if there are other symptoms such as fatigue, photosensitivity and Raynaud's phenomenon. It is important to distinguish fibromyalgia achiness and pain from arthralgia and arthritis, since the latter two complaints are more likely to be consistent with a diagnosis of lupus.

S.M. Helfgott, M.D. (✉)
Division of Rheumatology, Brigham and Women's Hospital,
75 Francis Street, Boston, MA 02115, USA

Harvard Medical School, Boston, MA, USA
e-mail: shelfgott@partners.org

Arthralgias

Arthralgias are the most common musculoskeletal complaint. Joint pain and stiffness are often described, involving the hands, wrists, shoulders and occasionally the large joints.

The symptoms may persist for long periods, prompting medical attention and subsequent laboratory testing. In contrast to rheumatoid arthritis, the absence of objective joint swelling does not rule out the diagnosis of SLE.

Arthritis

Arthritis may be either symmetric or asymmetric. It can develop at any time during the course of the disease. It tends to involve small joints such as the hands and feet as well as the wrists. In contrast to rheumatoid arthritis, frank synovitis is typically not seen at the onset; boggy synovitis is uncommon. Instead, the swelling may be subtle. There may be associated complaints of morning stiffness and fatigue. A common observation is that the degree of joint pain typically exceeds that which would be expected from the limited objective evidence of joint inflammation. Symptoms may be evanescent, resolving within hours or days but they may recur and eventually become chronic. As symptoms become more persistent, the large joints such as the knees, shoulders, and elbows may become involved.

The development of an oligo- or monoarticular arthritis in an immune compromised patient warrants careful evaluation. Since the differential diagnosis includes septic arthritis, a careful evaluation including appropriate diagnostic testing may be indicated.

SLE and the use of corticosteroids therapies may predispose patients to the development of osteonecrosis (see below). Atypical infections such as fungal and mycobacterial can present as a monoarthritis. Synovial fluid culture and even tissue biopsy may be required to establish the diagnosis. Osteonecrosis may be a risk factor for the development of septic arthritis in SLE. The commonest agents include *Escherichia coli*, *Staphylococcus aureus*, *Neisseria gonorrhoeae*, Pneumococcus species and, in particular, Salmonella.

The treatment of SLE-related arthritis is similar in many ways to the management in other inflammatory arthritides, with some exceptions. For mild disease, analgesics such as acetaminophen or low doses of nonsteroidal anti-inflammatory drugs (NSAIDs) may be considered. For more significant disease, short-term use of low doses of corticosteroids may provide relief. Hydroxychloroquine is often prescribed for longer term management. The use of other immunosuppressive drugs and biologically based therapies is discussed below.

The Synovium

The appearance of the synovium in SLE arthritis is fairly nonspecific. In contrast to RA, where there is an intense degree of synovial proliferation and lymphocytic infiltration, the changes in SLE including vascular congestion, with proliferation of small blood vessels, some perivascular mononuclear cell infiltration with surface fibrin deposits, and edema.

When present, joint effusions tend to be small. The fluid appearance ranges from clear to slightly cloudy. A more turbid appearance should alert the clinician to underlying infection Synovial fluid may be mildly inflammatory with the white blood cell counts ranging from a few hundred cells to about 18,000 cells with a predominance of lymphocytes. There may be reduced synovial fluid complement levels compared to serum. Prior to the advent of automated laboratory testing, the LE cell prep test was often performed on synovial fluid in patients suspected of having SLE. Though the test was highly specific for lupus, it is not sensitive and was very labor intensive.

Jaccoud's Arthropathy

A key clinical observation has been that, unlike rheumatoid arthritis, lupus arthritis is often related to periarticular inflammation, particularly of the tendon sheaths. This was first described by Osler in 1895. Nearly four decades later, Tremaine described the synovial histopathology as featuring" articular, and periarticular inflammatory synovial villous hypertrophy with the resultant "swan-neck fingers." Subsequently, Friedberg first reported a deforming arthritis and observed that the onset of lupus could simulate rheumatic fever. This observation was noted by other authors. For example, Zvaifler described the features of joint deformity seen in patients with rheumatic fever. There was ulnar displacement of the extensor tendons and a mild hyperextension deformity without swelling pain or tenderness with joint motion of the metacarpophalangeal (MCP) joints. Bywaters highlighted the similarity between the deforming arthropathy of SLE and that originally described in 1869 by Jaccoud for recurrent rheumatic fever. The clinical picture of Jaccoud's syndrome is characterized by chronic nonerosive deformities that superficially resemble those of rheumatoid arthritis. Furthermore Bywaters described the formation of "hooks" and cysts of the metacarpal heads in later stages of the disease, which he interpreted to be the result of bone remodeling to accommodate altered stress caused by extreme laxity of the tendons along with periarticular fibrosis (Fig. 7.1).

Although Jaccoud's arthropathy is most often observed in patients with SLE, it has been described in a variety of other disorders as well as other autoimmune diseases such as scleroderma, dermatomyositis, and juvenile rheumatoid arthritis, chronic lung disease, sarcoidosis, hypermobility syndrome, and hypocomplementaemic urticarial vasculitis syndrome.

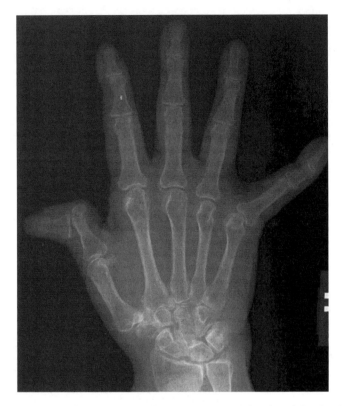

Fig. 7.1 Multiple reducible swan-neck deformities. Marked deformity of the thumb and fifth MCP joint. Unlike RA, the cartilage space is preserved and no erosions are seen

This condition presents with hand joint deformities predominately involving the MCP, proximal interphalangeal joints (PIP), the wrists and less commonly the knees. Ulnar deviation is the earliest of these features. Thumb deformities begin as passively correctable flexion deformity at the MCP joint with hyperextension at the interphalangeal joint. Later, if the carpometacarpal joint becomes unstable, and subluxation or dislocation and adduction of the thumb metacarpal occur, flexion develops at the intraphalangeal joint with hyperextension at the MCP joint. This is important because treatment will require stabilization of the carpometacarpal joint before other joints are addressed.

In severe cases, the ulnar deviation and subluxation resemble that seen in patients with rheumatoid arthritis. The key distinction between Jaccoud's arthropathy and rheumatoid arthritis is the absence of rheumatoid-like erosions on imaging studies. Unlike rheumatoid arthritis where the loss of bone and joint stability are secondary to destructive arthritis, the deformity of Jaccoud's arthropathy appears to be the consequence of ligament and tendon pathology. This is confirmed by a magnetic resonance study (MRI) of patients with Jaccoud's arthropathy which demonstrated joint capsule swelling, tenosynovitis with edema but no changes of an active synovitis. The histopathology of this lesion reveals

Fig. 7.2 Marked valgus angulation at the MTP joints. Note preservation of the joint spaces and lack of erosions. Patient sustained ankle fracture requiring a pin placement

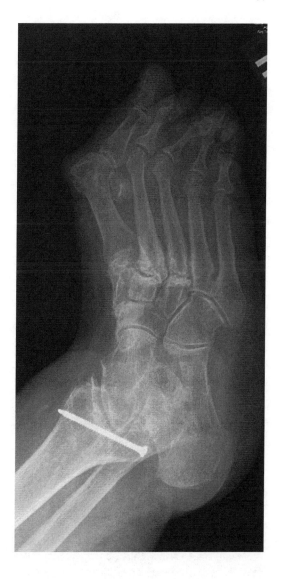

fibrin deposition, scant cellular infiltrates, and microvascular changes but without any pannus (Fig. 7.2).

The treatment options for Jaccoud's arthropathy are limited. The condition is due to noninflammatory periarticular rather than synovial-based tissue changes. Thus there is no role for the use of the standard disease-modifying antirheumatic drug (DMARD) regimens that are used in RA and other inflammatory arthritides. Perhaps the key issue in making a diagnosis of JA is to separate this hand deformity from other entities that require aggressive anti-inflammatory therapy. Conservative measures including the judicious use of NSAIDS and mild analgesics for joint discomfort along with intermittent splinting of joint subluxations that become painful can be offered.

Intra-articular joint injections provide little benefit and should be avoided. Referral for customized splinting and hand exercises to preserve function may be required for patients who continue to lose function.

Tendon Involvement

In addition to the ligament laxity that is seen with Jaccoud's arthropathy, other forms of tendon involvement can also be observed in SLE. Tenosynovitis of the hand was noted in 44 % of SLE patients in an ultrasound study. In one study comparing hand magnetic resonance imaging (MRI) findings, the pattern of tenosynovitis in SLE was nearly indistinguishable from RA. Though uncommon, tendon rupture can occur, particularly in patients with Jaccoud's arthropathy. In one retrospective study, almost one-third of the SLE patients with tendon rupture also had Jaccoud's arthropathy suggesting this arthropathy should be recognized as a risk marker for tendon rupture. The most frequently involved areas include the patellar and Achilles tendons. Biopsy of these tendons has revealed degeneration, mononuclear cell infiltration, neovascularisation, and vacuolar myopathy.

The treatment of tendonitis includes rest, ice, and intermittent immobilization. Formal physical therapy may alleviate symptoms. Mild analgesics may provide some pain relief.

Since there has been an association between the use of quinolone antibiotics and tendon rupture, the use of this class of antibiotics in SLE with tendonitis or tendon rupture should be carefully considered.

Nodules

Lupus profundus represents a firm nodular lesion with or without an overlying cutaneous lesion. The nodules are often painful and consist of perivascular infiltrates of mononuclear cells with panniculitis, manifested as hyaline fat necrosis with mononuclear cell infiltration and lymphocytic vasculitis. These nodules may appear on the scalp, face, arms, chest, back, thighs, and buttocks. They usually resolve but may leave a depressed area. Ulcerations are uncommon. Some patients with lupus profundus exhibit no other manifestations of SLE, thereby resembling the clinical findings seen in Weber–Christian disease.

Erosive Arthritis

Some patients with lupus may demonstrate features of an erosive arthritis. The localization of erosions at the finger joints is similar to those seen with patients with RA, primarily involving the second and third MCP joints. It has been debated whether these patients have an overlap of RA and SLE commonly referred to "rhupus". The first reports of coexistence of SLE and RA were made by Toone, who described the presence of LE cells in the serum of 15 patients with RA. The incidence of coexistent SLE with RA has been estimated at 0.01–2 % without establishing if this association corresponds to a clinically and immunologically distinctive entity, the coincidence of two diseases, or a subgroup of patients with lupus.

In a British study of 104 patients with lupus, an erosive arthritis was identified in 11 % of patients. The presence of erosive arthritis was significantly associated with anti-citrulline antibodies and more weakly with rheumatoid factor. HLA-DQB1*0302 was associated with erosive arthritis with similar trends for HLADRB1*0401 and two copies of the shared epitope (SE). There were trends for associations of HLADQB1*0302 and two SE copies with anti-CCP antibody production. In another study, the association of antibodies to cyclic citrullinated peptides (anti-CCP) was studied in 34 systemic lupus erythematosus patients with a deforming arthritis. The frequency of anti-CCP antibodies was 5 and 7 % in patients with lupus nondeforming or deforming arthritis, respectively. There was a higher frequency of positive rheumatoid factor (RF) in SLE patients with deforming arthritis (65 %) than in those without it (15 %).

The treatment of erosive arthritis resembles the treatment of RA, up to a point. For example, disease-modifying anti-rheumatic drug (DMARDs) such as methotrexate (in the patient with normal renal function) or azathioprine can be used. For treatment of refractory disease, the biological therapies including anti-TNF alpha blockade has been considered. However, there is the theoretical risk that these drugs may induce a lupus flare, since clinical trial data has shown the development of positive ANA tests in about 15–20 % of patients. It is not clear whether anti-B cell therapy is therapeutic.

Fasciitis

Necrotizing fasciitis (NF) is a limb- and life-threatening infection of the subcutaneous tissue and superficial fascia. Characterized by a rapid and progressive clinical course, this infection is often fatal despite the use of appropriate measures to treat and control the underlying process. The clinical presentation of patients with NF may be deceptively benign, and at onset it may not be possible to clearly distinguish NF from minor soft tissue infections. Initially infection spreads widely along subdermal fascial planes with destruction occurring in fascial and subcutaneous tissues, while little or no abnormality is evident in the skin. It is this relatively normal appearance of the skin that often causes delay in diagnosis. Later, occlusion of nutrient vessels results in ischemia, blistering, and eventually, gangrene. A recent review described a series of 21 patients with SLE and NF. It occurred in 8 of 449 SLE patients followed at their institution. A history of nephritis and corticosteroid use heightened the risk for NF. The commonest organisms included staphylococcal and streptococcal species.

There is a 33 % mortality in those patients with NF described in the literature; prompt intervention with appropriate antibiotic coverage along with surgical debridement is required.

Spine

There have been a few reports of cervical spine subluxation at the atlanto axial joint level. For example, subluxation, ranging from 3.5 to 7.0 mm, was seen in 5 of 59 unselected lupus patients (8.5 %). It was associated with Jaccoud's arthropathy, longer disease duration, renal disease with increased serum parathyroid hormone levels.

Unlike RA, cervical spine fusion is rarely required and patients can be managed conservatively. Because of the ubiquitous use of corticosteroids, patients with SLE have a greater risk for developing osteoporosis of the vertebral bodies and compression fracture. The development of acute back pain in the lupus patient may herald this diagnosis. If there is an associated fever, the possibility of an epidural abscess needs to be considered, since these patients may be immune compromised by their disease or their treatment.

Osteonecrosis

Osteonecrosis (ON) [also known as avascular necrosis (AVN)] is characterized by death of bone marrow and trabecular bone as a result of compromised blood supply to the bone. It results in collapse of the architectural bone structure leading to joint pain, bone destruction, and loss of function. The interruption of the vascular supply may be traumatic or non-traumatic. Non-traumatic ON is now a well-recognized complication in systemic lupus erythematosus, having first been described by Dubois and Cozen. The reported prevalence in SLE is between 4 and 15 % but can be up to 40 % when asymptomatic patients are included.

Several factors have been associated with the development of ON in SLE but corticosteroid therapy has been the most consistent association. One study sought to determine factors that predisposed to, or protected from, the development of ON in lupus patients when cumulative oral corticosteroid doses were matched between cases and controls, thereby removing presence of corticosteroid therapy and cumulative dose as risk factors. Of the 570 patients seen within the first year after diagnosis 65 (11.4 %) developed ON. None of the variables examined were found to confer additional ON risk in multivariate analysis. It appears that the major factor associated with the development of ON is corticosteroid therapy. Factors that may protect patients on corticosteroids from developing ON have not been identified.

The commonest joints to be affected are the hips although the shoulder, knees, and scaphoid navicular can also be affected. ON may be uni- or bilateral or may affect several joints in the same individual. It may be an symptomatic radiographic finding or it may present with acute joint pain and loss of function. In the acute case of ON, the plain radiographs of the affected joint may be misleading—there may be no abnormalities found for up to several weeks. The pathognomonic "crescent sign" or subchondral radiolucency may be evident weeks to months later and is evidence of subchondral collapse.

MRI is the most sensitive test to detect ON. MRI of affected joints may demonstrate a geographic focus of heterogeneous signal surrounded by low signal on T1-weighted images and by a double line on T2-weighted images. A Japanese study utilized MRI to document the long-term natural history of asymptomatic osteonecrosis associated with corticosteroid therapy in SLE patients. Two hundred and one SLE patients treated with high-dose corticosteroids were prospectively observed for 11 years. During this time all patients received periodic MRI examinations of their hip and knee joints. Five hundred and thirty-seven joints (251 hips and 286 knees) were identified in 144 patients. Osteonecrosis developed in 238 (44 %) of 537 joints. At final follow-up, 117 (49 %) of these 238 joints demonstrated spontaneous repair in the necrotic area. Fifty-two joints (22 %) had collapsed. Osteonecrosis completely disappeared in 21 joints. Enlargement of osteonecrosis was noted in 35 joints (15 %) following increased corticosteroid dosage required to treat active SLE.

Corticosteroids use is the greatest risk for the development of ON in lupus patients. Other risk factors for ON include Raynaud's phenomenon, and hyperlipidemia. There are conflicting data on the role of antiphospholipid (aPL) antibodies in lupus; some data support an association while other data do not. The pathophysiology of osteonecrosis in patients with APS has not been entirely established; however, many mechanisms have been proposed. These mechanisms revolve around two main ideas: First, anticardiolipin antibodies antibodies have been associated with thrombophilia and second, anticardiolipin antibodies have been associated with avascular necrosis of bone. Therefore, osteonecrosis may be caused by thrombosis in the setting of a hypercoagulable state caused by the presence of aPL antibodies. These proposed mechanisms revolve around the idea that a hypercoagulable state predisposes a patient to vascular pathology resulting in bone death. The thrombophilic and hypofibrinolytic states generated by APS predispose patients to venous thrombi. The resulting venous occlusion of the bone by fibrin clots leads to venous sinusoidal hypertension within the cancellous bone. The venous sinusoidal hypertension increases to the point that arterial blood flow to the region is no longer able to deliver adequate oxygen to the bone. The resulting cellular hypoxia presumably gives way to bone and marrow cell death, thereby causing osteonecrosis.

Additional associations between lupus and ON have been suggested including African-American origin, Cushingoid habitus, vasculitis, pleuritis, and CNS involvement.

The treatment for ON involves the avoidance of full weight-bearing activities to allow for healing of the lesion. Despite this approach, the bone remodeling that ensues may be less than optimal, resulting in more advanced cartilage loss and bone damage. Clinically, this situation will usually present with worsening or persistent pain that interferes with daily activities. Joint arthroplasty may be required to correct this problem. In fact, ON is the most common reason for a lupus patient to require joint replacement. Core decompression procedures have been attempted with limited success. Bone marrow grafting is a relatively new procedure that has not yet been fully evaluated.

Withdrawal or reduction of corticosteroids should be a focus of treatment. The use of crutches or a cane to achieve a degree of non-weight-bearing status should be encouraged. This is especially important for the first several weeks after the diagnosis is made, in order to allow for optimal bone remodeling. Other treatment options for osteonecrosis are limited. Core decompression surgery was advanced on the belief that reducing core pressures within the shaft of the bone would eliminate the key driver of bone necrosis. However, this procedure has fallen out of favor because of its lack of long-term efficacy and high risk for secondary fracture due to the procedure. For patients with severe pain and loss of joint function, standard joint arthroplasty is recommended.

Medications that have been used to treat osteonecrosis include bisphosphonates and statins. There are no clinical trials to support either of these agents.

Myositis

Myalgias, muscle tenderness, or muscle weakness occur in up to 70 % of patients with SLE, and may be the major presenting complaint. Severe weakness, muscle atrophy, and myositis are all fairly uncommon, seen in about 10 % of patients. Muscle biopsies from affected areas show perivascular and perifascicular mononuclear cell infiltrates. Other histologic findings include muscle atrophy, microtubular inclusions, mononuclear infiltrate, fiber necrosis, and occasionally vacuolated muscle fibers.

Glucocorticoids and antimalarial drugs can cause muscle weakness. Serum levels of creatine kinase (CK) and/or aldolase are usually normal in patients with glucocorticoid-induced myopathy. Muscle biopsy reveals an increase in the number of sarcolemmal nuclei, rowing and centralization of the nuclei, vacuolization and loss of fiber cross-striations, and phagocytosis, but no inflammation. Similarly in patients with antimalarial-induced myopathy, muscle biopsy may reveal vacuolar changes without inflammation. Similar to polymyositis, lupus-associated myositis generally responds to corticosteroids and when necessary, steroid-sparing agents such as azathioprine or methotrexate.

Fractures

Osteopenia and osteoporosis may account for much of the increased risk of fracture seen in patients with SLE. The magnitude of the fracture risk was illustrated in a retrospective, cohort study of approximately 700 women with SLE and an equivalent number of age-matched controls; a fivefold increase in fracture among those with SLE was noted. Risk factors for fracture development included older age at the time of diagnosis of SLE, longer disease duration, longer duration of glucocorticoid use, less use of oral contraceptives, and menopause status.

The presence of aPL may be associated with an increased risk of non-traumatic fractures. This was illustrated in one study that linked aPL to an increased risk of metatarsal (stress) fractures in patients with SLE. Vertebral fractures, found in up to 20 % of patients with SLE, have been associated with intravenous use of methylprednisolone at any time and with male sex.

Sources

1. Fries J, Holman H. Systemic lupus erythematosus: a clinical analysis. Philadelphia: WB Saunders; 1975.
2. Dubois EL, Tuffanelli DL. Clinical manifestations of systemic lupus erythematosus. Computer analysis of 520 cases. JAMA. 1964;190:104–11.
3. Pekin TJ, Zvaifler NJ. Synovial fluid findings in systemic lupus erythematosus. Arthritis Rheum. 1970;13:777.
4. Osler W. On the visceral complications of erythema exudativum multiforme. Am J Med Sci. 1895;110:629–46.
5. Zvaifler N. Chronic post-rheumatic fever (Jaccoud's) arthritis. N Engl J Med. 1962;267:10–5.
6. Alarcon-Segovia D, Abud-Mendoza C, Iglesias-Gamarra A. Deforming arthropathy of the hands in systemic lupus erythematosus. J Rheumatol. 1988;15:65–9.
7. Weissman BN, Rappoport AS, Sosman JL, Schur PH. Radiographic findings in the hands in patients with systemic lupus erythematosus. Radiology. 1978;126:313–7.
8. Potasman I, Bassan HM. Multiple tendon rupture in systemic lupus erythematosus: case report and review of the literature. Ann Rheum Dis. 1984;43(2):347–9.
9. Van Vugt RM, Derksen RH, Kater L, Bijlsma JW. Deforming arthropathy or lupus and rhupus hands in systemic lupus erythematosus. Ann Rheum Dis. 1998;57:540–4.
10. Panush RS, Edwards L, Longley S, et al. 'Rhupus' syndrome. Arch Intern Med. 1988;148: 1633–6.
11. Kamran M, Wachs J, Putterman C. Necrotizing fasciitis in systemic lupus erythematosus. Semin Arthritis Rheum. 2008;37:236–42.
12. Gladman DD, Urowitz MB, Chaudhry-Ahluwalia V, Hallet DC, Cook RJ. Predictive factors for symptomatic osteonecrosis in patients with systemic lupus erythematosus. J Rheumatol. 2001;28:761–5.
13. Prasad R, Ibanez D, Gladman D, Urowitz M. The role of non-corticosteroid related factors in osteonecrosis (ON) in systemic lupus erythematosus: a nested case-control study of inception patients. Lupus. 2007;16:157–62.
14. Miyakis S, Lockshin MD, Atsumi I, et al. International consensus statement on an update of the classification criteria for definite antiphospholipid syndrome (APS). J Thromb Haemost. 2006;4:295–306.

Chapter 8
Cardiac and Vascular Disease in SLE

Robert A. Sands

Systemic lupus may have highly significant effects upon the heart, both as a direct result of the disease and as a result of the side effects of the medications used to treat the illness. Since the first descriptions of heart disease in lupus by Osler, more than a hundred years ago, it has become clear that lupus may affect all parts of the heart: pericardium, myocardium, endocardium, conduction system, and coronary arteries. While heart disease is often subclinical, in the past several decades, it has become clear that cardiac disease is a major source of morbidity for lupus patients.

Pericarditis

The most commonly seen form of lupus heart disease is pericarditis. This may occur in 20–30 % of patients clinically but is more commonly noted on echocardiogram (38 %) and at pathologic exam (up to 66 %) in several clinical reports. Typical symptoms include dyspnea and anterior chest pain that is often worse with inspiration and when supine and improved by sitting up. Physical exam is often normal, but a pericardial rub and resting tachycardia may be noted, and jugular venous distension may be seen when effusions are large. Pericardial tamponade is very rare but may occur in 1–2 % of patients with pericarditis. Constriction and purulent pericarditis are other even more rare complications of pericardial inflammation. Pericarditis is often seen when there is evidence for lupus being active elsewhere, and in particular, pleural effusions are more common in patients with pericarditis.

R.A. Sands, M.D. (✉)
Division of Rheumatology, Brigham and Women's Hospital,
75 Francis Street, Boston, MA 02115, USA

Harvard Medical School, Boston, MA, USA
e-mail: rsands@partners.org

There is nothing specific about pericarditis in patients with lupus. It is thus important to keep in mind the differential diagnosis of chest pain in these patients including pneumonia, cardiac ischemia, pulmonary hypertension, and pulmonary embolus. Characteristic EKG findings are often noted, with PR depression and ST segment elevation. Echocardiographic findings include pericardial effusion and pericardial thickening. Pericardial fluid has been reported to have a variable protein content, elevated white blood cell count, a normal or low glucose level, antinuclear antibodies, and low complement components. Hemorrhagic fluid has also been reported.

Treatment of pericarditis is directed most often toward controlling pain due to inflammation. Small, asymptomatic effusions seen on echocardiogram do not need medical intervention. In patients who do not respond rapidly to treatment with nonsteroidal medication, or who are not able to take these medications due to renal disease or other contraindication, prednisone is usually quickly effective in doses between 20 and 80 mg/day. Patients with tamponade need to be hospitalized and undergo drainage of the pericardial fluid, with consideration for possible creation surgically of a pericardial window. For patients with recurrent pericarditis, colchicine has sometimes been used, based on a report of its effectiveness in treating idiopathic recurrent pericarditis, but its helpfulness in this context is unknown.

Valvular Heart Disease

Valvular heart disease was first described nearly a century ago by Libman and Sacks and is perhaps the best known cardiac manifestation in lupus. These small, flat, or raised vegetations occur principally along valve rings and commissures and most commonly involve the mitral valve, though any valve may be involved. The lesions may spread to involve adjacent structures including the papillary muscles. Definitive diagnosis of these lesions is made at autopsy with pathologic findings consisting of fibrin, immune complexes, and chronic inflammatory cells. The prevalence of these lesions varies in autopsy series between 10 % and 74 % and is felt to have decreased in frequency since steroid therapy was introduced. Transthoracic echocardiography has been found to be less sensitive than transesophageal imaging in detecting Libman–Sacks endocarditis. Complications of these endocardial growths include embolism, superimposed bacterial infection, and valve dysfunction.

Multiple echocardiographic studies have shown an increased frequency of valvular heart disease in lupus patients compared with controls, with between 38 % and 74 % of lupus patients having valvular disease on echocardiogram. It is, however, important to remember that murmurs may occur due to anemia or fever in patients without any valve disease. Regurgitant lesions are seen far more frequently than stenotic ones. In one observational study over a period of 5 years, these valvular lesions changed or resolved, or new lesions developed in one series. No relationship between lupus disease activity and echocardiographic findings has been noted.

The pathogenesis of the valvular lesions seen in lupus patients is not clear. It has been suggested that the verrucous lesions of Libman–Sacks endocarditis and the valve thickening and dysfunction seen frequently on echocardiogram have a shared pathogenesis. There are multiple reports of an association between antiphospholipid antibodies and valvular heart disease seen in patients with SLE as well as in patients who have primary antiphospholipid antibody syndrome, but two investigators were not able to find that phospholipid antibody positivity conferred an increased risk for valve disease. Examination of valve tissue has revealed the deposition of immunoglobulins, complement, and anticardiolipin antibodies, though it is not fully clear if the latter are playing a causative role. However, it has been theorized that these antibodies promote local thrombosis or interact directly with valve tissue promoting injury.

Though common, valvular heart disease is only clinically important in about 10 % of patients with SLE. These patients are at increased risk for progressive valve insufficiency and resulting CHF. There also appears to be an increased risk for SBE, stroke and embolus formation in these patients. Patients with significant valve disease should be followed by a cardiologist who can also help assist with advice about monitoring, decisions about anticoagulation, and potential role for surgery. These patients should also be considered for antibiotic prophylaxis during invasive procedures that may lead to bacteremia, especially if on immunosuppressive therapy.

Myocarditis

Myocardial involvement has been noted in up to 50 % of SLE patients in autopsy series, but myocarditis is only rarely seen clinically. Biopsies have shown chronic inflammatory cells in the interstitium and fibrosis. While CHF has been reported in between 5 % and 44 % of patients with SLE, it is difficult to separate out the contribution of hypertension and renal disease to heart failure from the effects of lupus itself. The diagnosis of lupus myocarditis is based on a clinical picture of resting tachycardia, nonspecific ST changes on EKG, CHF, arrhythmia, and cardiomegaly. Fever and pericarditis are also seen commonly in this context. Echocardiography may show global abnormalities in systolic and diastolic function. A strong association was noted in one report in lupus patients with myocarditis, peripheral myositis, and positive RNP antibodies. Antimyocardial antibodies have also been described. The differential diagnosis includes viral and medication-induced myocarditis. Endomyocardial biopsies can be done to help clarify diagnosis and may be useful in particular in ruling out heart involvement from hydroxychloroquine, an agent that causes a characteristic vacuolar myopathy. In addition to standard agents for treating heart failure, the treatment for lupus patients with suspected myocarditis includes high-dose steroid, and in addition, immunosuppressive agents may also be needed.

Conduction System Disease

Conduction system disease and arrhythmia may occasionally be seen in patients with lupus, on the order of about 10 %. All degrees of AV block have been noted, and this may occur in up to 5 % of patients. Structural damage to the conduction system has been identified with inflammation, scarring, and arteritis and often associated with adjacent pericarditis. Conduction system disease is, however, best described in the infants of mothers with anti-Ro and anti-La antibodies, who have an approximate 3 % chance of developing heart block in utero. Also, a dysautonomia has also been described in patients with lupus leading to abnormalities in heart rate variability.

Coronary Artery Disease

In the past 30 years, it has become clear that coronary artery disease occurs with a troublingly high frequency and that it is a leading cause of mortality in patients with established lupus. This is in the large majority of cases due to atherosclerosis, with only rare reports of coronary arteritis or embolism. Data from several centers indicate a prevalence of clinically apparent coronary artery disease in between 6 % and 15 % of patients with SLE.

Women with SLE have a five- to sixfold increased risk for coronary artery disease compared to healthy controls. However, when asymptomatic patients with SLE are looked at with either myocardial perfusion canning or electron beam CT, the prevalence of coronary artery disease is far greater, between 28 % and 38 %. These data are particularly impressive when one considers that the majority of these patients are young. When stratified for age, lupus patients between the ages of 35 and 44 had a 50-fold increased risk for coronary artery disease compared to normal controls in the Framingham study.

The causes for premature coronary artery disease in SLE has been felt to be the result of the added effects of traditional coronary risk factors, steroid medications, and aspects of the inflammatory process intrinsic to SLE. It has been shown in a number of studies that lupus patients have an increased risk for the traditionally recognized disorders that predispose to atherosclerosis: hypertension, hyperlipidemia, diabetes, insulin resistance, and inactivity. Compared with controls, lupus patients were shown to have a nearly threefold increased risk for metabolic syndrome, 32 % vs. 11 %.

Steroids have been recognized to promote the development of a number of these traditional risk factors, including hypertension, hyperglycemia, and hyperlipidemia with weight gain. They have thus long been felt to have played a significant role in promoting atherosclerosis in patients with lupus. Bulkley's classic autopsy report done more than 30 years ago offers strong support for that association: of the 16 patients on steroid medication for a year or more, 42 % had at least 50 % narrowing of a coronary artery compared to none of the 17 patients who had not been on steroids for that long a duration. Duration of prednisone therapy and cumulative steroid dose have also been found to be predictors of coronary artery disease in lupus. However, traditional risk factors have not been felt to be able to explain all of the accrued risk for coronary artery disease in lupus patients.

A large number of other factors have been identified that may be intrinsic to the lupus disease process itself or to individual patient factors that may play a role in adding to this high risk for coronary disease. Male gender carries an added risk for patients with lupus to develop coronary disease. Lupus nephritis may predispose to hypertension, a clotting tendency, as well as hyperlipidemia, thereby increasing the risk for atherosclerosis. Premature menopause may lead to a loss of the protective effects of estrogen on developing atherosclerosis. Other factors reported by some, but not all, authors to augment the risk of developing coronary include increased disease activity, serologic markers of inflammation, renal disease, inflammatory lung disease, and phospholipid antibodies.

The latter may promote vascular disease by virtue of their procoagulant activity, but they have an added direct effect on components of the vessel wall. Beta-2 glycoprotein may have a physiologic effect of preventing uptake of oxidized LDL by vascular macrophages. Antibodies to that protein may interfere with that protective function. In addition, phospholipid antibodies have the ability to cross-react with antibodies directed against HDL and against Apo-A-1, the main component of HDL, with resultant low levels of HDL, and a possible added risk for developing atherosclerosis. Not all studies have supported a role for antiphospholipid antibodies in the development of coronary artery disease, but they have been found to be associated with the development of carotid plaque formation.

In the past several years, it has become abundantly clear that atherosclerosis has an inflammatory pathogenesis. This is reviewed in depth by Bruce, but there is much laboratory evidence to support the role of inflammatory cells, complement activation, immune complex deposition, and cytokine release or suppression with the development of atherosclerosis. In recent years, it has also become apparent that in other inflammatory rheumatic diseases, especially RA and psoriatic arthritis, there is an increased risk for coronary artery disease. This has led to the sense that suppressing inflammation should be a key part of decreasing the risks for atherosclerosis in patients with autoimmune disease.

Given the extraordinary high risk for coronary artery disease in lupus, it is clear that physicians caring for lupus patients need to assume the complex and time-consuming task of helping reduce the chance for a heart attack for their patients. Having an actively involved primary care physician is also very important in this regard. Patients need to be informed about this subject, reeducated at follow-up visits, and need to play an active role in leading a healthy lifestyle, avoiding obesity, with healthy diet, regular exercise, and avoidance of tobacco. Blood pressure, glucose, and lipid levels need to be monitored and abnormalities minimized. A low-dose coated 81 mg aspirin is worth considering for all lupus patients, in the absence of a contraindication to its use. As hydroxychloroquine has a disease-modifying effect on lupus as well as anti-inflammatory properties, and a beneficial effect on lipids in patients with lupus, it too should be used in all patients with lupus as a rule.

Limiting steroid exposure while at the same time working to control the manifestations of lupus so as to limit the role of inflammation in promoting atherosclerosis is an ongoing goal. Statin therapy is indicated in the context of hyperlipidemia but may have an added benefit of being anti-inflammatory. To date, there are no guidelines to use for making decisions about screening for asymptomatic patients with lupus with regard to exercise testing or other noninvasive techniques to identify those already with coronary artery disease, though studies are clearly needed to help define the optimal approach to patients.

Cerebrovascular Disease

Patients with lupus have been shown to be at an increased risk for cerebrovascular accidents, with between 3 % and 20 % of patients developing this complication. The relative increased risk for stroke is variably reported at being between 1.5 and 8 times greater than normal controls. Strokes tend to be severe in up to 77 % of patients and may be more commonly be fatal than in non-lupus patients. Strokes often occur during the first 5 years if disease and may be recurrent in up to 67 % of patients. Studies have varied in their identification of predisposing factors for stroke, but these have been reported to include disease activity, the traditional risk factors for atherosclerosis. The pathogenesis of stroke in lupus patients is complex and includes accelerated atherosclerosis, thrombosis with positive antiphospholipid antibody testing, spasm, and rarely arteritis.

Attempts to control disease activity and to maintain ideal blood pressure, lipid, and glucose levels are key to the ongoing care for lupus patients. To date, there are no guidelines for the management of patients who have had a stroke. In addition to the previously mentioned measures, anticoagulation with aspirin and Coumadin needs to be started on an indefinite basis to help decrease the chance of recurrent stroke. Those with risk factors for stroke, such as valvular heart lesions or antiphospholipid antibodies, are probably best treated with a more intensive regimen than aspirin alone, i.e., Coumadin.

Peripheral Vascular Disease

Peripheral vascular disease is less well studied than coronary artery disease in lupus. However, this is not a rare occurrence in lupus, and up to 28 % of patients may have either venous or arterial disease. Multiple risk factors have been identified but not all agreed upon by different reports in the literature, including age, extravascular organ injury, disease activity, homocysteine level, and the traditional risk factors for atherosclerosis. Severe digital ischemia has been reported in patients with antiphospholipid antibody positivity and vasculitis. In any single patient, it may be difficult to separate out the separate contributions of atherosclerosis, vasculitis, thrombosis, and spasm. Early recognition is important to optimal therapy. This may include not only anticoagulation but also high-dose steroid therapy if vasculitis is felt to be present.

Sources

1. Mandell B. Cardiovascular involvement in systemic lupus erythematosus. Semin Arthritis Rheum. 1987;17:126–41.
2. Doherty N. Cardiovascular manifestations of systemic lupus erythematosus. Am Heart J. 1985;10:1257–63.
3. Kahl L. The spectrum of pericardial tamponade in systemic lupus erythematosus. Arthritis Rheum. 1992;35:1343–9.
4. Guido J, et al. Recurrent pericarditis. Relief with colchicine. Circulation. 1990;82:1117.
5. Moder K, et al. Cardiac involvement in systemic lupus erythematosus. Mayo Clin Proc. 1999;74:275–84.
6. Hojnik M, et al. Heart valve involvement (Libman-Sacks endocarditis) in the antiphospholipid syndrome. Circulation. 1996;93:1579–87.
7. Galve E, et al. Prevalence, morphologic types and evolution of cardiac valvular disease in systemic lupus erythematosus. N Engl J Med. 1988;319:817–23.
8. Roldan C, et al. Transthoracic versus transesophageal echocardiography for detection of Libman-Sacks endocarditis: a randomized controlled study. J Rheumatol. 2008;35:224–9.
9. Nihoyannopoulos P, et al. Cardiac abnormalities in systemic lupus erythematosus. Circulation. 1990;82:369–75.
10. Roldan C. An echocardiographic study of valvular heart disease in systemic lupus erythematosus. N Engl J Med. 1996;335:1424–30.
11. Perez-Villa F, et al. Severe valvular regurgitation and antiphospholipid antibodies in systemic lupus erythematosus: a prospective. Long-term follow up study. Arthritis Rheum. 2005;53:460–7.
12. Ong ML, et al. Cardiac abnormalities in systemic lupus erythematosus: prevalence and relationship to disease activity. Int J Cardiol. 1992;34:69–74.
13. Evangelopoulos ME, et al. Mitral valve prolapse in SLE patients: clinical and immunological aspects. Lupus. 2003;12:308–11.
14. Gabrieli F, et al. Cardiac involvement in systemic lupus erythematosus and primary antiphospholipid antibody syndrome: lack of correlation with antiphospholipid antibodies. Int J Cardiol. 1995;51:117–26.
15. Roldan C, et al. Systemic lupus erythematosus valve disease by transesophageal echocardiography and role of antiphospholipid antibodies. J Am Coll Cardiol. 1992;20:1127–34.
16. Bidani A, et al. Immunopathology of cardiac lesions in fatal systemic lupus erythematosus. Am J Med. 1980;69:849–58.
17. Ziporen L, et al. Libman-sacks endocarditis in the antiphospholipid antibody syndrome. Lupus. 1996;5:196–205.
18. Bornstein D, et al. The myocarditis of systemic lupus erythematosus: association with myositis. Ann Intern Med. 1978;89:619–24.
19. Schur, P, Costenbader, K. Non-coronary cardiac manifestations of systemic lupus. Up To Date in Rheumatology.
20. James TN. Pathology of the cardiac conduction system in systemic lupus erythematosus. Ann Intern Med. 1965;63:402–10.
21. Stein KS, et al. Heart rate variability in patients with systemic lupus erythematosus. Lupus. 1996;4:44–8.
22. Urowitz M, et al. Bimodal mortality in systemic lupus erythematosus. Am J Med. 1976;60:221–5.

23. Schattner A, Liang M. The cardiovascular burden of lupus. Arch Intern Med. 2003;163: 1507–10.
24. Bruce N. "Not only…but also": factors that contribute to accelerated atherosclerosis and premature coronary heart disease in systemic lupus erythematosus. Rheumatology. 2005; 44(12):1492–502.
25. Manzi S, et al. Age specific incidence of myocardial infarction and angina in women with systemic lupus erythematosus: comparison with the Framingham Study. Am J Epidemiol. 1997;145:408–15.
26. Yu A, et al. Premature coronary artery atherosclerosis in systemic lupus erythematosus. N Engl J Med. 2003;349:2407–15.
27. Nikpour M, et al. Myocardial perfusion imaging in assessing risk of coronary events in patients with systemic lupus erythematosus. J Rheumatol. 2009;36:288–94.
28. Chung C. High prevalence of the metabolic syndrome in patients with systemic lupus erythematosus: association with disease characteristics and cardiovascular risk factors. Ann Rheum Dis. 2007;66:208–14.
29. Petrie M, et al. Risk factors for coronary artery disease in patients with lupus. Am J Med. 1992;93:513–9.
30. Bulkley B, et al. The heart in systemic lupus erythematosus and the changes induced in it by corticosteroid therapy. Am J Med. 1975;58:243–64.
31. Manger K. Factors associated with coronary artery calcification in systemic lupus erythematosus. Ann Rheum Dis. 2003;62:846–50.
32. Esdaile JM, et al. Traditional Framingham risk factors fail to fully account for accelerated atherosclerosis in systemic lupus erythematosus. Arthritis Rheum. 2008;26:32.
33. Lee A, et al. Traditional risk factor assessment does not capture the extent of cardiovascular risk in systemic lupus erythematosus. Arthritis Rheum. 2001;44:2331.
34. Pons-Estel G, et al. Predictors of cardiovascular damage in patients with systemic lupus erythematosus: data from LUMINA (LXVIII), a multiethnic US cohort. Rheumatology (Oxford). 2009;48:817–22.
35. Pineau LA, et al. Lupus disease activity and coronary artery disease (abstract). Athritis Rheum. 2001;44:S287.
36. Petrie M, et al. Thrombosis and systemic lupus erythematosus: the Hopkins Lupus Cohort perspective. Scand J Rheumatol. 1996;25:191.
37. Maroni G, et al. Cardiologic abnormalities in patients with long-term lupus nephritis. Clin Nephrol. 1995;43:20.
38. Bruce N. The natural history of hypercholesterolemia in systemic lupus erythematosus. J Rheumatol. 1999;26:2137–43.
39. Nojuma J. Arteriosclerosis obliterans associated with beta 2 glycoprotein 1 antibodies as a strong risk factor for ischemic heart disease in patients with systemic lupus erythematosus. Rheumatology (Oxford). 2008;47:684–9.
40. Svenungsson E, et al. Risk factors for cardiovascular disease in systemic lupus erythematosus. Circulation. 2001;104:1887–93.
41. Roman MJ. Prevalence and correlates of accelerated atherosclerosis in systemic lupus erythematosus. N Engl J Med. 2003;349:2399–406.
42. Ahmad Y, et al. Antiphospholipid antibodies contribute to atherogenesis in systemic lupus erythematosus. Arthritis Rheum. 2004;50:S191.
43. Hansson G. Inflammation, atherosclerosis and coronary artery disease. N Engl J Med. 2005;352:1685–95.
44. Petrie M, et al. Effect of prednisone and hydroxychloroquine on coronary artery disease risk factors in systemic lupus erythematosus: a longitudinal data analysis. Am J Med. 1994;96: 254–9.

Chapter 9
Pulmonary Manifestations of Systemic Lupus Erythematosus

Hilary J. Goldberg and Paul F. Dellaripa

Dyspnea

Patients with systemic lupus erythematosus (SLE) may present with dyspnea from a variety of causes, as described below. The initial evaluation of the patient with SLE and dyspnea should involve a comprehensive medical history, including duration of symptoms, acuity of symptom progression, sputum production and hemoptysis, systemic symptoms, comorbid conditions, and exposure history. Physical examination, detailing oxygen needs at rest and on exertion, presence and location of crackles on examination, pleural or pericardial friction rub, supportive evidence for pulmonary hypertension on cardiac examination, and the presence of clubbing and edema, is vital to the initial formulation of a differential diagnosis. Functional status should also be assessed, as deconditioning, resulting from limitations related to joint disease, pulmonary symptoms, or other systemic manifestations of disease, may contribute to the patient's dyspnea.

Chest X-ray should be considered as the initial screening tool, but in general, a high-resolution CT (HRCT) scan of the chest will be better able to define the underlying parenchymal process, if present. Full pulmonary function testing, including

---

H.J. Goldberg, M.D., M.P.H. (✉)
Division of Pulmonary and Critical Care Medicine, Brigham and Women's Hospital,
75 Francis Street, Boston, MA 02115, USA

Harvard Medical School, Boston, MA, USA
e-mail: hjgoldberg@partners.org

P.F. Dellaripa, M.D.
Division of Rheumatology, Brigham and Women's Hospital, Boston, MA, USA

Interstitial Lung Disease (ILD) Clinic, Brigham and Women's Hospital,
Boston, MA, USA

spirometry with and without bronchodilators, lung volumes, and diffusing capacity of carbon monoxide, is also helpful in determining the etiology of dyspnea. Bronchoscopy with bronchoalveolar lavage should be considered if focal infiltrates are noted on imaging, and in select cases, lung biopsy may be necessary.

Acute Parenchymal Disease

Pulmonary Infections

Lung infections constitute the most common pulmonary complications in patients with SLE. While patients with lupus have abnormal immune function, including altered delayed hypersensitivity, T cell function, and alveolar macrophage function, the primary risk factor for the development of infection in such patients is exposure to immune-modulating agents as part of disease treatment.

Patients with SLE are at risk for infection with routine community-acquired organisms, nosocomial bacterial infections, as well as opportunistic infections. Opportunistic infections may be caused by *Pneumocystis jirovecii*, *Aspergillus*, and cytomegalovirus, among other opportunistic organisms. Mycobacterial infection may also be seen, with a higher than average frequency of tuberculosis infections observed in patients with SLE from endemic areas. In addition, nocardial infections have been reported in patients with SLE. While lung infection with nocardia is most common, central nervous system infection is also observed.

Some have suggested that patients with SLE who receive treatment with 1 month or more of intermediate- to high-dose systemic corticosteroids (>10–20 mg/day prednisone or its equivalent) should be considered for PCP prophylaxis. In general, trimethoprim/sulfamethoxazole is the preferred agent for such prophylaxis, with alternatives including dapsone and atovaquone. However, given the significant risk of allergic reactions and flares of disease associated with the use of trimethoprim/sulfamethoxazole in SLE patients, we recommend that alternatives such as atovaquone be strongly considered. All patients with parenchymal lung disease should be vaccinated against influenza and pneumococcus, unless contraindicated.

In addition, infection should be considered in the differential diagnosis for all patients with respiratory signs or symptoms and new pulmonary infiltrates. Institution of broad spectrum antibiotic coverage, particularly for patients on immunosuppressive medication or at risk for nosocomial pneumonia, should be considered, with a plan for narrowing or discontinuation of coverage once the infectious agent is defined or infection is ruled out. The evaluation of infection often requires bronchoscopy with assessment of bronchoalveolar lavage fluid for microbiologic and virologic cultures. Transbronchial biopsies can be considered to assist in diagnosis, particularly in the setting of chronic infiltrates unresponsive to standard antibiotics. Nodular or peripheral infiltrates may be amenable to fine needle aspiration when bronchoscopy is unlikely to yield significant information.

Acute Noninfectious Lung Disease

Acute noninfectious parenchymal pathology seen in SLE includes acute lupus pneumonitis (ALP), diffuse alveolar hemorrhage (DAH), and acute respiratory distress syndrome (ARDS). The identification of ALP as a distinct entity remains controversial, and some authors postulate that all three of these processes are interrelated, with each representing a point on a spectrum of acute noninfectious, SLE-related illness.

Acute Lupus Pneumonitis

ALP is an uncommon complication of SLE, and its designation as a process distinct from other acute pulmonary complications, such as alveolar hemorrhage, is controversial. The exact prevalence of ALP is not well defined but is estimated at 2–12%. ALP typically presents earlier in the disease course than does chronic interstitial lung disease (ILD) in SLE. ALP is often seen in conjunction with other acute complications of the disease, such as acute lupus nephritis, arthritis, pericarditis, and pleuritis. ALP can, however, serve as the presenting manifestation of SLE.

Symptoms of ALP include dyspnea, cough, sometimes accompanied by hemoptysis, and pleuritic chest pain. Fever may accompany the symptoms. Examination may reveal crackles, and hypoxia can be observed. Radiographic imaging most commonly exhibits alveolar filling that is diffuse or bibasilar, and can be associated with pleural effusions. Occasionally, imaging can be normal.

PFT testing, if feasible, can help to assess for ALP (diminished diffusing capacity for carbon monoxide [DLCO]) as compared with pulmonary hemorrhage (elevated DLCO). Bronchoalveolar lavage should be performed to exclude acute infection, before concluding a diagnosis of ALP. In addition, cell count with differential on BAL fluid assessment may show lymphocytosis or granulocytosis, with a higher mortality rate associated with a predominance of neutrophils or eosinophils. Generally, lung biopsy with histopathologic assessment is required for definitive diagnosis. Pathology may demonstrate acute alveolar wall injury, hyaline membrane formation, and immunoglobulin and complement deposition. The most supportive finding is the evidence of vasculitis, with associated interstitial fibrosis, pneumonitis, alveolitis, or pleuritis.

As a result of the poor prognosis associated with this clinical presentation, the treatment is generally aggressive, despite the lack of controlled studies examining the efficacy of such an approach. Broad spectrum antibiotic coverage is recommended until acute infection can be fully ruled out and especially because the suggested treatment includes high-dose systemic corticosteroids (1–1.5 mg/kg daily of prednisone or its equivalent). If no clinical response is noted after 3–7 days, or if the patient presents with advanced disease (such as high oxygen requirement or respiratory decompensation with need for ventilatory support), IV corticosteroids (up to 1 g of methylprednisolone daily for 3 days) with or without cyclophosphamide could be considered. The mortality rate associated with this clinical presentation has been reported to be up to 50%, and patients who survive the acute illness may go on to develop chronic ILD. Alternative immunosuppressive agents and plasmapheresis have been considered in the treatment of ALP.

Diffuse Alveolar Hemorrhage

DAH is a rare complication of SLE, with a prevalence of 3.7% of hospitalized patients in one retrospective review. This complication can be recurrent. In the SLE population, DAH is most commonly observed in patients with a preceding diagnosis of SLE. In some cases, however, DAH can serve as the presenting manifestation of the disease. Patients may have evidence of active disease of other organs, such as glomerulonephritis, at the time when alveolar hemorrhage develops.

A triad of hemoptysis, decreased hemoglobin, and diffuse ground glass infiltrates by HRCT is highly suggestive of DAH. However, patients may not present with these findings, and, in particular, can present with alveolar hemorrhage in the absence of hemoptysis. Dyspnea and cough may be manifest. Imaging may demonstrate predominantly lower lobe abnormalities. Pleural effusions can also be seen in association with the infiltrates. If pulmonary function tests can be completed, an elevated DLCO is suggestive of DAH and can help to differentiate this from other acute parenchymal processes. In the absence of hemoptysis, diagnostic evaluation with bronchoscopy and bronchoalveolar lavage may reveal increasing sanguinous return on serial aliquots of lavage fluid. Rarely, surgical lung biopsy will be required for definitive diagnosis. Infection should be considered in the differential diagnosis and may be identified in conjunction with DAH. As the treatment of this disorder involves immunosuppression, a full assessment of infection should be completed.

The diagnosis of DAH is strongly supported by the finding of increasingly sanguinous return on serial aliquots during bronchoalveolar lavage. BAL fluid assessment can also assist with the diagnosis in the presence of hemosiderin-laden macrophages, and can also be of benefit in assessing for the presence of infection. Surgical lung biopsy is only rarely required for diagnosis, and the risk of complications should be weighed against the benefits of such a procedure given the tenuous clinical status of most patients with DAH. Pathologic examination in DAH has demonstrated capillaritis with immune complex deposition in some patients, while in others, hemorrhage has been observed without any evidence of active inflammation.

The prognosis in the setting of DAH is poor in the absence of treatment, with some studies quoting a mortality rate of up to 50%. The need for mechanical ventilation portends a worse prognosis, as does the presence of concomitant infection. As a result of the high reported mortality, initial treatment is typically aggressive. This treatment typically consists of high-dose systemic corticosteroids (methylprednisolone 500–2,000 mg daily IV) with or without intravenous cyclophosphamide. Plasmapheresis has also been considered in patients with DAH if no response is seen to the above therapy after 3–7 days or prior to the initiation of cyclophosphamide if concern for acute infection exists. No controlled data is available to define the preferred combination of interventions. Mortality has, however, appeared to decrease with aggressive treatment regimens.

Acute Respiratory Distress Syndrome

ARDS is a pulmonary parenchymal process most often seen as a complication of infection. Patients typically present with acute onset of dyspnea and tachypnea. Fever may result from the underlying disease process. Patients often suffer from respiratory compromise, including high oxygen requirements and/or the need for ventilatory support. The most common infectious etiology for ARDS is pneumonia, though any major infection can be associated with this process. ARDS is diagnosed in the setting of the acute onset of respiratory decompensation, diffuse alveolar infiltrates, a normal pulmonary capillary wedge pressure (less than or equal to 18 mmHg), and a ratio of oxygen tension to fraction of inspired oxygen (P/F ratio) of less than or equal to 200 mmHg.

Risk factors for the development of ARDS in patients with SLE include the use of systemic corticosteroids and the presence of antiphospholipid antibody syndrome. ARDS can be seen in association with acute infection in patients with SLE, most commonly gram negative bacilli. The presence of ARDS confers a poor prognosis. Treatment of ARDS in the setting of SLE is similar to that associated with other etiologies, including supportive care and treatment of the underlying process, if one is identified.

Chronic Parenchymal Disease

Chronic Interstitial Lung Disease

Interstitial changes are often observed on HRCT scanning of the chest, with some reports suggesting these findings are seen in one-third to two-thirds of patients. However, the prevalence of clinically significant ILD in patients with SLE is much less common than in those with rheumatoid arthritis, scleroderma, or other autoimmune disorders. Reported prevalence rates range from 0% to 13%. ILD may be seen sporadically or subsequent to ALP. Patients with chronic ILD generally have had SLE for longer periods of time than those who present with acute parenchymal disease.

Patients with clinically significant interstitial disease may present with dyspnea on exertion, cough, and pleuritic chest pain. Physical examination findings may include hypoxia, basilar crackles, and digital clubbing.

Evaluation of suspected ILD generally requires detailed imaging provided by the HRCT, which can assist not only in identifying the presence of ILD but also in suggesting the contribution of inflammation and fibrosis. The presence of ground glass abnormalities on imaging is suggestive of a more cellular process, often correlating with the histologic finding of cellular nonspecific interstitial pneumonitis (NSIP) on pathology. In contrast, fibrotic changes with honeycomb formation are more suggestive of a predominance of fibrosis on biopsy specimens consistent with either fibrotic NSIP or usual interstitial pneumonitis (UIP). The distinction of cellular NSIP from fibrosis is helpful in deciding upon the use of immunosuppression as well as in prognostic assessment.

Patients with suspected ILD should complete full pulmonary function tests, including spirometry, lung volumes, and DLCO. PFT abnormalities, like HRCT changes, can be observed in asymptomatic patients with SLE. As in other forms of ILD, a decrease in DLCO may be the earliest manifestation of disease and may be observed only on exertion in early disease. Most patients with clinically significant ILD will manifest a symmetric decline in forced expiratory volume in 1 second (FEV1) and forced vital capacity (FVC), and the presence of restrictive lung disease will be confirmed by a decrease in total lung capacity.

The correlation between severity of PFT abnormalities and severity of imaging changes is not clearly defined, with some studies suggesting correlation and others showing none. We propose that imaging with HRCT be used in the initial diagnosis of ILD, with support from PFT abnormalities, in particular to determine the clinical significance of the findings. Given the risks of radiation exposure, pulmonary function assessments can be utilized on a more frequent basis to assess the progression of disease, with the support of less frequent follow-up imaging.

When clinically significant ILD is suspected, bronchoscopy with bronchoalveolar lavage assessment can be used to exclude infectious causes and alveolar hemorrhage, especially for those already on immunosuppressive therapy. The utility of transbronchial lung biopsies in the diagnosis of ILD is limited, and in general, a definitive pathologic assessment would require a surgical lung biopsy to assure large enough sampling of distinct areas of lung for diagnosis. In light of the details provided by HRCT scanning, however, an accurate assessment of the disease can be made in most cases in the absence of a pathologic diagnosis.

Treatment generally consists of systemic corticosteroid treatment, often in combination with an additional immunosuppressive agent, with the goal of eventual tapering of steroids to low doses. Rapidly progressive ILD is less common in SLE than in other autoimmune disorders. In patients with severe or progressive disease, high-dose corticosteroids and cyclophosphamide may be initiated, with the goal of eventual management with alternative immunosuppressive medications such as azathioprine or mycophenolate once disease has stabilized. No clinical trial information is available to demonstrate the effectiveness of immunomodulation in SLE-associated ILD.

Airway Disease

Obliterative Bronchiolitis

Obliterative bronchiolitis is the pathologic finding of granulation tissue that obstructs the distal airway lumen. Presenting symptoms include cough and dyspnea. OB is rarely seen as an isolated abnormality in patients with SLE. Plain chest radiograph is often normal, and the most common finding on HCRT is air trapping, best observed when both inspiratory and expiratory images are obtained. Ground glass infiltrates may also be observed. Pulmonary function tests demonstrate an obstructive ventilatory defect. OB has a poor prognosis, with variable response to immunomodulation. Immunosuppressive therapy with steroids, azathioprine, and/or mycophenolate has been utilized, with limited response.

Cryptogenic organizing pneumonia (COP), formerly known as bronchiolitis obliterans organizing pneumonia (BOOP), while more common than isolated OB, is another rare parenchymal process seen in association with SLE. Presenting symptoms include cough and dyspnea. In COP, OB is seen in association with chronic inflammation of the surrounding alveoli. HRCT changes seen in association with COP are variable and include alveolar consolidation, nodular infiltrates, and ground glass infiltration. Restriction is more commonly seen than obstruction on pulmonary function testing. In general, COP is more responsive to treatment than OB, and management typically involves systemic corticosteroids at moderate dosage with a gradual taper to low dose or off. Alternative immunosuppressants may be employed for refractory diseases or to allow for steroid sparing.

Other Airway Diseases

Asymptomatic obstructive changes can be seen on pulmonary function testing in SLE but are rarely clinically significant. Rare reported upper airway abnormalities include laryngeal inflammation, epiglottitis, subglottic stenosis, and vocal cord paralysis.

The Pleura in Systemic Lupus Erythematosus

Pleuritic chest pain is frequent in SLE and may be due to chest wall or musculoskeletal pain, inflammation of the pleura, or pulmonary embolism. Chest pain of musculoskeletal origin may increase with deep breaths or may worsen with change of position. Palpation of a specific area of the chest such as the costochondral joints may illicit pain. Symptoms may be alleviated by use of nonsteroidal anti-inflammatory agents, acetaminophen, topical analgesics, or local corticosteroid injections. Caution must be taken to ascertain that chest wall pain does not represent underlying infection or pulmonary embolism.

Pleuritis or inflammation of the pleura occurs in greater than 50% of patients with SLE. The presence of concomitant positive Sm and RNP antibody, prolonged disease duration, and younger age at onset appear to predisposed to pleuritis. While the presence of a pleural friction rub or effusion is helpful in identifying this as the cause, pleurisy may be present in the absence of either. However, in this situation, pleurisy is a diagnosis of exclusion, and alternative diagnoses should be investigated. Effusions that are visible on radiography may be bilateral or unilateral and are typically small, though occasionally can be large. The pleural fluid in SLE is exudative with a WBC count under 5,000 mm^3 in most cases. Differentiation between pleural effusions in SLE and RA may be difficult, but generally, the cell counts in SLE are lower, the glucose concentration is higher, and the protein concentrations are lower compared to RA. The use of ANA, RF, complement, or LE prep testing has been largely abandoned for clinical purposes. Most importantly, pleural fluid analysis should include gram stain and culture to assess for infection, and cytologic examination if malignancy is suspected. When a diagnostic dilemma exists and infection with such organisms as mycobacteria is a consideration, a pleural biopsy can help identify features that are consistent with SLE, which include chronic mononuclear cell infiltration and complement deposition.

Treatment for pleuritis in SLE includes NSAIDs in mild cases and if needed short courses of steroids in moderate doses for 2–4 weeks. Rarely, steroid sparing agents such as methotrexate, leflunomide, and azathioprine and mycophenolate mofetil may be considered. The use of decortication due to entrapment or talc pleurodesis for recurrent effusions has been described but only in recalcitrant cases.

Pulmonary Vascular Disorders in Systemic Lupus Erythematosus

Pulmonary Arterial Hypertension

Pulmonary vascular disease is uncommon in SLE but can have a significant impact on morbidity and mortality. Pulmonary hypertension occurs in about 4% of SLE patients based on prospective data. Patients with PAH complain of dyspnea, chest pain, nonproductive cough, and fatigue. Later findings include jugular venous distension, a fixed split and prominent S2, a right ventricular S3, prominent A and V venous pulsations, ascites, peripheral edema, and hepatomegaly. Laboratory findings include a decreased DLCO, desaturation with activity, and evidence of right ventricular hypertrophy on EKG. Pathologic examination of the parenchymal vasculature may show luminal narrowing, thickening of the muscular wall, and plexiform angiomatous lesions. In rare cases, evidence of vasculitis may be present, and immunoglobulin and complement deposition may be found within vessel walls. The presence of antiphospholipid antibodies and lupus anticoagulant may portend a greater risk for the development of PAH in SLE. Diagnostically, echocardiography can be useful to detect elevated pulmonary pressures, though evidence of pulmonary hypertension must be confirmed by right heart catheterization. It is important to note that tricuspid regurgitation is present to calculate pulmonary artery pressure in only 60–80% of patients, and therefore, right heart catheterization may be necessary when PAH is clinically suspected. In SLE patients with evidence of PAH, other diagnoses besides SLE/PAH should be considered including chronic pulmonary embolism, especially in the setting of antiphospholipid antibodies, and ongoing ILD. Mixed connective tissue disease and overlap syndrome with features of SLE and scleroderma should be considered.

Treatment for pulmonary hypertension includes endothelin antagonists, phosphodiesterase inhibitors, and prostacyclins, which can be delivered intravenously, via inhalation, and transdermally. Advances in drug delivery have revolutionized the treatment of PAH. The relative efficacy of these agents in connective tissue diseases such as SLE compared to idiopathic PAH is unknown. While anecdotal evidence suggests that treatment may not be as effective as in primary pulmonary hypertension, outcomes in SLE/PAH are likely to be better than in scleroderma. Finally, there have been reported cases of PAH in SLE that may respond to immunomodulating therapy such as cyclophosphamide and Rituxan, suggesting a vasculitic cause for PAH, though identifying which group of patients may benefit from this approach or therapy is challenging.

Pulmonary Veno-Occlusive Disease

PVOD is a rare cause of PAH and is characterized histologically by diffuse occlusion of pulmonary veins by fibrous tissue. Patients may present with dyspnea and hypoxemia similar to PAH, and CT scanning may show nodular ground glass opacities and lymph node enlargement. Initially, the patient may appear to have a form of inflammatory ILD and evidence of PAH, but the histologic changes are distinct and the treatment options differ from treatment for either ILD or PAH. In fact, the diagnosis can only be confirmed by biopsy, which shows preferential occlusion and thickening of post-capillary venules and pulmonary vessels. Standard treatment for PAH, such as vasodilating agents such as epoprostenol, may actually promote pulmonary edema, and therapies in general for PAH are unsatisfactory. Anticoagulation is often utilized, and in severe cases, lung transplantation may be necessary.

Other Pulmonary Disorders in Systemic Lupus Erythematosus

Antiphospholipid Antibodies and the Lung

APL can induce a variety of clinical syndromes that affect the lung, including PE, pulmonary infarction, pulmonary hemorrhage, pulmonary hypertension, and ARDS. Therapy for this disorder is discussed elsewhere.

Acute Reversible Hypoxemia

Acute reversible hypoxemia is a rare phenomenon noted in SLE, characterized by unexplained hypoxemia, and normal radiography. Evaluation for pulmonary embolism is negative. This process is thought to be related to leukoaggregation and complement activation within pulmonary capillaries associated with upregulation of the adhesion molecules E selectin, VCAM 1, and ICAM 1. C3a levels are markedly elevated in most cases. Corticosteroids are effective in this disorder, and some have suggested that aspirin may be helpful.

Shrinking Lung Syndrome

Shrinking lung syndrome is rare in SLE and should be suspected in patients with dyspnea, pleuritic chest pain, and progressive decrease in lung volume. Patients with this disorder present with a clear chest X-ray but elevated diaphragms and markedly decreased diffusion capacity, which partially or nearly completely corrects for volume. In such cases, there is no evidence of interstitial disease or thromboemboli. It is unclear whether this disorder is secondary to diaphragmatic muscle dysfunction or whether lung compliance is reduced. Esophageal balloon manometry may be helpful to distinguish the specific deficit. Proposed treatments include steroids, mycophenolate mofetil, azathioprine, and rituximab, though many patients may develop only a limited decline in function regardless of treatment.

Conclusion/Summary

The thoracic manifestations of SLE are diverse, and limited data exist regarding the management and prognosis of patients with these complications of disease. Diagnosis and management depend upon accurate historical information, a comprehensive physical assessment, and supporting data from imaging, pulmonary function testing, and, when appropriate, cardiovascular evaluation and invasive testing. Treatment of noninfectious complications often relies upon immunomodulation. Preventive strategies, including appropriate vaccination and prophylaxis, are important in the setting of immunosuppressive intervention.

Sources

1. Eisenberg H, Dubois EL, Sherwin RP, et al. Diffuse interstitial lung disease in systemic lupus erythematosus. Ann Intern Med. 1973;79:37–45.
2. Matthay RA, Schwartz MI, Petty TL, et al. Pulmonary manifestations of systemic lupus erythematosus: review of twelve cases of acute lupus pneumonitis. Medicine. 1975;54:397–409.

3. Isbister JP, Ralston M, Hayes JM, et al. Fulminant lupus pneumonitis with acute renal failure and RBC aplasia. Successful management with plasmapheresis and immunosuppression. Arch Intern Med. 1981;141:1081–3.
4. Weinrib L, Sharma OP, Quismorio FP. A long term study of interstitial lung disease in systemic lupus erythematosus. Semin Arthritis Rheum. 1990;20:48–56.
5. Zamora MR, Warner ML, Tuder R, et al. Diffuse alveolar hemorrhage and systemic lupus erythematosus: clinical presentation, histology, survival and outcome. Medicine. 1997;76:192–202.
6. Murin S, Wiedemann HP, Matthay RA. Pulmonary manifestations of systemic lupus erythematosus. Clin Chest Med. 1998;19:641–66.
7. Keane MP, Lynch JP. Pleuropulmonary manifestations of systemic lupus erythematosus. Thorax. 2000;55:159–66.
8. Cheema GS, Quismorio FP. Interstitial lung disease in systemic lupus erythematosus. Curr Opin Pulm Med. 2000;6:424–9.
9. Strange C, Highland KB. Interstitial lung disease in the patient who has connective tissue disease. Clin Chest Med. 2004;25:549–59.
10. Swigris JJ, Fischer A, Gilles J, et al. Pulmonary and thrombotic manifestations of systemic lupus erythematosus. Chest. 2008;133:271–80.
11. Jais X, Launay D, Yaici A, et al. Immunosuppressive therapy in lupus and mixed connective tissue disease associated pulmonary arterial hypertension. Arthritis Rheum. 2008;58:521–31.
12. Montani D, Achouh L, Dorfmuller P, et al. Pulmonary veno occlusive disease: clinical, functional, radiologic and hemodynamic characteristics and outcome of 24 cases confirmed by histology. Medicine. 2008;87:220–33.
13. Prabu A, Patel K, Yee CS, et al. Prevalence and risk factors for pulmonary arterial hypertension in patients with lupus. Rheumatology. 2009;48:1506–11.
14. Cefle A, Inanc M, Sayarlioglu M, et al. Pulmonary hypertension in systemic lupus erythematosus: relationship with antiphospholipid antibodies and severe disease outcome. Rheumatol Int. 2011;31(2):183–9.
15. Schur PH, Dellaripa PF. Pulmonary manifestations of systemic lupus erythematosus in adults. UpToDate. http://www.uptodate.com/online/content/topic.do?topicKey=lupus/7797&selectedTitle=10%7E150&source=search_result. Accessed 19 Oct 2010.
16. Mittoo S, Gelber AC, Hitchon CA, et al. Clinical and serologic factors associated with lupus pleuritis. J Rheumatol. 2010;37:747–53.
17. Chung L, Li J, Hasssoun PM, et al. Characterization of connective tissue disease associated pulmonary arterial hypertension from the REVEAL registry. Chest. 2010;138(6):1383–94.
18. Ernest D, Leung A. Ventilatory failure in shrinking lung syndrome is associated with reduced chest compliance. Intern Med J. 2010;40:66–8.

Chapter 10
Hematologic Manifestations of SLE

Ami S. Bhatt and Nancy Berliner

Hematologic problems are common and often clinically significant in patients with systemic lupus erythematosus (SLE). The purpose of this chapter is to provide an overview of potential hematologic complications of SLE, with a focus on the prognostic significance, pathophysiology, workup, and treatment options for lupus-associated anemia, thrombocytopenia, immunological defects, and coagulopathies.

The prevalence of hematologic problems is estimated at ~59% in one survey and ranges from ~50% to well over 70% in some series. Thus, the majority of patients with SLE will have at least one, and often more than one, clinically significant hematologic abnormality. All three of the major blood cell lines can be affected by SLE. Associated platelet disorders include thrombocytopenia related to either immune-mediated destruction of platelets or thrombotic thrombocytopenic purpura (TTP). Red cell disorders include anemia of chronic inflammation (ACI) (previously termed the anemia of chronic disease), iron-deficiency anemia, aplastic anemia, and autoimmune hemolytic anemia (AIHA). White blood cell disorders include asymptomatic lymphopenia, autoimmune neutropenia, and lymphadenopathy/splenomegaly. Lymphoma is a rare but clinically important complication.

A.S. Bhatt
Harvard Medical School, Boston, MA, USA

Clinical Fellow in Hematology and Oncology, Brigham and Women's Hospital and Dana Farber Cancer Institute, Boston, MA, USA

N. Berliner, M.D. (✉)
Division of Hematology, Brigham and Women's Hospital,
75 Francis Street, Boston, MA 02115, USA

Harvard Medical School, Boston, MA, USA
e-mail: nberliner@partners.org

Thrombocytopenia

Thrombocytopenia, defined as a total platelet count of $<100 \times 10^9/L$, is a common manifestation of SLE. The presence of thrombocytopenia has been associated with decreased survival in SLE patients, suggesting that its presence may serve as a prognostic indicator of more severe disease. The incidence at diagnosis has been reported to be 15–20% in recent population studies from various geographic regions, and the prevalence has been estimated at 15–30%. The incidence of thrombocytopenia has been noted to vary significantly both geographically and among different ethnic populations within the same geographic location. In two studies, thrombocytopenia was significantly correlated with increased mortality, while neutropenia, anemia, and lymphopenia were not. In one of these studies, thrombocytopenia was associated with a relative risk (RR) of mortality of 45.4 (95% confidence interval 2.4–862, $p=0.01$).

Thrombocytopenia can precede development of SLE by many years, and patients who have a positive ANA and thrombocytopenia should be monitored closely for the development of other symptoms and signs consistent with the disease. While modest declines in platelet count are fairly common in patients with SLE, a subset of patients will develop clinically significant thrombocytopenia with a platelet count of $<50 \times 10^9/L$. At a platelet count of $<20 \times 10^9/L$, clinically significant mucosal bleeding (such as gingival bleeding and epistaxis) and the presence of petechiae and ecchymoses can occur, necessitating treatment. A platelet count of $<10 \times 10^9/L$ constitutes a medical emergency requiring the initiation of immediate treatment.

Immune Thrombocytopenic Purpura

As previously noted, there are two predominant mechanisms of thrombocytopenia in patients with SLE. The vast majority of thrombocytopenic patients with SLE have immune thrombocytopenic purpura (ITP), an immune-mediated destruction of platelets that may, in some cases, be accompanied by central hypoproduction of platelets. Antiplatelet antibodies and antibodies directed at cytokine receptors critical for megakaryopoiesis have both been identified in these patients. Bone marrow studies of patients with ITP typically demonstrate a "reactive megakaryocytosis," but in a subset of cases where central hypoproduction is evident, megakaryocytopenia in the marrow with abnormal, hypolobated, and pyknotic megakaryocytes is observed. Antiplatelet antibodies in ITP are commonly directed against GPIIb–IIIa in patients with and without SLE. In the setting of SLE, patients may also have anticardiolipin antibodies, AIHA, and renal involvement. The final site of destruction of the antibody-bound platelets is the spleen where splenic macrophages destroy opsonized platelets by phagocytosis. Splenomegaly is rarely, if ever, seen in ITP, and its presence should prompt a search for another etiology of thrombocytopenia.

ITP is an immune-mediated process, and therefore, the majority of successful medical therapies for the condition are directed at immune modulation and suppression. The choice of therapy is based on several factors. These include the severity of thrombocytopenia, the rapidity of the required response to therapy, the SLE drug regimen of the patient, and comorbid illnesses. Corticosteroids are the mainstay of therapy. In the setting of emergent, life-threatening thrombocytopenia, physicians may opt to treat with high-dose intravenous methylprednisolone. Steroid response is rapid, and the platelet count usually begins to rise within 12–24 h. Patients requiring rapid response may also benefit from administration of intravenous immunoglobulin (IVIG), which has a short duration of effect (on the order of weeks) and is very costly, but produces a quick response. The mechanism of IVIG is complex. It is hypothesized to work, in part, by inhibiting phagocytosis of antibody-coated platelets by overwhelming the Fc receptor-bearing splenic and hepatic macrophages by high circulating levels of IVIG. However, several other mechanisms have been proposed, including activation of inhibitory receptors on macrophages and/or dendritic cells, modulation of cytokine levels, and modulation of dendritic cell activity. IVIG should be given with concomitant steroids to initiate definitive therapy. In the setting of life-threatening bleeding, platelet transfusions may also provide transient increases in platelet count, but the half-life of transfused platelets is extremely short and again should only be used as an accompaniment to definitive therapy. As most of the antibodies that mediate this disease are IgG, plasmapheresis is of little clinical value.

For patients who have less severe disease without significant mucocutaneous bleeding, oral steroids should be administered as the first line of therapy when the platelet count falls below 20×10^9/L. For many years, the standard initial dose of steroids has been 1 mg/kg in prednisone equivalents, although several dosing comparisons have failed to establish the optimal initial dose. Therapy at this level is continued until a response is seen, usually for 1–2 weeks. Once a response has been observed, the steroid dose can be tapered with frequent platelet monitoring. Again, there is no evidence that the duration of steroids or the rapidity of tapering has an impact on the durability of response. In patients who relapse during steroid tapers or who are unresponsive to steroid therapy, other medical therapies should be considered.

Most patients treated with prednisone will relapse at some time following discontinuation of steroids. More recent studies have suggested that 4–8 doses of pulse high-dose dexamethasone (40 mg/day for 4 days) induce similar remission rates (85–90%) and better long-term responses than historical controls treated with prednisone (70–75% of responding patients). Although a direct comparison to prednisone is still in process, this is far superior to the results with historical controls and suggests that pulse dexamethasone may be the treatment of choice for the initial therapy of ITP. In that study, patients with autoimmune disease were excluded, so the efficacy of this regimen in SLE patients remains to be established. Pulse dexamethasone avoids the long-term complications of prolonged prednisone and is likely to become established as the initial therapy of choice for ITP.

For those in whom tapering of the steroid dose is difficult, a steroid-sparing agent such as cyclophosphamide, cyclosporine, danazol, and azathioprine has been considered. More recently, rituximab, the anti-CD20 antibody that targets B lymphocytes, has been used successfully in ITP, returning platelet counts to normal levels in case studies and small case series. Splenectomy is a traditional therapeutic alternative that is becoming less commonly used but remains highly effective. In three single-center studies of patients with SLE, a small subset of patients with steroid-resistant thrombocytopenia were treated with splenectomy, and resolution or improvement of thrombocytopenia was observed in >60–70% of patients. Infrequently, patients relapsed and required additional medical therapy. The surgical morbidity and mortality associated with splenectomy was low. The incidence of subsequent infections was not reported, though based on other reports of infectious complications in splenectomized patients, the mortality associated with postsplenectomy infections is approximately 1–2%.

Several additional novel therapies are under investigation for use in ITP. Double filtration plasmapheresis has been reported to be successful in a case of severe ITP when combined with corticosteroids and IVIG. More recently, the thrombopoietin mimetic, romiplostim, was FDA approved for the treatment of chronic idiopathic ITP. While it has not been studied specifically in patients with SLE-associated ITP, this may be a reasonable rescue therapy in patients with refractory ITP, especially in those who are steroid resistant and have failed splenectomy. As with any new agent, the long-term safety of this agent has yet to be established in this patient population, and it is therefore premature to consider it as long-term therapy in patients who have not failed better-established interventions. It is administered as a weekly subcutaneous injection, and platelet counts typically rise within 1–2 weeks. Platelet counts fall precipitously after withdrawal of the drug, so patient compliance with regular visits for administration of the drug is of great importance. Concerns have been raised that long-term therapy may be complicated by increased reticulin deposition in the bone marrow, as well as other complications. An oral thrombopoietin mimetic agent, eltrombopag, is awaiting approval.

Thrombotic Thrombocytopenic Purpura

While the majority of cases of thrombocytopenia in SLE patients are attributable to ITP, TTP accounts for a small subset (<1–2%) of all cases of SLE-related thrombocytopenia and should be considered especially in cases of acute, new thrombocytopenia, usually associated with other acute findings. TTP is potentially rapidly fatal and early diagnosis and treatment is essential to prevent morbidity and mortality. A deficiency in ADAMTS13 activity has been identified as the causative defect in most cases of TTP. ADAMTS13 is a metalloproteinase responsible for the processing of large von Willebrand factor multimers into small- and medium-sized proteins. A decrease in ADAMTS13 activity can be attributed to inherited mutations in the ADAMTS13 gene, leading to familial TTP that is frequently recurrent. More commonly, decreased activity results from acquired antibody inhibitors to the enzyme.

TTP is rare but appears to be somewhat more common in patients with SLE, probably reflecting the autoimmune etiology of both diseases. The hallmarks of TTP are fever, thrombocytopenia, hemolytic anemia, and evidence of microangiopathy on the peripheral smear (schistocytosis). End-organ dysfunction, manifested as renal failure and neurological abnormalities with altered mental status, completes the classic pentad of findings in TTP, although with increased recognition of the disorder, TTP is now often diagnosed before these end-organ manifestations become obvious. Laboratory studies are remarkable for an elevated lactate dehydrogenase (LDH), low haptoglobin, and indirect hyperbilirubinemia, as well as microangiopathic hemolysis and thrombocytopenia.

It is important to distinguish TTP from disseminated intravascular coagulation (DIC), in which evidence of a microangiopathic hemolytic anemia may also be present. DIC is associated with most of the same laboratory abnormalities as TTP, with elevated LDH, indirect bilirubin, and low haptoglobin. The important differentiating factor is evidence of coagulopathy in DIC, which manifests as prolonged prothrombin and partial thromboplastin times (PTTs). There is also evidence of hypofibrinogenemia (low fibrinogen levels). DIC is usually a manifestation of severe underlying illness, such as sepsis or shock, and its treatment is directed at eliminating that underlying cause. Treatment of TTP, however, is directed at restoring the presence of small- and medium-sized von Willebrand factor and ADAMTS13 activity by (a) provision of small- and medium-sized von Willebrand factor and ADAMTS13 enzyme by administration of fresh frozen plasma, and (b) removal of inhibitors directed at ADAMTS13. This is accomplished in the short term by plasmapheresis with plasma exchange but may require immunosuppression to achieve durable response. While it is generally agreed that early initiation of plasmapheresis prevents morbidity and mortality associated with TTP, the necessity for and time of incorporation of immunosuppressive agents such as corticosteroids and novel agents such as rituximab remains controversial. Current practice favors addition of immunosuppressive agents in the setting of TTP refractory to plasmapheresis. Pheresis should be carried out on a daily basis, and patients should be monitored closely when weaning pheresis. Response time to plasmapheresis is remarkably rapid, often with full recovery of platelet counts within days of initiation of therapy. In clinical settings where plasmapheresis is not readily available, patients should be treated with large volumes of fresh frozen plasma and transferred to a facility with plasmapheresis capability. Most cases of TTP are self-limited, but 10–30% of patients with TTP relapse, with a higher rate of relapse in patients with severe ADAMTS13 deficiency and patients with autoimmune disease.

Antiphospholipid Antibody Syndrome

Antiphospholipid antibody syndrome is a constellation of findings that includes the presence of one or more antiphospholipid antibodies (classically the lupus anticoagulant antibodies or anticardiolipin antibodies) and evidence of arterial or venous thrombosis. Evidence of these antibodies was first obtained when it was noted that the PTT was prolonged in a subset of patients with SLE. Initially called an "anticoagulant" antibody, it is now clear that the presence of these antibodies is associated with a hypercoagulable state. The incidence of antiphospholipid antibody presence in SLE is approximately 20–35%, and the syndrome of hypercoagulability is explored in detail in the chapter dedicated to this important and often devastating clinical syndrome.

Anemia

Anemia is the most common hematologic consequence of SLE and is likely to affect most SLE patients at some point in their disease course. Both iron-deficiency anemia and ACI (formerly termed the anemia of chronic disease) are common in patients with SLE. Other disorders such as AIHA happen with some frequency; AIHA is, in fact, one of the 11-point criteria for entry into SLE research studies. Less commonly, bone marrow failure syndromes due to aplastic anemia (usually secondary to drugs used to treat SLE) and pure red cell aplasia can occur in patients with SLE.

The most common type of anemia in SLE is a normochromic, normocytic anemia resulting from chronic inflammation. The "ACI" is characterized by an inappropriately low or normal reticulocyte count and normocellular bone marrow with normal or increased iron stores. Recently, the mechanism of anemia in chronic inflammatory states was elucidated with the discovery of hepcidin. Hepcidin is a secreted protein that is a critical regulator of iron metabolism. This liver-derived polypeptide down-regulates the activity of the iron transporter ferroportin, thereby decreasing iron absorption from the gastrointestinal tract and blocking iron release from macrophages. In settings of iron overload, hepcidin is appropriately repressed to prevent continued iron accumulation. However, hepcidin is also potently induced by inflammatory cytokines, notably IL-6, and it is expressed at inappropriately high levels in chronic inflammatory states. Therefore, in the setting of chronic inflammation, increased hepcidin expression induces iron-limited erythropoiesis despite adequate iron stores, leading to anemia. Treatment of ACI is directed at the underlying immunoinflammatory process. With resolution of the overwhelming inflammatory state, normal erythropoiesis can be restored. Iron therapy is of no utility in this setting. Erythropoietin is of little clinical value in these patients, unless the erythropoietin response is documented to be inadequate, as in the setting of associated renal insufficiency.

As with the general population, iron-deficiency anemia is fairly common in patients with SLE. Iron deficiency is typically the result of iron loss secondary to GI bleeding or menorrhagia, although prolonged ACI can also lead to iron deficiency through the inhibition of intestinal iron absorption. Treatment with corticosteroids and NSAIDs can predispose to upper GI blood loss that is often clinically inapparent until iron-deficiency anemia is diagnosed. Early iron deficiency can present with a normocytic, hypochromic anemia that may progress to a microcytic, hypochromic anemia over time. Hypoferritinemia and a reduced iron level in the setting of elevated total iron-binding capacity (TIBC) are also observed. Treatment of iron-deficiency anemia should be directed at the source of bleeding and at a correction of iron stores to normal levels.

AIHA can present with a spectrum of severity in SLE patients and is estimated to occur with an incidence of 10–20% and a prevalence of as high as ~25%. Mediated by antibodies directed at red blood cells, AIHA can be one of the most dramatic and catastrophic anemias associated with SLE. Red cell destruction can be mediated by either IgG or IgM antibodies, although IgG antibodies are more common. IgG antibodies are referred to as "warm" antibodies because they bind to red cells at body temperature. IgM antibodies are referred to as "cold" antibodies because they tend to bind poorly at body temperature. Cold antibodies bind in cooler, distal regions in the body and fix complement; the IgM frequently then falls off as the blood returns to the central circulation, leaving only complement on the red cell surface. Cold antibodies are frequently clinically silent. AIHA should be suspected in SLE patients with new-onset anemia with elevated markers of hemolysis including LDH, indirect bilirubin, and a depressed haptoglobin in the setting of normal or baseline coagulation parameters. Unlike ACI and iron-deficiency anemia, AIHA is associated with brisk reticulocytosis. Classically, the peripheral blood smear demonstrates spherocytes. AIHA can be associated with thrombocytopenia in setting of ITP (Evans syndrome) or a microangiopathic process such as TTP or DIC.

The exact prevalence of AIHA is controversial, as some physicians may overdiagnose AIHA when a patient with autoimmune disease develops unexplained anemia. Identification of the antibody responsible for mediating hemolysis can be achieved by performing a direct Coombs' test and further isotype characterization. In some cases, a cold agglutinin antibody may require additional special testing by the blood bank. Warm AIHA is much more common than complement-mediated cold AIHA.

As with the platelet destruction seen in ITP, antibody-coated red blood cells are recognized and destroyed by splenic macrophages. Erythrophagocytosis can occur, but more commonly, a portion of the red blood cell phospholipid bilayer is removed by the splenic macrophage, leading to a conformational changed of the red blood cell shape from a biconcave disc to a sphere. The spherical red blood cell is less resistant to shear stress and hemolyzes under osmotic stress in the spleen or the liver. AIHA, like ITP, occurs with an increased frequency in SLE patients who have antiphospholipid antibodies. In one study of 41 consecutive patients with SLE and AIHA, patients with AIHA were more likely to have elevated titers of IgG anticardiolipin antibodies with an OR of 5.8 (95% CI 1.4–24). AIHA typically occurs at the onset of symptoms of SLE and is independently associated with thrombocytopenia and SLE-related renal involvement. The mainstay of treatment for AIHA is corticosteroids at a prednisone equivalent of 1–2 mg/kg/day based on the severity of disease. A response can be observed within a week in most patients, and after maintaining the prednisone dose at a stable level for a period of weeks, the dose can be tapered slowly while carefully monitoring the hematocrit and hemolysis parameters. Patients who cannot be tapered off steroids can be transitioned to steroid-sparing immunosuppressive agents such as azathioprine. In most cases, the addition of steroid-sparing immunosuppressive agents allows steroids to be tapered completely, but on occasion, low-dose steroids must be continued to avoid hemolysis. In that setting, alternate day low-dose steroids are often effective and are associated with less steroid-related complications than daily steroids. IVIG has been studied and is felt to be efficacious in the adjunctive setting but has insufficient therapeutic effect to be used as monotherapy. As in ITP, the anti-CD20 (anti-B cell) rituximab has been reported to be effective in case studies or small case series. A large, randomized trial has yet to be performed, but early reports are encouraging, suggesting that rituximab is a highly effective and durable therapy of refractory AIHA. Most patients do not relapse after successful treatment of AIHA with one trial reporting a recurrence rate of only 4 per 100 person-years.

Sickle cell anemia, caused by point mutations in the beta globin gene, is prevalent in patients of African, Mediterranean, and Arabian descent. There is no convincing evidence of an increased prevalence of SLE in patients with sickle cell disease. It is, however, important to note that there is considerable overlap between the organ dysfunction that results from sickle cell anemia and that observed in SLE. This can confound the diagnosis of SLE. Pure red cell aplasia, defined by a severe decrease or absence of red cell precursors in the bone marrow, is a rare but known syndrome that can occur in SLE. It is unknown whether the incidence of this disease is above the baseline incidence in the general population. Aplastic anemia, a trilineage bone marrow failure syndrome, characterized by anemia, thrombocytopenia, and leucopenia, is a very rare disease that can occur in association with SLE, either de novo or as a result of cytotoxic therapy used to treat SLE. Treatment of aplastic anemia is directed at suppression of cell-mediated immunity with agents such as anti-thymocyte globulin derived from animal sources (horse, rabbit). Patients also require transfusional support. Patients who are not responsive to immunomodulatory therapy may go on to receive high-dose chemotherapy followed by allogeneic stem cell transplant.

Leukopenia

Leukopenia, defined as a total white blood cell count of $<4 \times 10^9/L$, has been estimated to occur with an incidence of ~20–25% at the time of diagnosis of SLE and occurs with a prevalence as high as 35%. Both major circulating lines of leukocytes, lymphocytes, and neutrophils can be affected in SLE. Lymphopenia, defined as $<1.5 \times 10^9/L$, occurs in most SLE patients in contrast to the very low prevalence of this finding in patients with other autoimmune diseases. Neutropenia occurs in about 50% of patients, though severe neutropenia, defined as a neutrophil count of $<1 \times 10^9/L$, is quite rare. Agranulocytosis, or the absence of neutrophils, is exceedingly uncommon and, when it does occur in SLE, is most often secondary to toxic drug effects.

The neutropenia associated with SLE has been attributed to the presence of circulating anti-granulocyte antibodies. To date, immunoglobulins directed at both neutrophil membrane antigens and soluble growth factors such as G-CSF have been detected. More recent studies have shown serum TNF-related apoptosis-inducing ligand (TRAIL) to be elevated in patients with SLE-associated neutropenia. The neutropenia in SLE is usually mild, rarely symptomatic, and reflective of overall disease activity. Infections related to neutropenia are distinctly uncommon, and most infections are probably more attributable to the immunosuppression used to control active disease than to neutropenia itself. Some authors have suggested that high circulating levels of endogenous G-CSF and soluble Fc receptor III are predictive of the risk of infection. Clinically significant neutropenia complicated by infection can be successfully treated with exogenous administration of G-CSF, although it is rarely necessary.

Severe neutropenia, and especially agranulocytosis, is most commonly drug induced. Chronic therapy with cytotoxic agents, such as azathioprine, cyclophosphamide, and even rituximab, has been associated with both immediate and more delayed-onset severe neutropenia and agranulocytosis. In particular, therapy with rituximab can lead to the rare complication of late-onset neutropenia up to 6 months after exposure to the agent.

A rare cause of severe neutropenia or agranulocytosis is large granular lymphocyte (LGL) leukemia. LGL is more commonly seen in rheumatoid arthritis, where it has significant overlap with Felty's syndrome (FS). In fact, the striking overlap in manifestations of the disease, coupled with the finding that nearly all patients with LGL and FS in the setting of rheumatoid arthritis are positive for HLA-DR4, has led to the hypothesis that these two diseases fall along a spectrum of a single disease. Although much rarer in SLE, LGL and profound neutropenia have been observed in that setting. LGL is a clonal lymphoproliferative disease that tends to be very indolent and responds to low-dose MTX or other immunomodulatory drugs.

Lymphopenia occurs in a majority of patients with SLE and tracks with clinical activity of the disease. Most commonly, patients with SLE show a significant decrease in T cells with either a relative preservation or mild decrease in B cells. Severe lymphopenia with a lymphocyte count of $<1.5 \times 10^9/L$ occurs in many SLE patients, with estimates of prevalence of ~25%. Patients who present with severe lymphopenia at diagnosis have a higher frequency of fevers, polyarthritis and CNS involvement, but a lower incidence of thrombocytopenia and AIHA. The relative lymphopenia may be associated with subtle defects in cell-mediated immunity seen in SLE patients. Lymphocytotoxic antibodies have been identified in patients with SLE, and in a study of patients with SLE and rheumatoid arthritis, those patients with SLE were found to have more lymphocytotoxic antibodies. These cytotoxic antibodies appear to have a dose–response relationship with lymphopenia. While both IgG and IgM antibodies to lymphocytes have been identified in the serum of SLE patients, the most clinically significant is likely to be an IgM antibody, active only at cold temperatures. This cold antibody, interestingly, has been identified both in SLE patients and in household contacts of these patients, suggesting that the antibody may be induced by an environmental or transmissible agent. In a recent study, investigators identified another aspect of the mechanism of lymphocytotoxicity in SLE patients. Two cell surface antigens, CD55 and CD59, which are known to be compromised/deficient in patients with paroxysmal nocturnal hemoglobinuria (a complement-mediated red cell disorder), are also downregulated in SLE patients. This may play a role in lymphopenia by increasing the susceptibility of these cells to complement-mediated lysis.

While lymphopenia is one of the most common hematologic manifestations of SLE, it is typically not treated aggressively, and patients with profound T-cell depletion do not seem to be at risk of the same types of opportunistic infections as are patients with other T-cell depleting conditions (such as the acquired immunodeficiency syndrome).

Macrophage-Activation Syndrome

Macrophage-activation syndrome (MAS) is a disorder characterized by unexplained fever and cytopenias with associated hyperferritinemia in the setting of systemic autoimmune disease. It is caused by a defect in NK cell regulation associated with excessive proliferation and activation of macrophages and T lymphocytes, leading to widespread phagocytosis and high levels of circulating cytokines. The disease is manifested by hemophagocytosis (blood cells engulfed by macrophages) on bone marrow examination, although it can often be difficult to visualize; detection is facilitated by specific staining for macrophages. It is clinically similar to hemophagocytic lymphohistiocytosis (HLH), a rare inherited childhood disorder caused by mutations in the perforin gene or other signaling intermediates required for normal NK cell granule secretion and function. Paradoxically, intact NK cell activity is required for down-modulation of the immune response. Hence, these congenital abnormalities lead to a failure of target cell killing and loss of appropriate feedback on the immune response. This lack of immunomodulation is manifest by constitutive T-cell and macrophage activation, exuberant cytokine production, and a fulminant clinical syndrome with high mortality unless treated with hematopoietic stem cell transplantation.

Adult HLH is usually seen in the setting of infection (especially EBV), T-cell malignancy, and autoimmune diatheses, and the term "macrophage-activation syndrome" is accepted as the designation for adult HLH developing in the setting of systemic autoimmune disease. The presentation of MAS can be variable, and many of the manifestations are nonspecific; consequently, diagnosis of the syndrome can be challenging. The diagnosis of HLH is based on the finding of five of eight clinical criteria based on clinical manifestations and laboratory signs. There are no established diagnostic criteria for MAS, but an international consortium is in the process of defining consensus criteria. A preliminary set of criteria were proposed for the diagnosis of MAS in the setting of active juvenile rheumatoid arthritis (JRA) based on meeting two of the following laboratory criteria: decreased platelet count, elevated AST, leukopenia, hypofibrinogenemia, and elevated soluble CD25 receptor levels. Clinical criteria are CNS dysfunction, clinically significant hemorrhage, and hepatomegaly. A recent consensus report has identified nine leading criteria for further study in establishing definitive diagnostic guidelines for MAS in the setting of JRA.

MAS occurs with the highest frequency in patients with JRA but is also prevalent in patients with adult-onset Still's disease and SLE. The applicability of diagnostic criteria for MAS in these settings will need to be further validated. While hyperferritinemia is not a part of the preliminary criteria for MAS, it is often associated with the disease and often over an order of magnitude above the baseline upper limit of normal.

MAS can be rapidly fatal, and the diagnosis should be considered early in any critically ill, febrile SLE patient. Several treatments including those aimed at immunomodulation and other cytotoxic approaches have been reported in case reports or small series in the literature. A hematology consultant should be contacted early in cases of suspected MAS, and treatment with agents such as cyclophosphamide, high-dose steroids, IVIG, and chemotherapeutic agents such as etoposide should be considered. Other approaches, including plasmapheresis, have also been reported to be successful in selected cases.

Workup of Lymphadenopathy

Lymphadenopathy is a common finding in SLE patients, present in 26% of SLE patients in one series and range as high as 69% in another. Patients with lymphadenopathy were found to have a higher incidence of so-called B symptoms of weight loss, fever, and fatigue, making differentiating between increased SLE disease activity and a potential malignancy difficult. This clinical dilemma is not well studied. We recommend that physicians monitor adenopathy regularly and consider referral to a hematologist and possible biopsy at the onset of progressive, localized adenopathy over a period of 4 weeks. Lymphadenopathy in patients who are clinically quiescent should also be considered worrisome for potential malignancy.

Lymphoproliferative Disorders

Patients with SLE are at increased risk of developing lymphoproliferative disorders as compared to the general population. Non-Hodgkin lymphomas predominate in this clinical setting, with a majority of patients presenting with an aggressive subtype, diffuse large B-cell lymphoma. Even in SLE patients, the prevalence of lymphoma is quite low with a prevalence in the range of <0.05%. To date, there are no convincing data to support an infectious cause of these lymphomas, such as EBV, though the involvement of a viral pathogen in transformation remains an attractive hypothesis. Standard chemotherapies for the treatment of NHL such as DLBCL are highly cytotoxic, and patients with active SLE who undergo cancer chemotherapy typically experience a period of quiescence of their underlying inflammatory disorder that can last up to a year or more.

Patients with SLE do not appear to be at increased risk for myeloid neoplasms, with the notable exception of patients who have been exposed to high doses of alkylating agents such as cyclophosphamide. For this reason, some practitioners avoid the long-term use of cyclophosphamide in the treatment of SLE patients, favoring therapies such as antimalarials, danazol, steroids, and azathioprine.

Sources

1. Aleem A, Al-Sugair S. Thrombotic thrombocytopenic purpura associated with systemic lupus erythematosus. Acta Haematol. 2006;115:68–73.
2. Berchtold P, Wenger M. Autoantibodies against platelet glycoproteins in autoimmune thrombocytopenic purpura: their clinical significance and response to treatment. Blood. 1993;81:1246–50.
3. Bernatsky S, Ramsey-Goldman R, Rajan R, et al. Non-Hodgkin's lymphoma in systemic lupus erythematosus. Ann Rheum Dis. 2005;64:1507–9.
4. Bussel JB, Cheng G, Saleh MN, et al. Eltrombopag for the treatment of chronic idiopathic thrombocytopenic purpura. N Engl J Med. 2007;357:2237–47.
5. Coon WW. Splenectomy for cytopenias associated with systemic lupus erythematosus. Am J Surg. 1988;155:391–4.
6. Cooper N. Intravenous immunoglobulin and anti-RhD therapy in the management of immune thrombocytopenia. Hematol Oncol Clin North Am. 2009;23:1317–27.
7. Cuker A. Toxicities of the thrombopoietic growth factors. Semin Hematol. 2010;47:289–98.
8. Davì S, Consolaro A, Guseinova D, et al. An international consensus survey of diagnostic criteria for macrophage activation syndrome in systemic juvenile idiopathic arthritis. J Rheumatol. 2011;38(4):764–8.
9. Ehrenfeld M, Shoenfeld Y. Hematologic manifestations. In: Schur PH, editor. The clinical management of systemic lupus erythematosus. Philadelphia: Lippincott-Raven Publishers; 1996. p. 95–108.
10. Giannouli S, Voulgarelis M, Ziakas PD, Tzioufas AG. Anaemia in systemic lupus erythematosus: from pathophysiology to clinical assessment. Ann Rheum Dis. 2006;65:144–8.
11. Grom AA. Macrophage activation syndrome and reactive hemophagocytic lymphohistiocytosis: the same entities? Curr Opin Rheumatol. 2003;15:587–90.
12. Habib GS, Saliba WR, Froom P. Pure red cell aplasia and lupus. Semin Arthritis Rheum. 2002;31:279–83.
13. Henter JI, Horne A, Arico M, et al. HLH-2004: diagnostic and therapeutic guidelines for hemophagocytic lymphohistiocytosis. Pediatr Blood Cancer. 2007;48:124–31.
14. Janka GE. Hemophagocytic syndromes. Blood Rev. 2007;21:245–53.
15. King JK, Costenbader KH. Characteristics of patients with systemic lupus erythematosus (SLE) and non-Hodgkin's lymphoma (NHL). Clin Rheumatol. 2007;26:1491–4.
16. Kokori SI, Ioannidis JP, Voulgarelis M, Tzioufas AG, Moutsopoulos HM. Autoimmune hemolytic anemia in patients with systemic lupus erythematosus. Am J Med. 2000;108:198–204.
17. Kuter DJ, Rummel M, Boccia R, et al. Romiplostim or standard of care in patients with immune thrombocytopenia. N Engl J Med. 2010;363:1889–99.
18. Kuwana M, Kaburaki J, Okazaki Y, Miyazaki H, Ikeda Y. Two types of autoantibody-mediated thrombocytopenia in patients with systemic lupus erythematosus. Rheumatology (Oxford). 2006;45:851–4.
19. Lofstrom B, Backlin C, Sundstrom C, Ekbom A, Lundberg IE. A closer look at non-Hodgkin's lymphoma cases in a national Swedish systemic lupus erythematosus cohort: a nested case-control study. Ann Rheum Dis. 2007;66:1627–32.

20. Looney RJ, Anolik JH, Campbell D, et al. B cell depletion as a novel treatment for systemic lupus erythematosus: a phase I/II dose-escalation trial of rituximab. Arthritis Rheum. 2004; 50:2580–9.
21. Mazzucconi MG, Fazi P, Bernasconi S, et al. Therapy with high-dose dexamethasone (HD-DXM) in previously untreated patients affected by idiopathic thrombocytopenic purpura: a GIMEMA experience. Blood. 2007;109:1401–7.
22. Nakamura M, Tanaka Y, Satoh T, et al. Autoantibody to CD40 ligand in systemic lupus erythematosus: association with thrombocytopenia but not thromboembolism. Rheumatology (Oxford). 2006;45:150–6.
23. Nossent JC, Swaak AJ. Prevalence and significance of haematological abnormalities in patients with systemic lupus erythematosus. Q J Med. 1991;80:605–12.
24. Parodi A, Davi S, Pringe AB, et al. Macrophage activation syndrome in juvenile systemic lupus erythematosus: a multinational multicenter study of thirty-eight patients. Arthritis Rheum. 2009;60:3388–99.
25. Roy C. Anemia of inflammation. Hematology Am Soc Hematol Educ Program. 2010;2010: 276–80.
26. Sadler JE. Von Willebrand factor, ADAMTS13, and thrombotic thrombocytopenic purpura. Blood. 2008;112:11–8.
27. Shapira Y, Weinberger A, Wysenbeek AJ. Lymphadenopathy in systemic lupus erythematosus. Prevalence and relation to disease manifestations. Clin Rheumatol. 1996;15:335–8.
28. Sokol L, Loughran Jr TP. Large granular lymphocyte leukemia. Curr Hematol Malig Rep. 2007;2:278–82.
29. Starkebaum G. Chronic neutropenia associated with autoimmune disease. Semin Hematol. 2002;39:121–7.
30. Zandman-Goddard G, Levy Y, Shoenfeld Y. Intravenous immunoglobulin therapy and systemic lupus erythematosus. Clin Rev Allergy Immunol. 2005;29:219–28.

Chapter 11
Lupus Nephritis

Mary Anne Dooley

Introduction

Systemic lupus erythematosus (SLE) is a systemic autoimmune disorder characterized by the production of multiple autoantibodies, a striking female predominance, and the frequent development of immune complex-mediated glomerulonephritis.

Clinical Manifestations of Lupus Nephritis

The symptoms of nephritis in a patient with or without diagnosed lupus may be very subtle. These include changes in urination, weight gain, edema, and increased blood pressure. Symptoms may be more obvious with the development of overt nephrosis with peripheral or even generalized edema (e.g., periorbital edema) or acute renal failure with uremia. Patients with SLE, particularly African American and Hispanic patients, frequently develop nephritis during their first 3 years of illness, and thus, this is an important time to test frequently for renal function to facilitate early detection of lupus nephritis. Because nephritis can develop several years after the onset of SLE, it is prudent for the clinician to continue to monitor renal function. Ultimately, lupus nephritis is a diagnosis that evolves from the detection of proteinuria, an abnormal urinary sediment, and or azotemia.

M.A. Dooley, M.D., M.P.H. (✉)
Division of Rheumatology and Immunology,
University of North Carolina at Chapel Hill,
CB# 7280, 3330 Thurston Building, Chapel Hill, NC 27599, USA
e-mail: mary_dooley@med.unc.edu

Diagnosis

The diagnosis of lupus nephritis (LN) is a clinical diagnosis, based on combined clinical, histopathologic, and laboratory findings. Many parameters in frequent clinical use to define LN, such as hypocomplementemia and renal biopsy results, are not included in the ACR criteria—proteinuria and/or casts are the renal criteria. Clinical renal disease due to SLE affects close to 50 % of patients with SLE, although on biopsy most SLE patients have abnormalities. The diagnosis of clinical LN is usually made by renal biopsy prompted by significant proteinuria, hematuria, and/or casts or decreased renal function. The presence of renal disease remains the most important predictor of overall morbidity and mortality in patients with SLE. Despite advances in treatment for LN and accompanying comorbidities (diabetes, hypertension, hyperlipidemia), the proportion of patients requiring dialysis due to LN in the USA has not changed between 1996 and 2006.

Epidemiology

Several demographic, serologic, and genetic risk factors are associated with an increased risk of developing LN. Age at disease onset and sex are important: patients with onset of SLE under age 16 develop LN more frequently than adults (~85 % vs. 50 %) as do males compared to females. However, onset of SLE in older patients is not "milder." Race confounded initial reports that elderly patients were less likely to develop LN. The incidence and prevalence of LN differs significantly among different racial and ethnic groups. African Americans have a threefold increased incidence of SLE, develop the disease at younger age, more frequently develop LN and progress to end-stage renal disease. Hispanics also have greater frequency and severity of nephritis compared with Caucasians. Patients with LN are more likely than SLE patients without renal involvement to have a family history of SLE, anemia, high anti-dsDNA antibody titers, and hypocomplementemia. A family history of dialysis from any cause increases the risk of ESRD in lupus patients. The presence of anti-dsDNA and anti-nucleosome autoantibodies is associated with an increased risk of proliferative LN.

Pathogenesis

The major cause of lupus nephritis is the deposition on the glomerular basement membrane of immune complexes. These are mostly IgG, but IgA and IgM may also be found, as well as complement components, especially C1q, C4, and C3. Anti-dsDNA is the major antibody in these complexes, but antibodies to chromatin, nucleosomes, are also found. Immune complexes depositing in the mesangium may or may not cause nephritis. However, those immune complexes that deposit in the subepithelial space of the glomerular basement membrane activate the complement system, which generates the chemoattractants C3a and C5a, causing an influx of cells into glomeruli resulting in the classical proliferative pattern. By contrast, immune complexes that deposit in the subepithelium of the glomerular basement membrane do not appear to activate complement, even though one can demonstrate that complement components are present. This results in thickening of the glomerular basement membrane and membranous nephropathy. Other mechanisms of inflammation are also involved including antibodies to C1q, adhesion molecules, cytokines, chemokines, and other inflammatory mediators.

Laboratory Findings for the Diagnosis of LN

Routine tests of renal function facilitate the diagnosis of LN. These include serum creatinine, serum albumin, urinalysis with a careful evaluation of the sediment enumerating cellular casts, dysmorphic red blood cells, hematuria and pyuria, estimated GFR, spot urine protein/creatinine ratio, and/or 24 h urine for total protein.

Serologic test abnormalities may also suggest LN. Positive tests for anti-double-stranded DNA antibodies occur more frequently in patients with LN than SLE without nephritis. The total hemolytic complement (CH-50) and complement components C4 and C3 are typically low during active disease, especially LN. Because some patients with SLE have a genetic decrease in the synthesis of complement components (especially C4), a low C4 concentration does not always indicate active disease. Longitudinally repeated measurements of C3/C4 are more helpful in determining the relative state of disease activity of a patient

The Importance of Renal Biopsy

Lupus nephritis is an immune complex-mediated glomerulonephritis, varying in its expression from biopsy positive, but no clinical renal abnormalities, to mild, asymptomatic proteinuria to overt nephrotic syndrome or acute nephritis with rapidly progressing azotemia. Most patients with SLE have deposition of immunoglobulin and complement, even in the absence of clinically significant renal dysfunction. Location, quantity, and host response to the immune reactants result in a spectrum of renal lesions categorized into different classes of lupus nephritis. Despite these general correlations, there is overlap in the clinical presentation of patients with the various histopathologic findings, and it remains difficult to diagnose the type or severity of renal disease based on clinical grounds alone. Some patients, more frequently children, have what has been called "silent nephritis" with normal renal function but renal biopsy demonstrating class II, III, or even the more severe class IV nephritis. For this reason, a renal biopsy is essential in the management of patients with suspected LN and should be performed as promptly as possible. It provides an invaluable guide to therapy by clarifying the clinicopathologic syndrome and assessing the relative degrees of active inflammation and chronic scarring. It may also identify unsuspected causes for an acute, non-SLE-related worsening in renal function such as the development of a thrombotic microangiopathy or drug-induced tubulointerstitial nephritis.

Types of SLE Nephritis: The ISN/RPS Classification of Lupus Nephritis

The classification of LN into discrete classes has been a critical step in facilitating communication between and among pathologists and clinicians, as well as to define homogenous groups of patients enrolled in clinical trials. The initial classification of lupus nephritis was proposed in 1974 (WHO) and was modified in 1982 and 1995. An international panel of pathologists, rheumatologists, and nephrologists proposed a revision for the classification of lupus nephritis [International Society of Nephrology/Renal Pathology Society (ISN/RPS) classification of lupus nephritis 2003] (Table 11.1). WHO class I, normal renal histology, is not included in the 2003 classification. Class I is now characterized by immune complex deposition confined to the mesangium, without light microscopic abnormalities. Class II is characterized by varying degrees of focal to diffuse mesangial hypercellularity. Focal proliferative (class III) or diffuse proliferative (class IV) lupus nephritis remain defined as <50 % glomerular involvement vs. ≥50 % involvement, and descriptors of segmental vs. global involvement of the glomeruli are required. The subscripts A, C, S, and G are often added to class III or IV proliferative nephritis to denote the presence of active, chronic, segmental, and global lesions. Class V disease is characterized by diffuse thickening of the glomerular capillary wall. Patients with features of membranous and proliferative lesions are reported as having class V *in addition* to class III or IV lesions. Because of the typically relapsing pattern of LN, recurrent active proliferative nephritis (classes III and IV) and up to a third of membranous class V may eventually result in extensive glomerular sclerosis, adhesions, and fibrous crescents characterized as class VI.

Table 11.1 Indications for renal biopsy

Proteinuria >500 mg/24 h
Active renal sediment
Rising serum creatinine without other explanation
Confirmation of disease remission vs. remission on therapy

Transformation of Renal Biopsies

Transformation between classes of LN increases the complexity of managing patients with LN. Among biopsy comparison pairs from 88 patients within the Glomerular Disease Collaborative Network undergoing more than one renal biopsy, transformation to another WHO Class occurred in nearly 30% of biopsy pairs within a mean of 37 months. Transformations occurred from class II to IV in 4 %, class III to IV in 11 %, class V to IV in 6 %, and class IV and V progressed to class VI in 5 %. Four biopsies had thrombotic microangiopathy due to thrombotic thrombocytopenic purpura (TTP).

Differential Diagnosis of Lupus Nephritis

Immune complex-mediated glomerulonephritis may be due to viral infection as seen with HIV, hepatitis B or C, or due to syphilis. Some patients with SLE develop a thrombotic microangiopathy that may be associated with antiphospholipid antibodies, TTP, severe hypertension, or with an overlap syndrome with systemic sclerosis. Interstitial nephritis may be caused by drugs frequently used in patients with SLE. Postinfectious GN or acute tubulointerstitial nephritis may occur.

Guidelines for Repeat Biopsy

Guidelines for repeat biopsy include increasing proteinuria, development of an active urinary sediment, or rising serum creatinine without other explanation (Table 11.1). Repetitive clinical evaluations may not clearly define these changes, and repeated renal biopsies are sometimes needed. Another concern is the frequent relapses of LN shortly after discontinuation of immunosuppressive therapy despite clinical parameters suggesting remission. This raises the difficult issue of the role of repeat renal biopsy to define pathologic as well as clinical remission.

Laboratory Findings for Monitoring LN

Routine tests of renal function that facilitate in monitoring the activity of LN include serum creatinine, serum albumin, urinalysis with a careful evaluation of the sediment, estimated GFR, and spot urine protein/creatinine ratios (and/or 24 h urine for total protein).

In addition, levels of anti-double-stranded DNA antibodies may increase prior to renal flares and decrease as the patient improves. The total hemolytic complement (CH-50) and complement components C4 and C3 may decrease prior to an LN flare and are typically low during active disease, increasing as the patient improves. Longitudinally repeated measurements of C3/C4 are more helpful in determining the relative state of disease activity of a patient.

Treatment of SLE Nephritis

Therapeutic decisions for individual patients with lupus nephritis should be based on consideration of their clinical presentation, laboratory features, and histologic findings on biopsy. In general, patients with mesangial lupus nephritis (classes I and II) do not require immunosuppressive treatment beyond that for their extrarenal manifestations of disease. Adjunctive therapy to control hypertension, hyperglycemia, and hyperlipidemia is important to maintain renal function (see Table 11.2). In patients with advanced glomerulosclerosis (class VI), the risks of immunosuppression likely outweigh the potential of any benefits.

Table 11.2 Adjunctive therapy for lupus nephritis

Antihypertensive medication to maintain blood pressure to less than 130/80 and protein excretion to less than 500-1000mg/day, or at least 60% below baseline

Preference for angiotensin-converting enzyme inhibitors or angiotensin II receptor blockers given the preservation of renal function shown in diabetic and other renal diseases. Non-dihydropyridine calcium channel blockers, such as diltiazem and verapamil, have significant antiproteinuric effects in those individuals with >300 mg/day of proteinuria

Statin therapy

Control of hyperlipidemia: The ATP III guidelines published in 2001 recommended that the goal LDL cholesterol should be less than 100 mg/dL (2.6 mmol/L) in all high-risk patients including secondary prevention and in those with a coronary equivalent including diabetes. This goal for high-risk patients was also recommended by the 2006 AHA/ACC guidelines for secondary prevention. The modified ATP III guidelines published in 2004 recommended an optional goal LDL below 70 mg/dL (1.8 mmol/L) for patients at "very high risk" (Table 11.2), as did the 2006 AHA/ACC guidelines for secondary prevention. The 2007 ACC/AHA guidelines on the management of non-ST elevation acute coronary syndromes concluded that a goal of less than 70 mg/dL (1.8 mmol/L) was reasonable

Possible reduction in inflammation, though not demonstrated in pediatric lupus patients in the recently reported APPLE study

Control of hyperglycemia

Treatment to prevent or ameliorate osteoporosis

Bisphosphonates, though avoided in women of reproductive age and patients with estimated GFR <40 cc/min

Correction of vitamin D deficiency

Calcium intake 1,500 IU daily while on corticosteroids

Prevention of gonadal toxicity from cyclophosphamide therapy

Evaluation of individual risk by a reproductive endocrinologist is optimal

Men and boys at higher risk. No hormonal manipulation is helpful; sperm storage

Limited data suggests that gonadotrophin-releasing hormone agonist therapy decreases ovarian toxicity in women, but initial upregulation of estrogen levels incurs a thrombotic risk in nephrotic patients especially with APL

Therapy for Proliferative Lupus Nephritis

Patients with focal proliferative or diffuse proliferative glomerulonephritis (WHO class III and IV, respectively) are at high risk of progressive loss of renal function and warrant aggressive immunosuppressive therapy. In patients with proliferative lesions, the use of cytotoxic or immunosuppressive drugs (cyclophosphamide, mycophenolate mofetil, or azathioprine) in addition to corticosteroids has been shown to improve renal survival over treatment with corticosteroids alone. Delay of therapy is associated with an increase in renal scarring which is poorly responsive to immunosuppressive therapy.

The importance of reaching a complete clinical remission was during therapy became clear in the analysis of the Lupus Nephritis Collaborative Study Group. Complete remission was defined as an inactive urine sediment, a serum creatinine ≤ 1.4 mg/dL (124 µmol/L), and protein excretion ≤ 330 mg/day. Patients who reached a complete clinical remission with cyclophosphamide therapy had renal survival rates at 5 years of 94 % compared to those who did not attain remission, of only 46 %. At 10 years, the results were even more dramatic (94 % vs. 31 %). Improvement was also noted in overall patient survival (95 % vs. 60 % at 10 years). Compared with no response, partial remission was also associated with significantly higher renal survival (45 % vs. 19 %) as well as overall survival (76 % vs. 46 %). Patient survival at 10 years without renal failure was only 13 %.

Groundbreaking trials at the NIH demonstrated the superiority of immunosuppressive therapy added to corticosteroids over corticosteroids alone. This 2-year regimen of 6 monthly doses of cyclophosphamide followed by quarterly doses remained the standard of care for years. Nevertheless, remission had only occurred in 61 % after 5 years of follow-up. Thus, investigators began to look for better strategies. In 2005, the Contreras trial compared maintenance regimens in patients treated for induction with 6 monthly doses of cyclophosphamide. The trial showed convincing superiority of long-term maintenance with mycophenolate or azathioprine for 5 years compared with the quarterly dosing maintenance in the 2-year NIH regimen.

These observations led to a number of studies that compared different therapies to induce remission ("induction") followed by therapies that would maintain that remission ("maintenance"), ideally with less toxicity than observed with long-term cyclophosphamide therapy. Thus, currently, it is useful to conceptually divide the treatment of class III and class IV nephritis into induction and maintenance phases. The paradigm of "induction" therapy for lupus nephritis with a limited period of time (3–6 months) with aggressive immunosuppression with cyclophosphamide or mycophenolate mofetil therapy followed by a longer period of "maintenance" of 2–5 years with mycophenolate mofetil or azathioprine has been adopted for clinical trials. It is important to recognize that this paradigm has not been established in LN. There are no studies reporting distinct pathologic, physiologic, or clinical features defining these periods.

Induction

The ALMS clinical trial showed similar response to induction therapy with mycophenolate mofetil vs. 6 months therapy with intravenous cyclophosphamide. Patients with African ancestry were more likely to respond to mycophenolate than to cyclophosphamide. This trial was underpowered to show equivalence; however, a recent meta-analysis confirmed equivalence of mycophenolate mofetil to cyclophosphamide as induction therapy.

In a white population, the Euro-lupus trial demonstrated equal efficacy of low-dose cyclophosphamide (6–500 mg doses given at 2-week intervals) compared to the standard 2-year NIH regimen. Ten-year follow-up data confirms these results, with less toxicity in the low-dose cyclophosphamide arm.

In addition, recent clinical trials in lupus nephritis have produced sobering results with only slightly more than 50 % of patients showing complete or partial remission within 6 months with either mycophenolate mofetil or cyclophosphamide therapy. Furthermore, relapses, and thus a poorer prognosis, are more frequent in those patients with only a partial remission in the induction phase.

Maintenance

The original NIH maintenance protocol called for 2 years of cyclophosphamide therapy. This remained the standard of care for years. In 2005, the Contreras study demonstrated the superiority of continued immunosuppression beyond 2 years with either azathioprine or mycophenolate mofetil as compared to the NIH maintenance regimen of 2 years of quarterly doses of cyclophosphamide both in efficacy but more so in respect to less side effects. The Euro-lupus trial also has demonstrated the long-term efficacy and safety of azathioprine compared to the 2-year NIH maintenance regimen in a Caucasian European patient population followed for up to 10 years. Subsequently, this same group in the MAINTAIN LN trial demonstrated that MMF had equal efficacy as compared to azathioprine in maintaining remission, in a 4-year follow-up. However, there are still only limited data on the long-term relative efficacy and safety of the different maintenance regimes.

Risk Factors for Progressive Renal Failure

Risk factors for progressive loss of renal function include delayed therapy. The likelihood of response to therapy is greater if therapy is initiated early for LN. Additional factors increasing the risk of renal failure include the frequency and severity of renal relapses and failure to achieve either a complete or partial remission, elevated serum creatinine at the time of renal biopsy, hypertension, nephrotic range proteinuria, anemia (hematocrit less than 26), and Black and Hispanic race/ethnicity.

Treatment of Relapses

Relapses rates are said to occur about 5–15 per 100 patient years. There are no good trials. Experts have recommended corticosteroids plus MMF or azathioprine for mild relapses and steroids plus either cyclophosphamide (NIH protocol) or MMF for moderate to severe relapses. With failure of other therapies, more experimental therapies such as rituximab and cyclophosphamide or combined MMF and cyclosporine have been reported.

Renal Failure

Despite all of the above, some patients (up to 40 % of African Americans) do develop renal failure. They should be managed as any other patient with end-stage renal disease. They do as well with dialysis as any other patient with other causes for end-stage renal disease, despite being younger, more frequently female and less frequently diabetic. The mortality rate of patients on dialysis in the USA is 10 % per year. The survival rate among lupus patients on dialysis (i.e., 5-year survival rate of 60–70 %) is comparable with patients on dialysis who do not have SLE.

Hemodialysis is a better choice than peritoneal dialysis for lupus patients; several studies have reported higher anti-dsDNA levels, more thrombocytopenia, and higher steroid requirements in SLE patients who are on peritoneal dialysis. SLE is generally regarded as quiescent in patients on hemodialysis, although flares, including rash, arthritis, serositis, fever, and leukopenia, may occur, requiring treatment. Typically, hydroxychloroquine at reduced dose (200 mg daily) may be continued to prevent flares.

Lupus patients do well with renal transplantation, with recurrence of LN in the graft at <10 %. Graft survival for both cadaveric and living related donor organs is similar to patients with other causes of ESRD. Antiphospholipid antibodies increase the risk of thrombosis in the acute transplant period; if present, anticoagulation posttransplant is indicated.

Our Recommendations

Induction Therapy

Glucocorticoids. In patients with severe, active disease including acute renal failure, crescentic glomerulonephritis, or severe extrarenal disease should receive intravenous pulse methylprednisolone 500–1,000 mg given daily for 3 days followed by 1 mg/kg (not exceeding 60 mg) orally for the first month. Steroids may be tapered to 40 mg daily in the second month and 20 mg daily in the third month. Thereafter, tapering is done by smaller increments to <15 mg daily as needed for extrarenal disease.

Cyclophosphamide. In patients with severe proliferative LN, one of two regimens may be employed. The 6-month NIH regimen of 0.5–1 g/m^2 body surface area (the dose depending on neutrophil counts 10–14 days after the infusion) or the Euro-lupus dosing of 500 mg given at 2-week intervals for 6 doses, particularly for Caucasian patients. This regimen is being evaluated in US patients as part of the ongoing Immune Tolerance Network trial.

Mycophenolate mofetil. We recommend the ALMS study dosing 0.5 g twice daily × 1 week, then 1 g twice daily × 1 week then 1.5 g twice daily as tolerated. Patients could reduce to 1 g twice daily if intolerant to higher dosing. African ancestry and Hispanic patients were shown to respond more frequently to MMF than cyclophosphamide therapy. Cyclophosphamide may be preferred in those patients with a significantly decreased GFR or crescents on renal biopsy.

Maintenance

Mycophenolate mofetil. Patients who have responded to induction with cyclophosphamide or mycophenolate mofetil therapy may taper to 1 g twice daily of mycophenolate. The optimal duration of maintenance is not clear; however, the Contreras study showed good response in a high risk African ancestry and Hispanic cohort with immunosuppression continued for 5 years. At completion of 3 years therapy, the ALMS maintenance trial shows that mycophenolate mofetil is superior to azathioprine in reaching and maintaining renal response and preventing relapses of active lupus nephritis. This superiority was consistent regardless of induction treatment (cyclophosphamide or mycophenolate), race, or geographic region.

Azathioprine. 2 g/kg daily up to 150–200 mg daily. Patients responding to induction therapy with cyclophosphamide or mycophenolate mofetil may be treated with azathioprine as maintenance therapy, particularly if pregnancy is possible or planned.

Therapy for Membranous LN

The appropriate therapy for membranous LN is less clear. Immunosuppressive therapy (cyclophosphamide or cyclosporine) is indicated in patients with membranous LN with severe nephrotic syndrome (proteinuria >3.5 g in 24 h), an elevated serum creatinine, or the presence of crescents on renal biopsy. Patients without these indications may be treated with adjunctive therapy (Table 11.2) as indicated. Patients with proliferative and membranous findings on renal biopsy should be treated according to the proliferative features.

Sources

1. Appel GB, Cohen DJ, Pirani CL, et al. Long-term follow-up of patients with lupus nephritis. A study based on the classification of the World Health Organization. Am J Med. 1987; 83:877.
2. Austin 3rd HA, Boumpas DT, Vaughan EM, Balow JE. Predicting renal outcomes in severe lupus nephritis: contributions of clinical and histologic data. Kidney Int. 1994;45:544.
3. Contreras G, Pardo V, Cely C, et al. Factors associated with poor outcomes in patients with lupus nephritis. Lupus. 2005;14:890.
4. Schwartz MM, Lan SP, Bernstein J, et al. Role of pathology indices in the management of severe lupus glomerulonephritis. Lupus Nephritis Collaborative Study Group. Kidney Int. 1992;42:743.
5. Esdaile JM, Joseph L, MacKenzie T, et al. The benefit of early treatment with immunosuppressive agents in lupus nephritis. J Rheumatol. 1994;21:2046.
6. Faurschou M, Starklint H, Halberg P, Jacobsen S. Prognostic factors in lupus nephritis: diagnostic and therapeutic delay increases the risk of terminal renal failure. J Rheumatol. 2006; 33:1563.
7. Korbet SM, Lewis EJ, Schwartz MM, et al. Factors predictive of outcome in severe lupus nephritis. Lupus Nephritis Collaborative Study Group. Am J Kidney Dis. 2000;35:904.
8. Chen YE, Korbet SM, Katz RS, et al. Value of a complete or partial remission in severe lupus nephritis. Clin J Am Soc Nephrol. 2008;3:46.
9. Chan TM, Tse KC, Tang CS, et al. Long-term outcome of patients with diffuse proliferative lupus nephritis treated with prednisolone and oral cyclophosphamide followed by azathioprine. Lupus. 2005;14:265.
10. Korbet SM, Schwartz MM, Evans J, Lewis EJ, Collaborative Study Group. Severe lupus nephritis: racial differences in presentation and outcome. J Am Soc Nephrol. 2007;18:244.
11. Illei GG, Takada K, Parkin D, et al. Renal flares are common in patients with severe proliferative lupus nephritis treated with pulse immunosuppressive therapy: long-term followup of a cohort of 145 patients participating in randomized controlled studies. Arthritis Rheum. 2002; 46:995.
12. Moroni G, Quaglini S, Maccario M, et al. "Nephritic flares" are predictors of bad long-term renal outcome in lupus nephritis. Kidney Int. 1996;50:2047.
13. Dooley MA, Hogan S, Jennette C, Falk R. Cyclophosphamide therapy for lupus nephritis: poor renal survival in black Americans. Glomerular Disease Collaborative Network. Kidney Int. 1997;51:1188.
14. Alarcón GS, McGwin Jr G, Bastian HM, et al. Systemic lupus erythematosus in three ethnic groups. VII [correction of VIII]. Predictors of early mortality in the LUMINA cohort. LUMINA Study Group. Arthritis Rheum. 2001;45:191.
15. Adler M, Chambers S, Edwards C, et al. An assessment of renal failure in an SLE cohort with special reference to ethnicity, over a 25-year period. Rheumatology (Oxford). 2006;45:1144.
16. Valeri A, Radhakrishnan J, Estes D, et al. Intravenous pulse cyclophosphamide treatment of severe lupus nephritis: a prospective five-year study. Clin Nephrol. 1994;42:71.
17. Cheigh JS, Kim H, Stenzel KH, et al. Systemic lupus erythematosus in patients with end-stage renal disease: long-term follow-up on the prognosis of patients and the evolution of lupus activity. Am J Kidney Dis. 1990;16:189.
18. Appel GB, Contreras G, Dooley MA, et al. Mycophenolate mofetil versus cyclophosphamide for induction treatment of lupus nephritis. J Am Soc Nephrol. 2009;20:1103.
19. Contreras G, Pardo V, Leclercq B, et al. Sequential therapies for proliferative lupus nephritis. N Engl J Med. 2004;350:971.
20. Gourley MF, Austin 3rd HA, Scott D, et al. Methylprednisolone and cyclophosphamide, alone or in combination, in patients with lupus nephritis. A randomized, controlled trial. Ann Intern Med. 1996;125:549.

21. Illei GG, Austin HA, Crane M, et al. Combination therapy with pulse cyclophosphamide plus pulse methylprednisolone improves long-term renal outcome without adding toxicity in patients with lupus nephritis. Ann Intern Med. 2001;135:248.
22. Houssiau FA, Vasconcelos C, D'Cruz D, et al. Immunosuppressive therapy in lupus nephritis: the Euro-Lupus Nephritis Trial, a randomized trial of low-dose versus high-dose intravenous cyclophosphamide. Arthritis Rheum. 2002;46:2121.
23. Yee CS, Gordon C, Dostal C, et al. EULAR randomised controlled trial of pulse cyclophosphamide and methylprednisolone versus continuous cyclophosphamide and prednisolone followed by azathioprine and prednisolone in lupus nephritis. Ann Rheum Dis. 2004;63:525.
24. Houssiau FA, Vasconcelos C, D'Cruz D, et al. The 10-year follow-up data of the Euro-Lupus Nephritis Trial comparing low-dose and high-dose intravenous cyclophosphamide. Arthritis Rheum. 2010;69:61.
25. Houssiau FA, Vasconcelos C, D'Cruz D, et al. Early response to immunosuppressive therapy predicts good renal outcome in lupus nephritis: lessons from long-term followup of patients in the Euro-Lupus Nephritis Trial. Arthritis Rheum. 2004;50:3934.
26. Isenberg D, Appel GB, Contreras G, et al. Influence of race/ethnicity on response to lupus nephritis treatment: the ALMS study. Rheumatology. 2010;49:128.
27. Kamanamool N, McEvoy M, Attia J, et al. Efficacy and adverse events of mycophenolate mofetil versus cyclophosphamide for induction therapy of lupus nephritis: systematic review and meta-analysis. Medicine (Baltimore). 2010;89:227.
28. Chan TM, Tse KC, Tang CS, et al. Long-term study of mycophenolate mofetil as continuous induction and maintenance treatment for diffuse proliferative lupus nephritis. J Am Soc Nephrol. 2005;16:1076.
29. Lewis EJ, Hunsicker LG, Lan SP, et al. A controlled trial of plasmapheresis therapy in severe lupus nephritis. The Lupus Nephritis Collaborative Study Group. N Engl J Med. 1992;326:1373.
30. Ioannidis JP, Boki KA, Katsorida ME, et al. Remission, relapse, and re-remission of proliferative lupus nephritis treated with cyclophosphamide. Kidney Int. 2000;57:258.
31. Mosca M, Bencivelli W, Neri R, et al. Renal flares in 91 SLE patients with diffuse proliferative glomerulonephritis. Kidney Int. 2002;61:1502.
32. Moroni G, Gallelli B, Quaglini S, et al. Withdrawal of therapy in patients with proliferative lupus nephritis: long-term follow-up. Nephrol Dial Transplant. 2006;21:1541.
33. Grootscholten C, Berden JH. Discontinuation of immunosuppression in proliferative lupus nephritis: is it possible? Nephrol Dial Transplant. 2006;21:1465.
34. Renal Disease Subcommittee of the American College of Rheumatology Ad Hoc Committee on Systemic Lupus Erythematosus Response Criteria. The American College of rheumatology response criteria for proliferative and membranous renal disease in systemic lupus erythematosus clinical trials. Arthritis Rheum. 2006;54:421–32.
35. Houssiau FA, D-Cruz D, Sangle S, et al. Azathioprine versus mycophenolate mofetil for long-term immunosuppression in lupus nephritis: results from the MAINTAIN Nephritis Trial. Ann Rheum Dis. 2010;69:2083–9.
36. Falk RJ, Schur PH, Appel GB. Therapy of diffuse or focal proliferative lupus nephritis. In: Basow DS, editor. UpToDate. Waltham: UpToDate; 2011.

Chapter 12
Gastrointestinal Manifestations of Systemic Lupus Erythematosus

R.S. Kalman and J.L. Wolf

Introduction

Gastrointestinal (GI) manifestations are common in patients with systemic lupus erythematosus (SLE). Sir William Osler was the first organ systems to emphasize the importance of GI manifestations in SLE and stressed that GI symptoms associated with SLE could mimic nearly any abdominal condition. The GI tract is one of the most commonly affected systems in SLE. Incidence reports vary widely, but one autopsy study found that 60–70 % of SLE patients had evidence of previous peritonitis on post-mortem examination, even though only in 10 % of patients were the episodes clinically apparent while the patient was alive. Other studies estimate the incidence of GI symptoms in SLE patients to be somewhere between 25 and 40 %. Most GI manifestations are due to adverse reactions to potent medications and infection, while symptoms directly affecting the GI tract due to SLE are far less common than arthritis or nephritis in these patients.

Gastrointestinal Symptoms Due to Medications

Iatrogenesis is widely regarded as the most common cause of GI symptoms in patients with SLE. Since SLE is a chronic, multisystem disorder, toxic medications are often given for extended periods of time. GI toxicity is often ascribed to NSAIDs, corticosteroids, hydroxychloroquine, and immunosuppressive agents (see Table 12.1).

R.S. Kalman, M.D. (✉) • J.L. Wolf, M.D.
Beth Israel Deaconess Medical Center,
330 Brookline Ave, Deaconess 311, Boston, MA 02215, USA

Harvard Medical School, Boston, MA, USA
e-mail: rskalman@bidmc.harvard.edu

Table 12.1 Drugs causing GI manifestations in SLE

Azathioprine	Diarrhea, nausea/vomiting, hepatitis, pancreatitis
Cyclophosphamide	Nausea, mucositis, oral stomatitis
Corticosteroids	Dyspepsia, GI bleeding, pancreatitis, steatosis
Cyclosporine	Abdominal pain, anorexia, constipation, diarrhea, dyspepsia, flatulence, gingivitis, GI bleeding, nausea, vomiting, gingivitis, taste perversions, salivary gland enlargement, weight gain
Hydroxychloroquine	Abdominal pain, anorexia, diarrhea, hepatitis, nausea/vomiting, weight loss
Mycophenolate mofetil	Abdominal pain, anorexia, constipation, diarrhea, dyspepsia, nausea/vomiting
NSAIDs	Dyspepsia, GI bleeding, hepatitis, diarrhea
Rituximab	Abdominal pain, diarrhea, dyspepsia, inflammatory bowel disease, nausea/vomiting, weight loss

Table 12.2 Risk factors associated with NSAID-induced GI toxicity

Risk factor	Relative risk	Confidence interval
Age over 60	5.52	4.63–6.60
Prior GI event	4.76	4.05–5.59
High NSAID dose	10.1	4.6–22
Concurrent steroids	4.4	2.0–9.7
Concurrent anticoagulants	12.7	6.3–25.7

Adapted from American College of Gastroenterology. Lanza FL. A guideline for the treatment and prevention of NSAID-induced ulcers. Am J Gastroenterol 1998; 93:2037

NSAIDs commonly cause gastropathy, gastritis, and peptic ulcer disease. A postmortem review of patients taking NSAIDs for a variety of indications found that 21.7 % of patients taking NSAIDs in the 6 months prior to their demise had ulcers in the stomach or duodenum, compared with 12.3 % in patients not taking NSAIDs.

Mucosal damage to the stomach and duodenum from NSAIDs is due to inhibition of the COX-1 enzyme, which leads to a reduction in local prostaglandins. In addition to NSAID-induced peptic ulcer disease, some authors have suggested that SLE itself may cause peptic ulcers. The American College of Gastroenterology has identified the five most important risk factors for NSAID-related GI toxicity to be a prior history of a GI event (such as ulcer or hemorrhage), age greater than 60, high dose of NSAIDs (such as anti-inflammatory doses as opposed to analgesic doses), concurrent use of glucocorticoids, and concurrent use of anticoagulants (see Table 12.2). Patients with more than one of these risk factors may benefit from ulcer prophylaxis while taking NSAIDs. Misoprostol has been shown to reduce the risk of a serious GI event in patients with at least one of the above risk factors by 38–87 %. Proton pump inhibitors (PPIs) and Histamine receptor 2 (H2) blockers also have been shown to be effective, but H2 blockers may be less effective in preventing gastric ulcers. In addition, certain NSAIDs have been shown to cause less peptic ulcer disease than others. Ibuprofen, nabumetone, meloxicam, and etodolac have few GI side effects, while the risk for GI side effects is higher with sulindac, piroxicam, and ketorolac.

For mild symptoms related to NSAID use, such as low-grade discomfort, bloating, and nausea, most patients are treated with antacids and cessation of the drug. A more thorough workup may be warranted if symptoms are moderate to severe, such as intense pain, poor oral intake, and weight loss. This workup should include a serum hematocrit or hemoglobin, stool occult blood testing, serum or stool *Helicobacter pylori* testing (because infection doubles the risk of NSAID-related bleeding), and upper endoscopy. Most patients respond to NSAID withdrawal. For patients in whom NSAIDs must be continued, an H2 blocker or PPI should be added. Alternatively, changing therapy to a selective COX-2 inhibitor may be considered. Conservative measures such as alcohol reduction and tobacco cessation should be stressed.

Systemic corticosteroids are also potentially harmful to the GI tract. Their side effects include gastritis, ulcer formation, and GI bleeding. In one often cited nested case control trial of 1,415 case patients and 7,063 control patients, 2 % of case patients were currently using corticosteroids, with a history of peptic ulcer disease or upper GI bleed in comparison to 0.9 % of control patients giving an estimated relative risk of 2.0 (CI 1.3-3.1). The study authors felt that the risk of peptic ulcer disease in the case patients on corticosteroids was limited to patients on concurrent NSAIDs. Although the incidence of GI side effects is lower in steroid use than in NSAID use, when these medications are used in combination there appears to be a synergistic effect leading to a twofold increase in GI toxicity. Other GI toxicities from steroids include pancreatitis, visceral rupture, and hepatic steatosis. To detect GI toxicity in a patient on steroids, a high index of suspicion is required by the clinician because steroids may mask inflammation, thus causing only mild or minimal symptoms despite severe damage.

Hydroxychloroquine, like most anti-malarials, is associated with a high incidence of GI side effects. Nausea is the most common complaint, but diarrhea and vomiting may also occur. Peptic ulcer disease and gastritis do not often occur. When symptoms do occur, they are frequently dose related and may be improved with dose reduction followed by a slow upward titration. Medication administration at bedtime may also be of benefit in order to minimize nausea while the patient is awake.

Immunosuppressive medications are commonly used to treat SLE. Azathioprine can cause a wide variety of GI toxicities. Most often the side effects include nausea, vomiting, and malaise. These symptoms can occur in up to one quarter of patients, and usually arise within the first month of therapy. Dose-dependent liver dysfunction and dose-independent pancreatitis are also described, both of which usually require discontinuation of the drug. Cyclophosphamide may cause nausea and oral stomatitis. Hepatotoxicity is rare, but may be severe. Other side effects are far more common with this drug. Cyclosporine may also cause nausea and vomiting. Additionally gingival hyperplasia may occur with cyclosporine and is treated with metronidazole.

B cell targeted agents such as rituximab are more frequently being used to treat SLE. Although B cell agents carry many serious side effects, those involving the GI tract are rare. Mucocutaneous reactions, such as Stevens Johnson, are uncommon, and when they do occur often take place within the first 3 months of therapy.

Reactivation of viral hepatitis should be a concern for all practitioners prescribing immunosuppressants. Patients with a history of hepatitis B or at a high risk for hepatitis should be tested for hepatitis infection prior to any treatment with immunosuppressants by drawing a hepatitis B surface antigen and anti-hepatitis B core antibody according to the American Association for the Study of Liver Diseases. Patients at high risk for hepatitis B are people from endemic areas (such as Asia, Africa, and the Middle East), dialysis recipients, patients with a history of intravenous drug use, patients having sexual contact with a partner with hepatitis, patients with a personal history of a sexually transmitted disease, men who have sex with men and inmates at correctional facilities. If a patient is found to be a chronic hepatitis B carrier, then antiviral therapy should be considered while treating with immunosuppressants. Typically lamivudine or telbivudine is preferred if treatment with immunosuppressants will be less than a year. Alternatively tenofovir or entecavir can be used if longer immunosuppression is anticipated. At this time there is no consensus statement regarding screening for reactivation of hepatitis C or treating with prophylaxis for patients with chronic hepatitis C in the setting of immunosuppression.

Oral Cavity

The oral manifestations of SLE were first described by Bazin in the nineteenth century. Oral lesions are now considered so important to the identity of SLE that the American College of Rheumatology now includes oral ulceration as part of the diagnostic criteria for SLE. The prevalence of oral lesions is estimated to be between 7 and 52 %. There appears to be dramatic demographic differences in the incidence of oral lesions in SLE, as some studies have reported the incidence to be nearly 50 % in the English population but less than 20 % in the Brazilian and Swedish populations.

Lesions fall into one of three categories based on pathology and appearance: erythematosus, discoid, or ulcerative. Erythematosus lesions are painless, and edematous with associated petechial reddening. Discoid lesions are painful and are characterized by central areas of erythema surrounded by white striae and telangectasias. Ulcers are often noticed in groups of 1–2 cm lesions that extend into the pharynx. For all three lesions, the buccal mucosa, hard palate, and vermilion border are the areas typically affected.

Although controversial, some studies suggest that the presence of oral lesions corresponds to overall disease activity and that patients with oral lesions have a higher mortality. Discoid lesions and ulcerative lesions are described only in patients with active disease. Other oral lesions that may mimic those from SLE include lichen planus, steroid induced calcifications and gingivitis. At this time there are no evidence-based guidelines for systemic therapy, but surveys imply that oral lesions are most often treated with anti-malarials as first line agents, with steroids and azathioprine being used as a second line agent. Anti-leprosy drugs such as dapsone and clofazime have also been used with some success.

Since many SLE therapies and the disease itself cause reduced saliva, which increases the risk for tooth decay, preventative dental care is important. In addition, many patients consume a poor diet due to impaired taste, which further promotes tooth decay. In the setting of infection or pre-existing periodontal disease, chlorohexidine mouthwash and hydrogen peroxide mouthwash may provide some benefit. Anticholinergics such as tricyclic antidepressants (TCAs), antihistamines, and selective serotonin reuptake inhibitors (SSRIs) should be avoided when possible. Oral dryness may also be treated with sugar-free gum, artificial saliva or systemic pilocarpine to help increase salivary secretion. Finally, dental procedures should probably not take place during an active lupus flare, and patients with SLE and known valvular damage should be given prophylactic antibiotics prior to dental work to prevent endocarditis.

Esophagus and Stomach

Dysphagia

The incidence of esophageal involvement in patients with SLE is estimated to be between 1.5 and 25 %. Dysphagia, or difficulty with swallowing, occurs in 1–13 % of patients, and is most frequently due to esophageal hypomotility or gastroesophageal reflux disease (GERD). Although the exact mechanism of action is not known, authors have hypothesized that esophageal dysmotility is due to inflammatory damage to the esophageal muscles or Auerbach plexus. Hypomotility is most often found in the upper third of the esophagus, but the presence of abnormal esophageal manometry does not necessarily correlate with symptoms. In the subset of patients with systemic sclerosis, over 80 % had decreased pressure in the lower esophageal sphincter, whereas no patients with SLE alone had changes in the lower esophageal sphincter. GERD most often causes dysphagia via inflammation and may cause associated esophageal spasm or strictures. The American Gastroenterological Association has agreed upon guidelines for the workup of GERD. For typical symptoms that respond to therapy, such as a PPI, no further testing is required. Endoscopy should be pursued if an alternative diagnosis is suspected, if there is concern for complications from GERD, such as stricture, or if empiric therapy has failed.

Other etiologies of dysphagia aside from hypomotility and GERD are esophageal stricture, esophageal candidiasis (which should be suspected in the immunocompromised patient with dysphagia and odynophagia, or painful swallowing), esophageal viral infection (such as CMV and HSV), esophageal ulcerations and pill-induced esophagitis (especially in the patient taking bisphosphonates, NSAIDs, teteracyclines, or potassium supplements). A careful history is essential when evaluating dysphagia in the office or inpatient setting. If a patient has difficulty initiating a swallow, this most often indicates an oropharyngeal disorder, which is often associated with neurodegenerative disorders and myopathies. When a patient reports difficulty swallowing solid foods, this is likely due to a mechanical obstruction such as an esophageal ring or mass. If dysphagia presents with difficulty tolerating both solids and liquids, then a neuromuscular disorder should be suspected, such as achalasia or diffuse esophageal spasm.

Workup for dysphagia usually involves esophageal manometry, radiology studies, and upper endoscopy. Endoscopy and radiography may help differentiate esophageal dysmotility from the other above-mentioned etiologies of dysphagia. Adjunct studies that may help evaluate the differential diagnosis for dysphagia include pH probe monitoring (to diagnose acid reflux), barium swallow (to evaluate for obstructive or motility disorders of the esophagus), and video swallow (to rule out aspiration and evaluate causes of upper esophageal/oropharyngeal problems).

An interesting relationship between esophageal dysmotility and Raynaud's phenomenon has been established. This association was first noted in 1964, and further elucidated in the 1980s when a cohort of 30 patients with either SLE or mixed connective tissue disease was evaluated for dysphagia. A significant correlation was found between the patients reporting Raynaud's phenomenon and aperistalsis on esophageal manometry. Furthermore, an association was found between SLE patients with Raynaud's phenomenon and esophageal dysmotility with high titres of antibody to recombinant hn-RNP protein A1, perhaps identifying a subset of patients prone to antibody induced hypomotility.

The treatment of esophageal symptoms due to dysphagia is dependent on the specific etiology. There are no randomized controlled trials advocating one treatment over another. Interventions that may be of benefit include advocating slow meal ingestion, small meal size, avoiding post-prandial recumbent positions for 2–4 hours after eating and the use of PPIs and H2 blockers if there is concurrent reflux. No longer available in the United States due to an association with fatal arrhythmias, the prokinetic agent, cisapride was used in the past for treatment of hypomotility with success. Esophageal strictures should be treated with dilation, candidiasis with appropriate anti-fungal medication, and viral infections with appropriate antiviral medications.

Dyspepsia

The other common symptom related to SLE and the esophagus and stomach is dyspepsia, or more commonly referred to as indigestion. Dyspepsia may include symptoms of abdominal pain, nausea, bloating, early satiety, and belching. In the SLE population, symptoms of dyspepsia should raise suspicion for peptic ulcer disease. Although active peptic ulcer disease occurs in less than 25 % of patients with SLE, symptoms of dyspepsia occur in up to 50 % of patients. These symptoms are often secondary to concurrent NSAID and steroid use, as noted above. There should be a low threshold for evaluating such symptoms with endoscopy in order to determine if there is secondary infection or malignancy. Patients who present with odynophagia should be considered for urgent endoscopy to evaluate for infection. If peptic ulcer disease is demonstrated, then *Helicobacter pylori* must be ruled out and repeat endoscopy may be warranted to confirm resolution. On endoscopy, *Helicobacter pylori* infection can be diagnosed via pathology, culture or more rapidly via the Campylobacter-like organism (CLO) test that yields a diagnosis in minutes. Other methods are available for diagnosing *Helicobacter pylori* as a possible culprit for the patient's dyspepsia besides endoscopy. Serum antibody testing is widely available but can only determine whether the patient has been exposed to the bacterium, and not whether there is active infection. Therefore if a patient is known to have had *Helicobacter pylori* exposure in the past, then antibody testing should not be pursued. The urea breath test and stool antigen test are noninvasive methods of detecting active infection. The most common treatment in the USA is triple therapy consisting of a PPI, clarithromycin and amoxicillin or metronidazole for 14 days, or a PPI or H2 blocker, bismuth, metronidazole and tetracycline for 10–14 days.

Small and Large Intestines

Lupus Mesenteric Vasculitis

The small and large intestines are the sites of some of the most life-threatening complications of SLE in the GI tract. Lupus mesenteric vasculitis (LMV) is one of the most concerning causes of abdominal pain in the patient with SLE. This entity can be classified as an acute process of ischemic enteritis, which involves mainly the small intestine, or a chronic process which causes multiple ulcerations in the colon. Approximately 8–40 % of SLE patients with an active flare have abdominal pain, but the incidence of LMV is quite rare, estimated at 0.9 % in the USA and slightly higher in Asia (2.2 %). When LMV does occur, it almost always occurs in patients with active SLE elsewhere, such as in the skin, kidneys, cardiovascular system, or bone marrow.

Patients with LMV present with acute abdominal pain, nausea, vomiting, anorexia, dysphagia, cramps, diarrhea, ascites, gastrointestinal bleeding, and fever. Classically, the pain is diffuse, severe, and associated with rebound and guarding, thus mimicking the acute surgical abdomen. Symptoms may also be less malignant, including mild, nonspecific abdominal pain, diarrhea, and bloating. It is important to note that symptoms of peritonitis can be masked by corticosteroids, therefore the clinician must be vigilant with patients taking these medications. Metabolic acidosis, hypotension, abdominal distention and bowel dilation on X-ray, which is not otherwise explained, should be of particular concern. In severe cases, LMV can progress to bowel necrosis and perforation.

Risk factors for LMV include patients with peripheral vasculitis, central nervous system lupus, avascular necrosis, thrombocytopenia, and circulating rheumatoid factor, lupus anticoagulant, anticardiolipin antibody, and Beta 2 glycoprotein. Not very much is known about precipitating factors, but some authors hypothesize that bacterial infection, cytomegalovirus infection, eosinophilia, NSAIDs, helminth infection, caffeine, phosphodiesterase 4 inhibitors (such as sildenafil and tadalafil), and particular foods and herbal supplements may predispose one to LMV.

The pathophysiology of LMV is not entirely certain. It is presumed that antiphospholipid antibodies cause immune complex deposition and thrombosis in intestinal blood vessels. There is no macroscopic finding specific for LMV. Colonic ulcers may be seen on endoscopy but are neither sensitive nor specific. Microscopically, small vessel arteritis and venulitis are classic, with associated atrophy of the arterial media layer, fibrinoid necrosis of the vessel wall, as well as thrombosis, phlebitis, and monocyte infiltration within the lamina propria.

Rapid and accurate diagnosis of LMV is essential in order to avoid abdominal catastrophe. Given that clinical history and laboratory findings are nonspecific, imaging is the modality most relied upon to make the diagnosis of LMV. Abdominal computed tomography (CT) scan is the technique of choice at most institutions. The classic findings of LMV on CT are dilated bowel, bowel wall edema (including the "target sign," or abnormal bowel wall enhancement), ascites, mesenteric vessel edema or stenosis and mesenteric engorgement (also called the "comb sign"). A further finding supporting vasculitis is segmental sections of bowel wall inflammation, with alternating "normal" bowel. Arteriography may be pursued if CT imaging does not garner enough information for a diagnosis, but arteriograms are often negative because of the small arteries affected by LMV. In this situation, laparoscopy is required to make the diagnosis. Other imaging modalities that may be of use include plain X-ray films to rule out perforation, ultrasound to evaluate for ascites and bowel wall edema, and upper and lower endoscopy for tissue sampling. Of note, endoscopic biopsies are usually non-diagnostic because specimens are usually too superficial.

Treatment of LMV involves immunosuppression and bowel rest. Methylprednisolone (typically at a dose of 1–2 mg/kg/day) is first line therapy, but cyclophosphamide is occasionally used for nonresponders. Patients that do not respond to these measures within 24–48 hours should be considered for early laparotomy to evaluate for bowel perforation and ischemia. Surgical intervention within 48 hours for patients not responding to steroids has been shown to improve mortality in small studies. While small bowel ischemia is a surgical emergency, colonic ischemia may be treated with antibiotics and fluid resuscitation if the patient is stable. The overall prognosis for LMV is poor, with some mortality rates reported as high as 50 %. Patients with greater than 9 mm of bowel wall thickness on CT imaging have been shown to have a high risk of recurrence and should be monitored closely.

Inflammatory Bowel Disease

Ulcerative Colitis (UC) and Crohn's disease are autoimmune diseases that cause inflammation in the small and large bowel. UC is an inflammatory disease that involves the mucosal layer of the rectum and colon in a continuous fashion. Crohn's disease affects the entire GI tract and causes transmural inflammation, as well as fistulizing disease. Both diseases are associated with other autoimmune diseases, such as Hashimoto's thyroiditis and Wegener's granulomatosis. Not surprisingly, some authors have found that there may be an association between inflammatory bowel disease and SLE. Case reports have documented the presence of SLE prior to UC diagnosis, and several other case reports have found drug-induced SLE after administration of sulfasalazine for UC therapy. The estimated prevalence of UC in SLE patients is 0.4 %. Differentiating sulfasalazine-induced SLE from idiopathic SLE associated with UC can present a challenge. HLA status can be used to help differentiate the two entities. HLA DR3 is associated with idiopathic SLE, and HLA DR4 is linked to drug-induced lupus. Additionally, low complement levels, and the presence of autoantibodies such as anticardiolipin antibody, anti-Ro, and anti-La are more consistent with idiopathic SLE. Case reports link Crohn's disease and collagenous colitis with SLE. Finally, drug-induced colitis must be considered in patients receiving therapy with NSAIDs and antibiotics. Anti-TNF therapy, used to treat inflammatory bowel disease, has also been reported to cause SLE.

Celiac Disease

Celiac disease, also known as gluten sensitive enteropathy, is an autoimmune disease whereby antibodies to gluten cause small bowel villous atrophy and mucosal inflammation. Seventeen case reports have documented an association between SLE and celiac disease. This relationship was further strengthened when it was discovered that HLA B8 and DR3 were found in 70–90 % of patients with celiac disease, and are also found at higher rates in patients with SLE, which may indicate that these haplotypes carry a higher risk of patients developing both ailments. Further studies have shown the association of HLA DQ2 (which has a close linkage with HLA DR3) in 95 % of patients. A gluten-free diet is usually all that is necessary to treat celiac disease, but immunosuppressants and anti-inflammatories used to treat SLE likely also help quell the celiac disease process.

Protein-Losing Gastroenteropathy

Protein-losing gastroenteropathy (PLGE) is a rare condition associated with SLE characterized by hypoalbuminemia and edema. Hypoalbuminemia in SLE is most commonly caused by nephrotic syndrome. Reduced hepatic synthesis is another cause of hypoalbuminemia in patients with SLE. Approximately 60 case reports have confirmed the syndrome of PLGE related to SLE, which causes hypoalbuminemia secondary to loss of protein in the GI tract. There is a female predominance and a slightly higher incidence in Asia than in other parts of the world. PLGE is more common in patients with multi-organ SLE involvement. The pathophysiology is unknown, but may involve increased GI capillary permeability secondary to vasculitis and subsequent mucosal irritation. The main features of the disease are severe diarrhea, hypoalbuminemia without proteinuria, and profound pitting edema, often associated with ascites, and pleural and pericardial effusions. Diarrhea may be as frequent as 20 times daily but is absent in nearly 50 % of patients, and is classically without steatorrhea. Nausea and vomiting may also be present.

The diagnosis of PLGE is reliant on the exclusion of other causes of hypoalbuminemia, such as renal and hepatic disease. The diagnostic test of choice is fecal excretion of radio-labeled albumin via Technetium-99-m-albumin scintigraphy, which reveals loss of albumin from the blood to the intestinal lumen. Other diagnostic tests include a 4 day stool collection following indium-labeled albumin plasma infusion, and 24-h stool alpha 1-antitrypsin excretion. Endoscopic biopsy is usually unhelpful as half of patients are found to have nonspecific bowel wall edema, and 10 % of patients have normal biopsy specimens. When abnormal, biopsy specimens show villous atrophy, inflammatory infiltrate, and a lack of evidence of vasculitis.

PLGE is highly responsive to steroid therapy. More than 60 % of patients can expect a response from steroids alone. Intractable disease can be treated with the addition of azathioprine, cyclosporine, or cyclophosphamide. Antibiotics (such as metronidazole or tetracycline) are occasionally used when a component of bacterial overgrowth is suspected. Octreotide is sometimes employed to help reduce intestinal blood flow, thereby reducing protein loss. Some authors recommend prophylaxis for deep vein thrombosis in the setting of PLGE and antiphospholipid antibodies. Overall, outcomes are good but approximately 20–30 % of patients will relapse and may require maintenance steroid therapy.

Intestinal Pseudo-Obstruction

Intestinal pseudo-obstruction (IPO) manifests as symptoms suggestive of small bowel obstruction such as constipation, nausea, vomiting, and abdominal pain. IPO represents dysfunction of visceral smooth muscle and the autonomic nervous system. It occurs with ureterohydronephrosis in over 60 % of cases, and may rarely be associated with interstitial cystitis and biliary dilatation. Fewer than 30 cases have thus far been reported. The pathophysiology is not well established but is likely due to autoimmune damage to smooth muscle cells, perhaps with a contribution from circulating immune complexes. Involvement of the genitourinary and biliary tracts raises suspicion for a circulating antibody against both systems. Microscopic examination of the GI tract shows fibrosis and atrophy of the muscularis layer of the small bowel, an inflammatory infiltrate in the muscularis propria and a decrease in smooth muscle cells.

Symptoms of IPO are similar to that of intermittent small bowel obstruction, including nausea, vomiting, abdominal pain, distention, and constipation with intermittent diarrhea. X-rays and CT scans are consistent with small bowel obstruction showing dilated fluid-filled bowel loops with air–fluid levels. Ureter dilation may be noted if hydronephrosis is present. Manometry may demonstrate esophageal and intestinal hypomotility. No specific lab tests are helpful in distinguishing IPO from other causes of small bowel obstruction.

Treatment of IPO focuses on immunosuppressants, corticosteroids, antibiotics, and parenteral nutrition. Timely diagnosis and treatment is essential, as delay in therapy may cause reduced peristalsis in the future. Prokinetic agents such as erythromycin and octreotide (and cisapride prior to its withdrawal from the market in the USA) have been used with some efficacy.

Peritonitis

Serositis is an important diagnostic criterion for SLE. Serositis often presents as pericarditis, pleuritis, or peritonitis. A common but often overlooked cause of abdominal pain in the SLE patient is peritonitis. In autopsy studies, up to 70 % of patients with SLE have evidence of peritonitis. Often the diagnosis of peritonitis is not made until a thorough workup involving CT imaging and endoscopy has been negative. Clinical features consistent with peritonitis include abdominal pain with rebound tenderness, fevers, and the presence of ascites. Diagnosis should involve paracentesis to exclude infection. Other causes of ascites such as congestive heart failure, constrictive pericarditis, Budd–Chiari syndrome, nephrotic syndrome, cirrhosis, and hypoalbuminemia should be evaluated. In addition to ascites, other complications of peritonitis include adhesions, bowel perforation, and spontaneous bacterial peritonitis. Management often involves corticosteroids (often starting with prednisone 60 mg daily) if symptoms are severe and infection has been ruled out by paracentesis.

Infectious Diarrhea

Patients with SLE are prone to bacterial, viral, and parasitic infections because they are often treated with immunosuppressants or PPIs. Infectious diarrhea is no exception to this phenomenon. Other risk factors include functional asplenia, hemolysis, and low intra-abdominal compliment levels leading to decreased opsonization potential. Bacterial infections are the most frequently encountered GI infection. Salmonella infection has been documented in several case reports, and it appears that patients with SLE have a much higher risk of developing bacteremia than otherwise healthy patients with Salmonella. If a patient has traveled overseas, then amoebic colitis should be suspected. It is important to rule this out prior to starting immunosuppressant therapy, as high dose steroids can be fatal in this setting.

Pneumatosis Cystoides Intestinalis

Pneumatosis cystoides intestinalis is the presence of gas within the walls of the GI tract. This disease entity is associated with multiple rheumatic diseases. There are 14 case reports documenting SLE-associated pneumatosis cytoides intestinalis. Half of the cases were documented in the setting of LMV, and the pathophysiology is proposed to be mucosal injury secondary to vasculitis. On CT, the pathognomonic finding is many linear and cystic radiolucencies within the small bowel wall. Treatment may involve oxygen supplementation, and some have advocated hyperbaric oxygen. If asymptomatic, no treatment may be necessary. Bowel rest and antibiotics are also employed.

Pancreas

Pancreatitis is a potentially life-threatening complication of SLE. The presentation is identical to pancreatitis in the non-SLE setting, and includes epigastric abdominal pain radiating to the back, nausea, and vomiting. Chemistries reveal an elevated amylase and lipase. Anti-La antibody has been associated with SLE induced pancreatitis. The annual incidence of pancreatitis in the SLE population is 0.4–1.1 per 1,000 patients. Pancreatitis often occurs in the first years of diagnosis and is more common during an SLE flare. Iatrogenic pancreatitis in patients with SLE may be due to steroid and azathioprine use. Idiopathic SLE pancreatitis may be due to vasculitis, thrombi, or immune complex deposition in the blood vessels associated with the pancreas, but this hypothesis has never been formally proven.

The diagnosis of pancreatitis is based on clinical history, physical exam, elevated pancreatic enzymes, and CT findings suggestive of pancreatic inflammation. One should proceed with an evaluation of the biliary tree, a thorough infectious workup, medication reconciliation, serum calcium to rule out hypercalcemia, serum ethanol to rule out ethanol abuse and serum triglycerides to rule out hypertriglyceridemia. Treatment is similar to pancreatitis in the non-SLE setting (which includes bowel rest, analgesics, and intravenous fluids), but some authors advocate steroids, plasmapheresis and IV gammaglobulin in refractory disease.

Liver

Although hepatomegaly is common in patients with SLE, with some estimates as high as 50 %, the actual incidence of significant liver disease is less common. Over the course of their lifetimes, patients with SLE have a risk of 25–50 % of developing abnormal liver tests. However, the clinical consequences of these abnormalities are unknown. In a review of 206 patients with SLE, 124 patients had abnormal liver function tests, the vast majority of which could not be attributed to one distinct entity. Thirty-three patients went on to liver biopsy, and the spectrum of disease ranged from cirrhosis, chronic active hepatitis, granulomatous hepatitis, cholestasis, centrilobular necrosis, chronic persistent hepatitis, primary biliary cirrhosis (PBC), steatosis, fatty liver, and drug toxicity. Three of the patients died from liver disease.

Care should be taken to rule out secondary causes of liver disease and jaundice and a complete evaluation should include diagnostic tests to rule out intravascular hemolysis, The workup for abnormal liver function tests should include viral serologies (Hepatitis A, Hepatitis B, Hepatitis C, Hepatitis D and E if indicated, Cytomegalovirus, and HIV), ceruloplasmin (to rule out Wilson's disease), iron studies (to rule out hemochromatosis), and ultrasound (to evaluate for biliary pathology and signs consistent with cirrhosis). If a patient with SLE has a history of hepatitis B and has recently been treated with immunosuppressants (such as steroids or rituximab), then hepatitis B reactivation should be considered even if serologic clearance has been previously demonstrated. After other diseases have been ruled out, autoimmune hepatitis or lupoid-associated hepatitis may be considered. Autoimmune hepatitis was previously called lupoid hepatitis by Mackay in 1959, in order to describe SLE which predominantly affected the liver. The association between lupoid hepatitis and SLE was based on serologic similarities, such as a positive ANA, anticardiolipin antibody, and anti-smooth muscle antibody. Lupoid hepatitis has now been recognized as a distinct entity known as autoimmune hepatitis and is distinct from lupoid-associated hepatitis. Autoimmune hepatitis occurs in less than 2 % of patients with SLE, but may be more common in the juvenile population, with rates estimated as high as 10 %. Lupoid-associated hepatitis, or elevated liver enzymes secondary to underlying SLE, is a distinct entity from autoimmune hepatitis and is distinct from lupoid-associated hepatitis. Autoimmune hepatitis and lupoid-associated hepatitis can be distinguished based on pathology and clinical history. For example, the presence of anti-smooth muscle and antimitochondrial antibodies are more common in autoimmune hepatitis, whereas positive antiribosomal P protein antibody is more consistent with lupoid-associated hepatitis. In general, autoimmune hepatitis is considered to carry a worse prognosis if left untreated and shows more dramatic changes on pathology than lupoid-associated hepatitis.

The vast majority of patients with liver abnormalities in the SLE population will have no clinically relevant sequelae. In patients with hepatitis due to SLE, treatment often consists of steroids with the addition of azathioprine as necessary. It is rare for hepatitis due to SLE to progress to portal hypertension and cirrhosis.

Conclusion

SLE can affect nearly every portion of the GI tract, and it is essential for the practitioner caring for patients with SLE to be familiar with these manifestations. Although drugs used to treat SLE often cause GI distress, the disease itself can often cause life-threatening GI-related problems.

Sources

1. Osler W. On the visceral complications of erythema exudativum mulitforme. Am J Med Sci. 1895;110:629–46.
2. Wallace DJ. Gastrointestinal manifestations and related liver and biliary disorders. In: Wallace DJ, Hahn BH, editors. Dubois' lupus erythematosus. 4th ed. Philadelphia: Lippincott Williams & Wilkins; 1993. p. 410–7.
3. Hoffman BI, Katz WA. The gastrointestinal manifestations of systemic lupus erythematosus: a review of the literature. Semin Arthritis Rheum. 1980;9:237.
4. Jovaisas A, Kraag G. Acute gastrointestinal manifestations of systemic lupus erythematosus. Can J Surg. 1987;30:185.
5. Zizic TM, Classen JN, Stevens MB. Acute abdominal complications of systemic lupus erythematosus and polyarteritis nodosa. Am J Med. 1982;73:525.
6. Tian XP, et al. Gastrointestinal involvement in systemic lupus erythematosus. World J Gastroenterol. 2010;16(24):2971–7.
7. Allison MC, Howatson AG, Torrance CJ, et al. Gastrointestinal damage associated with the use of nonsteroidal anti-inflammatory drugs. N Engl J Med. 1992;327:749.
8. Ginzler EM, Aranow C. Prevention and treatment of adverse effects of corticosteroids in systemic lupus erythematosus. Baillieres Clin Rheumatol. 1998;12:495.
9. Lanza FL. A guideline for the treatment and prevention of NSAID-induced ulcers. Am J Gastroenterol. 1998;93:2037.
10. Simon LS, Hatoum TH, Bittman RM, et al. Risk factors for serious nonsteroidal-induced gastrointestinal complications: regression analysis of the MUCOSA trial. Fam Med. 1996;28:202.
11. Koch M, Dezi A, Ferrario F, Capurso I. Prevention of nonsteroidal anti-inflammatory drug-induced gastrointestinal mucosal injury. A meta-analysis of randomized controlled clinical trials. Arch Intern Med. 1996;156:2321.
12. Lancaster-Smith MJ, Jaderberg ME, Jackson DA. Ranitidine in the treatment of non-steroidal anti-inflammatory drug associated gastric and duodenal ulcers. Gut. 1991;32:252.
13. Piper JM, Ray WA, Daugherty JR, Griffin MR. Corticosteroid use and peptic ulcer disease: role of nonsteroidal anti-inflammatory drugs. Ann Intern Med. 1991;114(9):735–40.
14. Gabriel SE, Jaaklimainen L, Bombadier C. Risk for serious gastrointestinal complications related to use of nonsteroidal anti-inflammatory drugs: a meta-analysis. Ann Intern Med. 1991;115:787.
15. Moghadam-Kia S, Werth VP. Prevention and treatment of systemic glucocorticoid side effects. Int J Dermatol. 2010;49(3):239–48.
16. Taylor WR, White NJ. Antimalarial drug toxicity: a review. Drug Saf. 2004;27(1):25–61.
17. Weinshilboum RM, Sladek SL. Mercaptopurine pharmacogenetics: monogenic inheritance of erythrocyte thiopurine methyltransferase activity. Am J Hum Genet. 1980;32:651.
18. Wong W, Hodge MG, Lewis A, et al. Resolution of cyclosporin-induced gingival hypertrophy with metronidazole. Lancet. 1994;343:986.
19. Lok AS, McMahon BJ. Chronic hepatitis B: update 2009. Hepatology. 2009;50(3):661–2.
20. Bazin E. Lecons theoriques et cliniques sur la scrofula. 2nd ed. Paris: A. Delahue; 1861.

21. Tan E, Cohen A, Fries J, Masi A, McShane D, Rothfield N, et al. Special article: the 1982 revised criteria for the classification of systemic lupus erthematosus. Arthritis Rheum. 1982; 25:1271–7.
22. Sultan SM, Ioannou Y, Isenberg DA. A review of gastrointestinal manifestations of systemic lupus erythematosus. Rheumatology (Oxford) 1999;38:917.
23. Johnson A, Cavalcanti F, Gordon C, Nived O, Sturfelt G, Viner N, et al. Cross-sectional analysis of the differences between patients with systemic lupus erythematosus in England, Brazil and Sweden. Lupus. 1994;3:501–6.
24. Fries J, Holman HR. Systemic lupus erythematosus: a clinical analysis. Philadelphia: WB Saunders; 1975.
25. Vitali C, Doria A, Tincani A, Fabbri P, Balestrieri B, Galeazzi M, et al. International survey on the management of patients with SLE. I. General data on the participating centres and the results of questionnaire regarding mucocutaneous involvement. Clin Exp Rheumatol. 1996;14 Suppl 16:S17–22.
26. Jakes J, Dubois E, Quismorio FJ. Antileprosy drugs and lupus erythematosus. Ann Intern Med. 1982;97:788.
27. Luce E, Presti C, Montemayor I, Crawford M. Detecting cardiac valvular pathology in patients with systemic lupus erythematosus. Spec Care Dentist. 1992;12:193–7.
28. Chua S, Dodd H, Saeed IT, Chakravarty K. Dysphagia in a patient with lupus and review of the literature. Lupus. 2002;11(5):322–4.
29. Castrucci G, Alimandi L, Fichera A, Altomonte L, Zoli A. Changes in esophageal motility in patients with systemic lupus erythematosus: an esophago-manometric study. Minerva Dietol Gastroenterol. 1990;36:3–7.
30. Ramirez-Mata M, Reyes P, Alarcon-Segovia D, Garva R. Esophageal motility in systemic lupus erythematosus. Am J Dig Dis. 1974;19:132–6.
31. Lapadula G, Muolo P, Semeraro F, Covelli M, Brindicci D, Cuccorese G, et al. Esophageal motility disorders in the rheumatic diseases: a review of 150 patients. Clin Exp Rheumatol. 1994;12:512–21.
32. Kahrilas PJ, Shaheen NJ, Vaezi MF. American Gastroenterological Associations Institute technical review on the management of gastroesophageal reflux disease. Gastroenterology. 2008;135(4):1392–413. 1413.e1–e5.
33. Gutierrez F, Valenzuela J, Ehresmann G, Quismorio F, Kitridou R. Esophageal dysfunction in patients with mixed connective tissue diseases and systemic lupus erythematosus. Dig Dis Sci. 1982;27:592–7.
34. Montecucco C, Caporali R, Cobianchi F, Negri C, Astaldi-Ricotti G. Antibodies to hn-RNP protein A1 in systemic lupus erythematosus: clinical association with Raynaud's phenomenon and esophageal dysmotility. Clin Exp Rheumatol. 1992;10:223–7.
35. Saab S, Corr MP, Weisman MH. Corticosteroids and systemic lupus erythematosus. J Rheumatol. 1998;25:801.
36. Chey W, Wong B. American College of Gastroenterology guideline on the management of *Helicobacter pylori* infection. Am J Gastroenterol. 2007;102:1808–25.
37. Endo H, Kondo Y, Kawagoe K, Ohya TR, Yanagawa T, Asayama M, Hisatomi K, Teratani T, Yoneda M, Inamori M, Nakajima A, Matsuhashi N. Lupus enteritis detected by capsule endoscopy. Intern Med. 2007;46:1621–2.
38. Buck AC, Serebro LH, Quinet RJ. Subacute abdominal pain requiring hospitalization in a systemic lupus erythematosus patient: a retrospective analysis and review of the literature. Lupus. 2001;10:491–5.
39. Kwok SK, Seo SH, Ju JH, Park KS, Yoon CH, Kim WU, Min JK, Park SH, Cho CS, Kim HY. Lupus enteritis: clinical characteristics, risk factor for relapse and association with anti-endothelial cell antibody. Lupus. 2007;16:803–9.
40. Del Papa N, Guidali L, Sala A, Buccellati C, Khamashta MA, Ichikawa K, Koike T, Balestrieri G, Tincani A, Hughes GR, Meroni PL. Endothelial cells as target for antiphospholipid antibodies. Human polyclonal and monoclonal anti-beta 2-glycoprotein I antibodies react in vitro with endothelial cells through adherent beta 2-glycoprotein I and induce endothelial activation. Arthritis Rheum. 1997;40:551–61.

41. Medina F, Ayala A, Jara LJ, Becerra M, Miranda JM, Fraga A. Acute abdomen in systemic lupus erythematosus: the importance of early laparotomy. Am J Med. 1997;103:100–5.
42. Kim YG, Ha HK, Nah SS, Lee CK, Moon HB, Yoo B. Acute abdominal pain in systemic lupus erythematosus: factors contributing to recurrence of lupus enteritis. Ann Rheum Dis. 2006;65:1537–8.
43. Medeiros DA, Isenberg DA. Systemic lupus erythematosus and ulcerative colitis. Lupus. 2009;18:762–3.
44. Garcia-Porrua C, Gonzalez-Gay MA, Lancho A, Alvarez-Ferreira J. Systemic lupus erythematosus and ulcerative colitis: an uncommon association. Clin Exp Rheumatol. 1998;16:511.
45. Stevens HP, Ostlere LS, Rustin MH. Systemic lupus erythematosus in association with ulcerative colitis: related autoimmune diseases. Br J Dermatol. 1994;130:385–9.
46. Siurala M, Julkunen H, Tolvonen S, Pelkonen R, Saxen E, Pitkanen E. Digestive tract in collagen diseases. Acta Med Scand. 1965;178:13–25.
47. Rustgi AK, Peppercorn MA. Gluten-sensitive enteropathy and systemic lupus erythematosus. Arch Intern Med. 1988;148:1583–4.
48. Schuppan D. Current concepts in celiac disease pathogenesis. Gastroenterology. 2000;119(1):234–42.
49. Zheng WJ, Tian XP, Li L, Jing HL, Li F, Zeng XF, Tang FL. Protein-losing enteropathy in systemic lupus erythematosus: analysis of the clinical features of fifteen patients. J Clin Rheumatol. 2007;13:313–6.
50. Hung J, Wood CA, Woronik V, Vieira Jr JM, Barros RT. Protein-losing gastroenteropathy in a patient with systemic lupus erythematosus and antiphospholipid antibody syndrome simulating nephrotic syndrome. Nephrol Dial Transplant. 2006;21:2027–8.
51. Alexopoulou A, Andrianakos A, Dourakis SP. Intestinal pseudo-obstruction and ureterohydronephrosis as the presenting manifestations of relapse in a lupus patient. Lupus. 2004;13:954–6.
52. Park FD, Lee JK, Madduri GD, Ghosh P. Generalized megaviscera of lupus: refractory intestinal pseudo-obstruction, ureterohydronephrosis and megacholedochus. World J Gastroenterol. 2009;15:3555–9.
53. Ceccato F, Salas A, Góngora V, Ruta S, Roverano S, Marcos JC, Garcìa M, Paira S. Chronic intestinal pseudo-obstruction in patients with systemic lupus erythematosus: report of four cases. Clin Rheumatol. 2008;27:399–402.
54. Shahram F, Akbarian M, Davatchi F. Salmonella infection in systemic lupus erythematosus. Lupus. 1993;2:55–9.
55. Breuer GS, Baer A, Dahan D, Nesher G. Lupus-associated pancreatitis. Autoimmun Rev. 2006;5:314–8.
56. van Hoek B. The spectrum of liver disease in systemic lupus erythematosus. Neth J Med. 1996;48:244–53.
57. Miller MH, Urowitz MB, Gladman DD, Blendis LM. The liver in systemic lupus erythematosus. Q J Med. 1984;53:401–9.
58. Runyon BA, Larecque DR, Anuras S. The spectrum of liver disease in systemic lupus erythematosus. Report of 33 histologically proven cases and review of the literature. Am J Med. 1980;69:187.
59. Mackay IR, Taft LI, Cowling DC. Lupoid hepatitis and the hepatic lesions of systemic lupus erythematosus. Lancet. 1959;7063:65–9.
60. Irving KS, Sen D, Tahir H, Pilkington C, Isenberg DA. A comparison of autoimmune liver disease in juvenile and adult populations with systemic lupus erythematosus—a retrospective review of cases. Rheumatology (Oxford). 2007;46:1171–3.
61. Arnett FC, Reichlin M. Lupus hepatitis: an under-recognized disease feature associated with autoantibodies to ribosomal P. Am J Med. 1995;99:465–72.
62. Kaw R, Gota C, Bennett A, Barnes L, Calabrese L. Lupus-related hepatitis: complication of lupus or autoimmune association? Case report and review of the literature. Dig Dis Sci. 2006;51(4):813–8.
63. Hallegua DS, Wallace DJ. Gastrointestinal manifestations of systemic lupus erythematosus. Curr Opin Rheumatol. 2000;12:379–85.

Chapter 13
Neuropsychiatric Aspects of Lupus

S. Khoshbin

Systemic lupus erythematosus is one of the autoimmune disorders affecting the nervous system. However, in the field of clinical neuroimmunology, lupus presents a particularly complex problem in that it affects the nervous system at multiple levels, with a possible separate neuropathological process underlying each. Clinically, the neurologist and the psychiatrist have to consider SLE in the differential diagnosis of the commonest neuropsychiatric symptoms. In addition, both neurologists and psychiatrists are called upon in consultation to diagnose and manage nervous system complications due to the involvement of other organ systems, or secondary to therapy. Most of the neuropsychiatric symptoms seen in patients with lupus are a result of metabolic complications of the disease or hypertension, or opportunistic infections secondary to immunosuppressive therapy (or the side effects of therapy).

The prevalence of neuropsychiatric lupus has been the subject of multiple recent studies. Meta-analytic reviews have given a range of 10–80 % involvement. It appears that this wide range is primarily due to the different classifications. In 1999, the American College of Rheumatology, using case definitions, identified the 19 neuropsychiatric syndromes, 12 involving the central nervous system and 7 involving the peripheral nervous system (Table 13.1).

In addition, recognition was made of neuropsychiatric syndromes due to primary involvement of the nervous system, as opposed to neuropsychiatric syndromes secondary to the involvement of other organs first. Also, this nomenclature allowed identification of the most common syndromes, which includes cognitive dysfunction, headache, mood disorders, seizures, and cerebrovascular disease.

S. Khoshbin, M.D. (✉)
Department of Neurology, Brigham and Women's Hospital,
75 Francis Street, Boston, MA 02115, USA

Harvard Medical School, Boston, MA, USA
e-mail: skhoshbin@partners.org

Table 13.1 Neuropsychiatric syndromes in SLE

Central NP events	Peripheral NP events
Aseptic meningitis	Guillain–Barré syndrome
Cerebrovascular disease	Autonomic neuropathy
Demyelinating syndrome	Mononeuropathy
Headache	Myasthenia gravis
Movement disorder	Cranial neuropathy
Myelopathy	Plexopathy
Seizure disorders	Polyneuropathy
Acute confusional state	
Anxiety disorder	
Cognitive dysfunction	
Mood disorder	
Psychosis	

Source: The American College of Rheumatology nomenclature and case definitions for neuropsychiatric lupus syndromes. Arthritis Rheum. 1999; 42(4): 599–608

Historically, references to nervous system involvement started with M. Kaposi's descriptions in 1875. He published in a book edited by his father-in-law, von Hebra, who had described the butterfly rash. In a series of three articles between 1895 and 1903, Sir William Osler defined the disorder and in his third communication addressed the involvement of the nervous system, pointing out the association between seizures and psychiatric manifestations of lupus. In the 1920s and 1940s, a series of findings further elucidated etiologies of nervous system involvement, such as the description of Libman–Sacks endocarditis. As different tests for diagnosis became available, the association between nervous system disorders and diagnosis of SLE became clinically possible. In the 1950s, introduction of cortisone for the treatment of lupus by Herrick and Thorn started the modern age of treatment. In the last 20 years, identification of antibodies to nuclear elements in the neurons, identification of antiphospholipid antibodies, and the availability most recently of monoclonal antibodies in treatment, and research in other neuroimmunological disorders such as MS and CNS-AIDS have contributed to a more clear understanding of this complex picture.

Pathophysiology

Original assumptions that the nervous system pathology was mainly due to vasculitis were overturned after the landmark study of Johnson and Richardson, demonstrating that true vasculitis, although present, was a rare finding. When present, associated signs of peripheral vasculitis, such as Osler nodes and Janeway lesions, are seen. The modern view indicates vascular injury of intracranial vessels, with the prevailing pathology being that of lesions in the walls of small vessels and perivascular inflammation, and multiple microinfarcts. It was felt that the vasculopathy, in addition to direct damage, also affects the blood–brain barrier and alters "immunological privilege" of the nervous system. Also, the discovery of autoantibodies to neuronal antigens, phospholipid-associated proteins and ribosomes, such as antibodies to human neuroblastoma cells, lymphocytotoxic antibodies, and anti-ribosomal P antibodies has been associated with psychosis, cognitive dysfunction by some investigators, but not others. Antiphospholipid antibodies are associated with strokes and to some possible degree with other neuropsychiatric SLE features. In addition, intracerebral production of inflammatory mediators suggests a role for proinflammatory cytokines. Other mediators of inflammation, such as chemokines, APRIL, BAFF, neuropeptides, nitric oxide, and oxidative stress, also probably play a role in the pathogenesis of neuropsychiatric lupus. More recent studies have identified additional risk factors for neuropsychiatric lupus which in general include associated diabetes, older white patients, and the presence of active disease.

Clinical Syndromes

Cerebrovascular Disease

Ischemic cerebrovascular accidents, transient ischemic attacks, and hemorrhagic strokes are seen in patients with lupus. Like other neuropsychiatric manifestations, most strokes occur within the first 5 years of the illness. Autopsy studies show both small vessel disease and large vessel disease and embolic strokes such as infarcts seen in the context of Libman–Sacks endocarditis, and also both intracerebral and subarachnoid hemorrhages are seen. Stroke due to vasculitis is rare, and the syndrome of CNS vasculitis has a distinct picture of severe headaches, fever, confusional episodes, rapid progression to psychotic symptoms, onset of seizures, and coma. In these cases, evidence of activity of SLE is present, and the cerebrospinal fluid is abnormal. Additionally, most other stroke types are noted in the context of active lupus, and with the presence of risk factors, including advanced age, hypertension, smoking, renal disease, decreased albumin, decreased white cell count, low levels of high-density lipids, advanced age, cardiac valvular disease, and the presence of antiphospholipid antibodies.

The evaluation of patients requires imaging studies with MRI and diffusion-weighted images. Also, magnetic resonance angiography and CT angiography are available in most centers and should be done. Management of stroke in the lupus patient is similar to that of the general population—assessment for use of thrombolytic therapy in the first few hours, and/or endarterectomy and stenting done in the same manner as for other patients with stroke. The use of glucocorticoids or other immunosuppressive therapy is dependent on the activity of the lupus. In patients with antiphospholipid antibody syndrome, additional evaluation is required than just the test for lupus anticoagulants to include anticardiolipin/beta-2, glycoprotein-1, and anti-phosphatidylserine/prothrombin antibodies, the presence of which shows a greater association with cerebral infarction. In addition, these antibodies result in activation of platelets, thus contributing to a hypercoagulable state. Other risk factors such as elevated plasma homocysteine, hypertension, accelerated atherosclerosis (both associated with chronic glucocorticoid therapy), infections, and valvular heart disease increase stroke risk.

Small vessel disease and recurrent lacunes manifesting as stereotypic TIAs are common among lupus patients with or without antiphospholipid syndrome. A number of these patients would also show cognitive defects.

Stroke due to vasculitis is rare. There is usually evidence of active lupus with hypocomplementemia and elevated anti-dsDNA antibody. Imaging studies will show evidence of vasculitis. The electroencephalogram is usually abnormal, and so is cerebrospinal fluid. Rarely, there will be a need for conventional cerebral angiography or single-photon emission computed tomography (SPECT).

Management of Cerebrovascular Disease

In patients with antiphospholipid antibody syndrome with no stroke, treatment with low-dose aspirin (81 mg/day) is recommended. In patients with ischemic stroke, with no other risk factors, and MRI consistent with small vessel disease, also low-dose aspirin is recommended. However, in patients with lupus with moderate or high levels of antiphospholipid, anticoagulation with warfarin with an INR target of 2–3 is advisable. If there is an associated lupus flare, glucocorticoids and sometimes cyclophosphamide have been used, but not in the absence of active lupus.

Seizure Disorders

Seizures are considered a classification criterion for diagnosis of lupus, according to the American College of Rheumatology classification criteria. Generalized seizures are more commonly seen in CNS involvement as a secondary manifestation. However, partial seizures and complex partial seizures at times with secondary generalization are considered to be among the primary presentations of lupus. Seizures are reported in approximately 10–20 % of lupus patients. The etiologies are varied. Risk factors include history of acute inflammatory episodes; history of previous CNS damage, such as stroke and head trauma; and also metabolic causes such as uremia, hypertension, medication withdrawal, and drug toxicity. Studies have also shown an association with antiphospholipid, anti-50-kDA, and anti-SM antibodies. Like stroke, seizures occur within the first 5 years of the disease.

Vasculitis can present with seizures. However, in the absence of systemic vasculitis or other evidence of lupus flare, this is extremely rare. In our experience, complex partial seizures are more common than primary generalized seizures, and at times, they could be the initial manifestation of SLE. There is also a strong association with psychiatric aspects, particularly psychosis, and focal EEG abnormalities. Treatment with antimalarials has also resulted in a decrease in generalized seizures. The workup of patients who present with seizures is the same as for patients in the general populations. They should include imaging studies such as magnetic resonance imaging. An electroencephalogram should be done on all patients. In the absence of epileptogenic abnormalities on EEG, one may not need to initiate antiepileptic therapy in patients with a single seizure. However, patients at high risk for recurrence, such as two or more unprovoked seizures occurring in rapid succession, or within the first 24 h, and also the presence of structural abnormalities on brain MRI causally linked to the seizure, or the presence of focal neurological signs after a seizure or in a patient's general examination. An abnormal EEG showing focality or overt epileptogenic activity and a clinically focal seizure should be reason to initiate antiepileptic therapy. In patients with recurrent seizures, chronic antiepileptic therapy, usually monotherapy with one of the standard antiepileptics, is indicated. However, in complex partial seizures that are resistant to monotherapy, a second anticonvulsant is added. In the absence of active lupus, glucocorticoid or immunosuppressive therapy is not indicated. In seizures during lupus flare, however, that are resistant to therapy, glucocorticoids have been added to the regimen. Of the standard anticonvulsants, phenytoin and carbamazepine are the common treatments. The new anticonvulsants, including levetiracetam and lamotrigine, can be useful adjuncts to therapy.

Headaches

Using the American College of Rheumatology case definitions to establish the prevalence of neurologic and psychiatric manifestations, headaches are the commonest disorder next to cognitive dysfunction. Although meta-analysis studies using the criteria of the International Headache Society did not find a specific correlation with a headache type, and the same prevalence in the general population, clearly a greater majority of patients complain of symptoms suggestive of migraine, and next suggestive of tension headaches. No definite association of headaches was made with active lupus. Therefore, complaints of headache alone in patients with SLE do not seem to require additional investigation beyond evaluations performed for patients without SLE. However, rare known complications of lupus that may present with acute headaches have to be ruled out, particularly the question of venous thrombosis in patients with antiphospholipid antibodies, meningitis, or intracerebral or subarachnoid hemorrhage. The presence of focal neurological signs should alert the physician to the need for imaging studies. The presence of fever or meningismus would indicate the need for CSF evaluation. In the treatment of headaches, the same approaches as for patients without lupus should be used. Triptans for acute headaches and prophylactic medications such as tricyclics or some anticonvulsants such as valproate, topiramate, and gabapentin have been commonly prescribed with good result.

Cognitive Dysfunction

It is generally agreed that cognitive dysfunction is the most prevalent neuropsychiatric complaint among lupus patients. Patients complain of difficulty with short- and long-term memory, problems with executive function, evidence of cortical function difficulties such as dysphagias, apraxias, and agnosias have been seen in these patients. Multiple studies have showed a range of 20–80 % involvement based on neuropsychological evaluation. Although some associations with autoantibodies and the presence of cognitive dysfunction have been made, no definite association has been established, including association with vascular abnormalities, endocrine factors, matrix metalloproteinases, or cytokines. Also, as in headaches, there is no definite association with lupus flare. However, it has been noted more in patients with active disease on corticosteroids. In patients with complaints of memory dysfunction, a past history of CNS disease has been associated with long-term memory complaints, while difficulties with concentration, focusing, and short-term memory are noted with disease activity. In patients with small vessel disease and hypertension, and in patients with polypharmacy, cognitive dysfunctions are more common. For that reason, studies have indicated the beneficial effect of the use of aspirin to prevent cognitive decline in older patients. In general, the management involves reducing the number of medications in patients with polypharmacy. However, in patients with antiphospholipid antibody, and also in patients with antineuronal antibodies, a short course of steroids (0.5 mg/kg for a few weeks) has been considered beneficial. Neuropsychological evaluation, including standardized tests such as the Wechsler Adult Intelligence Scale, the Stanford–Binet Intelligence Test, pattern comparison tasks, and complex attention tasks, has been utilized. In our patients, using a battery of neuropsychological tests and electroencephalography, a predominance of left hemispheric EEG findings have been noted associated with word-finding difficulty in lupus patients. The American College of Rheumatology has recommended a neuropsychological battery for diagnosing cognitive dysfunction. This 1-h battery has shown high sensitivity and specificity. In young patients with rapid cognitive decline, imaging studies are indicated.

Psychiatric Manifestations

Delirium

Historically, Kaposi used the term "delirium" in describing changes in mental state in patients with lupus. However, the term has come to be used imprecisely to describe a host of CNS symptoms in patients with lupus. A review of the literature reveals that the term is used primarily to indicate an acute confusional state. It is important to recognize that acute confusional state and other agitated states may be the result of focal neurological damage, including stroke. Secondary encephalopathies are frequent in lupus, primarily metabolic encephalopathy due to hepatic or renal complications. However, toxic encephalopathies and also encephalitis and other autoimmune encephalopathies such as Hashimoto's disease and paraneoplastic syndromes, and also encephalitis (including HSV) may also occur in patients with lupus and may present with an agitated state. The EEG is very helpful in evaluating these different syndromes. Additionally, imaging studies and analysis of the CSF are mandatory for differentiating these syndromes. One may see generalized abnormalities or the presence of bitemporal or unilateral right or left abnormalities in patients with acute confusional state or agitated states.

Psychosis

Although not the most prevalent psychiatric symptom, psychosis is considered a classification criterion for diagnosis of lupus, according to the American College of Rheumatology classification criteria. Psychosis usually develops within the first 2 years of diagnosis. In one study, 61 % occurred within the first year, and some may have recurrent episodes. The classic pictures of delusional thinking and the presence of hallucinations, and also recurrent episodes of clouding of consciousness typically occurring at night are the cardinal manifestations. Patients also show easy distractibility, agitation, and illusions.

Complications of steroid therapy, "steroid psychosis," has to be ruled out. In most instances, if an increase in the steroid dose results in worsening of symptoms, and/or if auditory hallucinations are present, that is an indication of steroid psychosis. In lupus psychosis, visual and tactile hallucinations are more frequent. There has been an association made between the presence of psychosis in lupus and antibodies to ribosomal P protein in some but not all studies. Also, an association has been demonstrated to neuronal cells. Psychosis has been treated with corticosteroids (prednisone 1–2 mg/kg/day for a few weeks in divided doses). In the case of lack of improvement, pulse cyclophosphamide has been used. In resistant patients, in addition to oral cytotoxic drugs, IV pulse cyclophosphamide and even plasmapheresis have been tried. If long-term maintenance is required, azathioprine may be a safer alternative than long-term cyclophosphamide. In addition, the use of antipsychotic drugs to manage fluctuating symptoms should be used with careful monitoring of EKG as significant prolongation of q-t interval may occur with such medications as the new atypical antipsychotics (clozapine, quetiapine, ziprasidone) and the more traditional haloperidol, thioridazine, and risperidone. Also, tricyclic antidepressants, lithium, amphetamines, and SSRIs may cause prolonged QT syndrome. Additional risk factors for this complication are electrolyte imbalance and patients with hypothyroidism.

Depression

By far, a more common psychiatric complication is depression. It can be multifactorial, part of a reaction to chronic illness and lifestyle limitations. Additional risk factors are excessive fatigue caused by depression and/or causing depression, limited sun exposure, polypharmacy complicating other depression symptoms, and pregnancy. Associations have been made with autoantibodies, including anti-ribosomal P, and antibodies to NMDA receptors. There has also been an association made with secondary Sjogren's syndrome. In severe depression which is resistant to therapy, medical workup, including careful neurological examination, and obtaining imaging studies and EEG for focal neurological abnormalities, is indicated. The treatment in general is the same as that in the general population. Family and social support are an important part of the therapy. However, somatoform complaints including anorexia, insomnia, myalgia, arthralgia, and constipation are more common among lupus patients. Suicidal ideations and depression with psychotic features are rare and require formal psychiatric intervention and possible hospitalization.

Anxiety Disorders

These are usually seen early postdiagnosis, or with flares, and may be associated with depression. However, more so than the depressive syndromes, one is obligated to rule out the possibility of partial seizures, acute confusional state, and other encephalopathies. Therefore, careful neurological examination, imaging, and EEG in patients with prolonged symptoms of anxiety are recommended. Treatment is as for the general population. However, additional somatic symptoms such as hyperventilation, recurrent dizziness, palpitations, diarrhea, and, on rare occasions, the development of phobias, compulsive behavior, hypochondriasis, and, commonly, sleep disorders are noted in patients with lupus with anxiety disorders.

Rare Psychiatric Manifestations

Bipolar disorder and personality disorders, usually manifesting in irritability, insomnia, and marked increase in activity (mania), are also noted in lupus. However, side effects of steroids should be considered. Personality changes including development of apathy and emotional lability are noted. In patients with complex partial seizures, interictal personality dysfunctions hallmarked by religiosity, sexual indiscretion, and aggressivity have all been seen.

Imaging studies in the assessment of psychiatric disorders have low sensitivity and specificity. Only if focal neurological signs or other evidence of CNS disease is to be ruled out should imaging be used. On the other hand, an electroencephalogram may be helpful in differentiating other etiologies, such as partial seizures and encephalopathies.

In addition to psychopharmacological intervention, some studies have shown that cognitive therapy with biofeedback has been helpful. Recently, rituximab has been shown to improve psychiatric manifestations. In general, most psychiatric episodes resolve within a month. However, in persistent cases, continued treatment with SSRIs or tricyclics, especially when concomitant sleep abnormalities or pain syndromes are present is warranted. Continued treatment with SSRIs or benzodiazepines in the case of generalized anxiety is recommended.

Peripheral Nervous System Involvement in Lupus

This primarily manifests itself in the form of neuropathies. The etiology is presumed to be the involvement of vasa nervorum. However, axonal as well as demyelinating and autonomic neuropathies are also noted. The predominating picture is usually that of polyneuropathy and/or mononeuritis multiplex with sensory nerves involved more than the motor nerves. Patients complain of numbness and paresthesias, worse in the evenings. Painful neuropathy indicating small fiber involvement is also seen. Nerve conduction and electromyographic studies are helpful in patients with large fiber neuropathy. However, these studies may be negative in painful neuropathies of small fibers. Skin biopsies have been used for diagnosis of small fiber neuropathy. Neuropathies are usually noted late in the course of SLE.

Rarely, inflammatory polyradiculoneuropathy is also seen. Both Guillain–Barré syndrome and chronic inflammatory demyelinating polyradiculopathy (CIDP) have been reported in SLE patients. CIDP is characterized by abnormal sensory function in upper and lower extremities, and progressive weakness, usually in the lower extremities, along with loss of deep tendon reflexes and excessive fatigue. In patients showing acute onset of ascending areflexic motor weakness, glucocorticoids are used. In patients with recurrent symptoms suggestive of CIDP or recurrent mononeuritis multiplex, additionally intravenous gamma globulins and plasmapheresis have been utilized. In patients with axonal neuropathies that are resistant to therapy, nerve biopsy may show evidence of vasculitis, indicating the need for additional immunosuppressive therapy such as cyclophosphamide. Mild neuropathies may require glucocorticoids in moderate doses. Additionally, one can recommend symptomatic treatment with gabapentin in doses up to 1,800 mg/day and tricyclics such as amitriptyline.

Rare Neurologic Symptoms

Movement Disorders

A number of different dyskinesias are seen in lupus patients, including chorea, athetosis, dystonia, and hemiballismus. Rarely, akinesia in the form of dopamine-resistant Parkinsonism has been seen. Dyskinesias are usually seen during active disease. There has been some association with antiphospholipid antibodies, raising the question of the need for anticoagulant treatment. Imaging studies should be done in patients with movement disorders. Chorea is the most prevalent of these disorders. Imaging is needed in the evaluation of these patients in order to rule out infarcts and other focal neurological lesions. Chorea is usually self-limited. However, treatment with glucocorticoids and, in the case of resistance, with azathioprine or cyclophosphamide has been used.

Cranial Neuropathies

Although rare, the presence of cranial neuropathies as a presenting symptom creates a diagnostic dilemma in the differentiation of SLE from multiple sclerosis. Optic neuritis and internuclear ophthalmoplegia occur in both conditions. Additionally, transverse myelitis also occurs in both lupus and MS. In cases when MRI abnormalities are also suggestive of MS, the term "lupoid sclerosis" has been used. These patients may require CSF analysis and other studies to rule out Lyme disease, sarcoidosis, myasthenia gravis, meningitis, optic neuritis, internuclear ophthalmoplegia, and transverse myelitis. As with all cranial neuropathies, imaging studies to rule out brainstem and base-of-skull lesions should be done. In addition to optic nerve involvement, sensory neural hearing loss is more common in SLE than in the general population. Also, functional disorders with tunnel vision, monocular diplopia, and convergence spasm are rarely seen in neuropsychiatric lupus. In the treatment of cranial neuropathies, glucocorticoids are used (e.g., prednisone 0.5–1 mg/kg/day). If there is a risk of visual loss in optic neuritis, or persistent progressive cranial neuropathy, cyclophosphamide has been added. Of note, multiple ophthalmological disorders are seen among lupus patients, either as a result of the disease or complications of glucocorticoid or antimalarial treatment. Keratoconjunctivitis sicca presents with patients complaining of foreign body sensation and itching similar to Sjogren's syndrome. Anterior uveitis with complaints of photophobia and pain, and decreased vision, is common. Posterior segment involvement, usually retinal vasculopathy, with findings of cotton-wool exudates, indicating microangiopathy, is seen in lupus. Fluorescent angiography is indicated to rule out retinal vascular disease. Rare symptoms of autoimmune retinopathy have been noted.

As a complication of therapy, worsening glaucoma and cataract formation are seen with glucocorticoids. Fibrinous exudative retinal detachment has been seen. In addition, routine ophthalmological assessment in patients on antimalarial drugs for the corneal and retinal side effects is indicated. Caution is advised in patients with SLE in laser ablation for correction of refractive error, as increasing complications have been reported.

Transverse Myelitis

A sudden onset of paraparesis with sensory loss plus possible incontinence of bowel and bladder should make one suspect transverse myelitis. This usually occurs in active lupus. The pathophysiology is assumed to be that of an arteritis. Also association with antiphospholipid antibodies has been made in some but not all studies. Other causes of myelopathy such as disc herniation, hematomas, and infections have to be ruled out. Imaging studies are mandatory, and CSF analysis (typically showing marked protein elevation and pleocytosis) is strongly indicated. Myelitis may recur within a year. In addition, Devic's syndrome (neuromyelitis optica) has occurred in SLE and antiphospholipid syndrome. Transverse myelitis is recommended to be treated rapidly and aggressively. We and others have had success utilizing a combination of prednisone (1.5 mg/kg/day), cyclophosphamide, and plasmapheresis. In patients with antiphospholipid antibodies, warfarin has been added to glucocorticoid and immunosuppressive treatment.

Meningitis

Aseptic meningitis is noted in SLE. However, acute bacterial meningitis in SLE patients, especially those treated with corticosteroids and immunosuppressive agents, opportunistic infections such as cryptococcal meningitis, listeria, monocytogenes, and also reactivation of tuberculosis should be ruled out. Therefore, CSF analysis in patients with symptoms suggestive of meningismus, headache, and fever becomes mandatory. Aseptic meningitis has been noted in association with certain treatments, including azathioprine, ibuprofen, and other NSAIDs (excluding aspirin).

Cases of reversible posterior leukoencephalopathy have been reported with lupus. These patients present with headaches, visual disturbance, seizures, and mental status changes in the context of hypertension, renal failure, and immunosuppressive medication. The characteristic MRI finding of vasogenic cerebral edema is helpful in the diagnosis and differentiating from CNS infarct.

Dementia

In patients with lupus, with severe cognitive dysfunction, with impaired memory, judgment, and abstract thinking, progressive decline, the diagnosis of dementia usually reflects multiple small ischemic strokes and is associated with antiphospholipid antibodies. The symptoms may be worsened by high-dose corticosteroids and other treatments. Also, coexisting depression should be ruled out. The presence of livedo reticularis with antiphospholipid antibodies and ischemic small-vessel cerebrovascular disease best seen on MRI constitutes Sneddon's syndrome, which presents with a picture of vascular dementia. In cases with antiphospholipid antibodies, the treatment should be as for any antiphospholipid antibody-associated stroke with warfarin and glucocorticosteroids. In antiphospholipid-antibody-negative Sneddon's syndrome, clopidogrel has been used.

Evaluation

Serologic Testing

In diagnosing nervous system involvement in lupus, serologic studies used to establish the diagnosis of lupus are the first step. Antinuclear antibody titer (ANA), though very sensitive, is not specific. Patients with CNS symptoms and weakly positive ANA are often misdiagnosed as CNS lupus. Serum levels of anti-DNA and anti-SM antibodies, and low levels of complement, are more specific for the diagnosis of SLE. Antiphospholipid antibodies have been associated with stroke, dementia, seizures, chorea, transverse myelitis, and headaches. Anti-ribosomal P antibodies have been associated with psychosis and depression, although it has limited sensitivity and specificity. Anti-NMDA receptor antibodies and antineuronal antibodies are of uncertain importance but have been associated with cognitive dysfunction, depression, and other neuropsychiatric manifestations in some, but not all, studies. In patients with migraine, cognitive difficulty, and peripheral neuropathy, associations have been made with antiganglioside antibodies. Also, antibodies to microtubule-associated protein 2 have been associated with neuropsychiatric SLE.

CSF Analysis

In cases of suspected meningitis, transverse myelitis, and vasculitis, CSF abnormalities are required for diagnosis. A number of abnormalities in patients with lupus have been reported in CSF, including elevated anti-DNA antibodies, IgG oligoclonal banding, interleukin-6, and markers of B-cell activation. In a prospective study of 52 patients with neuropsychiatric disease, all 52 had abnormal CSF IgG index oligoclonal bands, increased antineuronal antibodies, and/or anti-ribosomal P antibodies. CSF levels of neurofilament triplet protein (NFL) are higher in patients with CNS lupus. This is also accompanied by higher intrathecal concentration of interleukin-6, interleukin-8, and oligoclonal immunoglobulins. However, at this time, these studies have little clinical usefulness because of low sensitivities and specificities and are still considered in the research phase.

Imaging Studies

Magnetic resonance imaging has revolutionized assessment of all neuroimmune disorders. However, in lupus patients without neuropsychiatric symptoms, nonspecific white matter changes and periventricular hyperintensities are seen. These are, as mentioned above, nonspecific and no action may be indicated. However, microvascular changes manifesting as nonspecific T2 signal abnormalities are now recognized, particularly in patients with migraine and in patients with lupus who have migraine. Some studies have correlated diffuse, high-signal intensity in the white matter on MRI with activity of lupus as assessed by the systemic lupus erythematosus disease activity index (SLEDAI). MRI scans also have been useful in detecting cerebral edema in lupus patients with seizures, psychosis, and encephalopathy. Advanced neuroimaging techniques are becoming available, including DTI (diffusion tensor imaging). Routine use of these studies has not been evaluated in lupus patients. However, the promise of more specific findings in diffusion tensor MRI, quantitative MRI, magnetic resonance spectroscopy, and magnetization transfer imaging in further evaluation of lupus patients is exciting.

Electroencephalography

Abnormalities of the EEG are present in 80 % of patients with lupus. Diffuse slow-wave activity is noted with encephalopathies, and electroencephalogram can be used to differentiate metabolic from hypoxic and toxic causes of encephalopathy. Focal changes in patients with stroke and seizures are important, and the presence of epileptogenic activity is helpful in initiating anticonvulsant therapy. EEG is sensitive but not specific. Additionally, quantitative EEG may increase the sensitivity. In our studies with quantitative EEG, we found a better correlation with neuropsychiatric lupus determined by other criteria.

Evoked potential studies are also quite helpful in detecting pathway lesions. Additionally, evoked potential mapping increases the sensitivity for detecting abnormalities. The EEG can be a useful tool in the differential diagnosis of psychiatric manifestations.

Sources

1. Khoshbin S, Glanz BI, Schur PH. Neuropsychiatric syndromes in systemic lupus erythematosus: a new look. Clin Exp Rheumatol. 1999;17:395–8.
2. Appenzeller S, Costallat LTL, Cendes F. Neurolupus. Arch Neurol. 2006;63:458–60.
3. Bertsias GK, Ioannidis JPA, Aringer M, et al. EULAR recommendations for the management of systemic lupus erythematosus with neuropsychiatric manifestations: report of a task force of the EULAR standing committee for clinical affairs. Ann Rheum Dis. 2010;69:2074–82.
4. The American College of Rheumatology nomenclature and case definitions for neuropsychiatric lupus syndromes. Arthritis Rheum 1999;42(4):599–608.
5. Kozora E, Ellison MC, West S. Reliability and validity of the proposed American College of Rheumatology neuropsychological battery for systemic lupus erythematosus. Arthritis Rheum. 2004;51:810–8.
6. Unterman A, Nolte JES, Boaz M, et al. Neuropsychiatric syndromes in systemic lupus erythematosus: a meta-analysis. Semin Arthritis Rheum. 2011;41(1):1–11.
7. Mikdashi J, Handwerger B, Langenberg P, et al. Baseline disease activity, hyperlipidemia, and hypertension are predictive factors for ischemic stroke and stroke severity in systemic lupus erythematosus. Stroke. 2007;38:281–5.

8. Krishnan E. Stroke subtypes among young patients with systemic lupus erythematosus. Am J Med. 2005;118:1415.e1–e7.
9. Roldan CA, Gelgand EA, Qualls CR, et al. Valvular heart disease as a cause of cerebrovascular disease in patients with systemic lupus erythematosus. Am J Cardiol. 2005;95:1441–7.
10. Mehta N, Uchino K, Fakhran S, et al. Platelet C4d is associated with acute ischemic stroke and stroke severity. Stroke. 2008;39:3236–41.
11. Andrade RM, Alarcon GS, Gonzalez LA, et al. Seizures in patients with systemic lupus erythematosus: data from LUMINA, a multiethnic cohort (LUMINA LIV). Ann Rheum Dis. 2008;67:829–34.
12. Climaz R, Meroni PL, Shoenfeld Y. Epilepsy as part of systemic lupus erythematosus and systemic antiphospholipid syndrome (Hughes syndrome). Lupus. 2006;15:191–7.
13. Appenzeller S, Cendes F, Costallat LTL. Epileptic seizures in systemic lupus erythematosus. Neurology. 2004;63:1808–12.
14. Mikdashi J, Krumholz A, Handwerger B. Factors at diagnosis predict subsequent occurrence of seizures in systemic lupus erythematosus. Neurology. 2005;64:2102–7.
15. Mitsikostas DD, Sfikakis PP, Goadsby PJ. A meta-analysis for headache in systemic lupus erythematosus: the evidence and the myth. Brain. 2004;127:1200–9.
16. Glanz BI, Venkatesan A, Schur PH, et al. Prevalence of migraine in patients with systemic lupus erythematosus. Headache. 2001;41:285–9.
17. Glanz BI, Schur PH, Lew RA, et al. Lateralized cognitive dysfunction in patients with systemic lupus erythematosus. Lupus. 2005;14:896–902.
18. McLaurin EY, Holliday SL, Williams P, et al. Predictors of cognitive dysfunction in patients with systemic lupus erythematosus. Neurology. 2005;64:297–303.
19. Goransson LG, Tjensvoll AB, Herigstad A, et al. Small-diameter nerve fiber neuropathy in systemic lupus erythematosus. Arch Neurol. 2006;63:401–4.
20. Birnbaum J, Petri M, Thompson R, et al. Distinct subtypes of myelitis in systemic lupus erythematosus. Arthritis Rheum. 2009;60:3378–87.
21. Glanz BI, Schur PH, Khoshbin S. EEG abnormalities in systemic lupus erythematosus. Clin Electroencephalogr. 1998;29:128–31.
22. Khoshbin S, Schur PH. Neurologic manifestations of systemic lupus erythematosus. In: Basow DS, editor. UpToDate. Waltham: UpToDate; 2011.
23. Khoshbin S, Schur PH. Neuropsychiatric manifestations of systemic lupus erythematosus. In: Basow DS, editor. UpToDate. Waltham: UpToDate; 2011.
24. Khoshbin S, Schur PH. Diagnostic approach to the neuropsychiatric manifestations of systemic lupus erythematosus. In: Basow DS, editor. UpToDate. Waltham: UpToDate; 2011.

Chapter 14
Systemic Lupus Erythematosus and Pregnancy

Bonnie L. Bermas

Systemic lupus erythematosus (SLE) disproportionally impacts women during their childbearing years. Thus, issues regarding birth control, fertility, pregnancy, and nursing commonly arise in the care of young women with SLE. For many years, contraceptive choices for SLE patients were limited due to concerns that hormone-containing methods would increase disease activity. Pregnancy itself was thought to exacerbate disease activity, and patients were often counseled that they should avoid becoming pregnant. Medication use during pregnancy and nursing were likewise thought to be limited which further complicated the management of the pregnant lupus patient. Fortunately, the past two decades have brought us a better understanding of how SLE disease activity responds during pregnancy. Newer treatment regimens have improved disease outcome and enabled more patients to contemplate pregnancy and parenthood. This chapter will discuss contraception, fertility, pregnancy, and nursing in women with SLE.

Contraception

Barrier methods, hormonal methods, and intrauterine devices can be used for contraception in SLE patients (Table 14.1). Barrier methods such as condoms and diaphragms, while less reliable than hormonal methods and intrauterine devices, have the advantage of having no impact on disease activity. Condoms in particular have the benefit of decreasing the incidence of sexually transmitted diseases, a distinct

B.L. Bermas, M.D. (✉)
Division of Rheumatology, Director, Lupus and Antiphospholipid Center,
Brigham and Women's Hospital, 75 Francis Street, Boston, MA 02115, USA

Harvard Medical School, Boston, MA, USA
e-mail: bbermas@partners.org

Table 14.1 Contraceptive methods for SLE patients

Barrier methods[a]
  Condoms
  Diaphragm
  Cervical cap

Hormonal methods
  Low-dose estrogen- and progestin-containing oral contraceptives[b]
  Progestin-only-containing IM or oral contraceptives
  Morning after pill

Intrauterine devices

[a] More effective if used in conjunction with a spermicide
[b] No available evidence for use with patients with moderately to severely active or renal disease

advantage in patients who may already be immunosuppressed. Nonetheless, their effectiveness is only 70–80 % because of compliance issues. Oral contraceptives are the most commonly employed hormonal contraceptive method. For years, practitioners avoided these medications in SLE patients because they were concerned that the estrogen contained in these medications could potentially trigger a flare. However, recent studies demonstrate that at least in the case of mild SLE, low-dose exogenous estrogens such as that contained in currently used oral contraceptives do not cause disease flares. Estrogens do increase the risk of thromboembolic events in those persons with antiphospholipid antibodies and should be avoided in individuals who have these antibodies and other risk factor for clotting. Whether oral contraceptives can be used safely in patients with more severe disease or lupus nephritis is unknown. Progestin-only-containing contraceptives do not cause disease flares and are considered safe for use in lupus patients. Intrauterine devices, while an effective form of birth control, can cause an increased incidence of infection in particular in those women that have multiple sexual partners and who are immunosuppressed.

Fertility

SLE itself does not impact fertility. Nonetheless, overall fertility rates in lupus patients are slightly decreased due to decreased fertility seen in those patients who have been treated with cyclophosphamide. Risk factors for ovarian failure after cyclophosphamide therapy include age over 30, cumulative doses of greater than 10 g of cyclophosphamide, and long duration of therapy. Whether some of the newer cyclophosphamide regimens, such as that used in the European cyclophosphamide regimens, have less of an effect on ultimate fertility is not clear. Techniques for preserving fertility include use of oral contraceptives and GNRH antagonists for the preservation of ovarian function. Less commonly, IVF with embryo cryopreservation or oocyte cryopreservation are used. This latter technique has the disadvantage of poor viability of oocytes upon thawing. Importantly, ovarian stimulation used in these methods can cause disease flares in some patients. Secondary infertility, defined as the ability to conceive but increased incidence of spontaneous abortion, is increased in women with SLE. This increase, however, is predominately related to antiphospholipid antibodies and the antiphospholipid syndrome. Management of this disorder during pregnancy is discussed in a separate chapter.

Pregnancy Changes

During pregnancy, the body undergoes immunologic and physiologic changes to support the fetus. Adjustments to usual immune surveillance that enable fetal survival occur because the fetus is a hemi-allograft. There is some evidence that the trophoblast does not respond to fetal HLA antigens. T-helper type 1 cytokines such as TNF alpha and interferon gamma involved in cell-mediated immunity are downregulated during pregnancy. This change in the immunologic milieu can impact disease activity. In addition to immunologic changes, the physiologic changes that happen with pregnancy can make assessment of disease flares challenging. Joint pain can occur with weight gain, postural changes, and the widening of the pelvis that occurs over the course of pregnancy. A physiologic anemia occurs with increased blood volume. Finally, pregnancy is a hypercoagulable state and predisposes to clotting events.

Some of the traditional markers of disease activity are also impacted by pregnancy. The erythrocyte sedimentation rate (ESR) is elevated during pregnancy and thus may not be an accurate reflection of disease activity. Complement component synthesis is also increased so that subtle drops in levels—often indicators of disease activity—may not be appreciated.

Disease Flares During Pregnancy

Significant controversy exists in the literature regarding whether or not SLE flares more frequently during pregnancy. There are several issues that make this topic difficult to assess. First, the existing studies often profile disparate patient populations or may lack appropriate control groups. Second, there is no consensus on what scale to use to define a disease flare. Moreover, items on standard disease flare assessment tools such as fatigue and achiness can be increased in pregnancy. Adjustments to standard disease activity scales have tried to compensate for these latter issues. Third, the existing case studies often do not correct for medication use. Finally, it is often difficult to predict how an individual patient will fare during pregnancy. What most experts agree upon, however, is that patients whose disease either begins during pregnancy or flares early in pregnancy tend to have complicated clinical courses. This is particularly true for systemic diseases in which multiple organ systems are involved.

Disease Flare

The disease flare rate in SLE in the nonpregnant state ranges from 0.2 to greater than 1 flare per patient-year. Therefore, during the 9 months of pregnancy, it can be expected that a certain percentage of SLE patients will flare. Some studies suggest that the flare rate during pregnancy rate is no higher than background. In several early case-controlled studies, flare rates were found to be similar to control groups. However, other studies, particularly in those done in patients with more severe disease, suggest that the flare rate is higher than background rate. In particular, those patients with active disease and renal disease are at greater risk of flaring. There does appear to be an increased flare rate in the postpartum period. Thromboembolic events in those patients with antiphospholipid syndrome also occur with higher frequency in the postpartum period. Thus, patients should be monitored closely in the first 6 weeks postpartum.

Prepregnancy Counseling

There are several tenets of management to keep in mind for patients with SLE who desire pregnancy. Ideally, pregnancies should be planned. Disease should be in remission on stable doses of medications compatible with pregnancy. Patients with a history of active disease or renal disease, prior poor pregnancy outcome or pregnancy complications, pulmonary hypertension, interstitial lung disease, current high doses of immunosuppressive therapy, presence of anti-Ro and anti-La antibodies, and other risk factors for high-risk pregnancies should be evaluated by a high-risk obstetrician prior to pregnancy. Pregnancy is contraindicated in those patients with recent lupus activity, antiphospholipid syndrome with a recent thrombosis, severe organ involvement, chronic renal failure, severe pulmonary hypertension, restrictive lung disease, or heart failure.

Prepregnancy Screening

In patients who have had a prior pregnancy, obstetrical history and outcome including medications that were used during pregnancy should be obtained. For all patients, either before conception or early during pregnancy, a careful review of the patients' medical history and medication (both past and present) is important. It is helpful to obtain some baseline testing in regard to disease activity. These baseline studies can be used as comparative points later during pregnancy and can be helpful in monitoring disease activity. Baseline labs including a complete blood count with differential, metabolic studies including renal and liver function, anti-dsDNA antibodies and complement levels, urinalysis, spot urine protein for creatinine, microalbumin, and protein, and uric acid levels should be obtained. In those patients with a prior history of renal disease or hypertension, 24-h urine excretion for protein, creatinine, and calcium is advised. Anti-Ro and anti-La, and anticardiolipin antibodies and a lupus anticoagulant should be assessed in patients who have not had these studies.

Pregnancy Monitoring

Pregnancy monitoring should be tailored to individual patients. In general, patients with mild disease can be evaluated every 6 weeks to 2 months. I generally recommend repeating the above studies once during the second trimester and once during the third trimester in patients with mild disease who are under good control. Patients with more severe disease should be seen more frequently in conjunction with a high-risk obstetrician. During the last 4 weeks of pregnancy, patients should be seen weekly. Often, I recommend that patients keep a home blood pressure cuff and scale to check their blood pressure and weight on a daily basis. Small changes in these parameters can indicate impending flare and enable the health-care provider to investigate and intervene earlier. Patients who have active disease or renal disease may need to be seen every week or two throughout the pregnancy. In these latter circumstances, it is important to work hand in hand with the obstetrician.

Patients with Anti-Ro and Anti-La Antibodies

Between 20 % and 30 % of persons with SLE have anti-Ro and anti-La antibodies. Women with these antibodies are at risk at having a child with congenital complete heart block and/or neonatal lupus. While that risk is small, less than 2% in those who have not had a child with these complications, congenital complete heart block has a fairly high morbidity and mortality and therefore is important to recognize in utero. A higher titer of anti-Ro antibody levels (greater than 50 U/ml) is associated with an increased risk CCHB and neonatal lupus. For those women who have given birth to a child with either neonatal lupus or CCHB, the risk of these events in subsequent pregnancies is 17–25 %. Fetal heart ultrasounds to assess for congenital complete heart block between 18 and 24 weeks are recommended for patients who have these antibodies. While there have been studies that have looked at the use of steroids or IVIG in the management of those fetuses that appear to be developing CCHB, no treatment has been shown to be clearly beneficial. One recent study suggests that hydroxychloroquine use in these patients may reduce the rate of CCHB, although further studies will need to be performed to confirm this finding. For those fetuses in which CCHB has been diagnosed, a pediatric cardiologist should be involved as often infants with CCHB will require a pacemaker at delivery. Those with neonatal lupus (skin rashes predominantly) generally have their symptoms resolve by 6 months.

Renal Disease

New-onset renal disease can be challenging to manage during pregnancy. Nonetheless, indications for renal biopsy are the same as in the nonpregnant state as biopsy is not contraindicated during pregnancy. It is often difficult to distinguish new-onset renal disease from preeclampsia (see below). High-dose or pulse steroids and immunosuppressive agents such as azathioprine and cyclosporine can be used in the short term for management. These medications, however, are associated with an increased incidence of pregnancy-induced hypertension, small for gestational age infants, and premature rupture of the membranes. In life-threatening cases, cyclophosphamide can be used in the second and third trimester.

Distinguishing Lupus Flare from Preeclampsia

Perhaps the biggest challenge in managing patients with SLE during pregnancy distinguishing a lupus flare from preeclampsia (Table 14.2). While symptomatically patients with these two disorders can similarly present with edema, renal insufficiency, thrombocytopenia, elevated creatinine, and hypertension, the underlying mechanism is different. Preeclampsia is essentially an intravascularly depleted state and is associated with increased or normal WBC, elevated complement components, increased uric acid levels, schistocytes, and relatively bland urine. Anti-dsDNA antibodies are not elevated on the basis of preeclampsia. Twenty-four-hour excretion of calcium is also diminished. On the other hand, SLE flare is associated with lowered WBC, decreased complement levels, increased dsDNA, low uric acid levels, and active urine sediment. While often difficult to distinguish these entities, it is important to do so as preeclampsia is often treated with immediate delivery while SLE flare is treated with medical management.

Table 14.2 Distinguishing SLE flare from preeclampsia

SLE flare	Preeclampsia
Hypertension	Hypertension
Edema	Edema
Low platelets	Low platelets
	Schistocytes
Normal LFTs	Abnormal LFTs
Cellular urine	Bland/acellular urine
Decreased complement levels	Elevated complement levels
Increased anti-dsDNA	Unchanged anti-dsDNA
Normal or low uric acid level	Elevated uric acid level
Normal 24-h urinary calcium	Decreased 24-h urinary calcium

The Effect of SLE on Pregnancy Outcome

Pregnancy outcome in lupus patients has improved in recent years. Reported live birth rates in women who have lupus range from 75 % to 85 %. There is an increased spontaneous abortion rate in individuals with SLE. The majority of this increase is secondary to coexisting antiphospholipid syndrome and not SLE itself. Women with SLE are at increased risk for developing preeclampsia and pregnancy-induced hypertension. They also have an increased risk of premature labor and premature rupture of the membranes in SLE patients. Small for gestational age infants and IUGR are also seen in higher frequency in SLE pregnancies. Other complications include stillbirth; neonatal death; gestational diabetes; pulmonary hypertension; renal failure; increased C-section rate; increased clotting events including strokes, pulmonary emboli, and DVTs; increased bleeding complications and increased infections; and increased maternal mortality. Risk factors for these complications include Raynaud's, antiphospholipid antibodies, anti-Ro antibodies, hypertension, nephritis, and active disease.

Disease Management (The Management of Antiphospholipid Syndrome During Pregnancy Is Discussed Elsewhere)

Lupus pregnancies tend to fare better if a few underlying guidelines are followed. Ideally, pregnancy should be planned. This allows for the adjustments in medication to occur prepregnancy. Second, disease should be in remission for 6 months prior to pregnancy. This is particularly important in individuals who have had prior renal disease or significant organ involvement. Lupus that is active at the time of conception tends to flare during pregnancy. In particular, individuals who have SLE with active renal disease at the start of pregnancy are particularly vulnerable to high pregnancy morbidity and even mortality. While not all patients need to be seen by a high-risk obstetrician, it helps if the patient, rheumatologist, and obstetrician all work together. In patients with a history of renal disease or significant organ involvement or who require immunosuppressive therapy during pregnancy, a high-risk obstetrician affiliated with a tertiary care facility is advisable. The patient and the rheumatologist should discuss acceptable treatment options in the case of a flare before or early in pregnancy. Patient preference and risk tolerance for medication use during pregnancy is highly individual and impacts and limits medication use.

During the postpartum period, there is an increased risk of disease flare and thromboembolic events especially in those patients with antiphospholipid syndrome. As with treatment during pregnancy, discussion regarding management in the postpartum period especially in conjunction with nursing should occur between the patients and their treating clinician.

Table 14.3 Summary of medications compatibility with pregnancy

Medications: compatible with pregnancy
NSAIDs—up to the third trimester
Glucocorticoids—risk of cleft palate (first trimester), pregnancy-induced hypertension and gestational diabetes (third trimester)
Hydroxychloroquine
Azathioprine—category D but substantial evidence from the transplant literature that this medication is compatible with pregnancy
Cyclosporine—category C but substantial evidence from the transplant literature that this medication is compatible with pregnancy
IVIG
Medications: incompatible with pregnancy
Cyclophosphamide—life threatening only—third trimester—otherwise incompatible with pregnancy
Methotrexate
Leflunomide
Mycophenolate mofetil
Medications: insufficient data
Rituximab
Belimumab
Abatacept

Medication Management of SLE During Pregnancy

Deciding whether a medication is safe during pregnancy can be challenging (Table 14.3). We commonly rely on the FDA "safety in pregnancy use classification"—a system that is often based on incomplete data. Some of the medications that are used in the treatment of SLE, such as methotrexate and leflunomide, are contraindicated during pregnancy (class X). Immunosuppressive agents such as glucocorticoids, cyclosporine A, and azathioprine despite their classification may be used cautiously. This section will discuss medication use during pregnancy.

Aspirin, Nonsteroidal Anti-inflammatory Drugs, and the Cyclooxygenase Inhibitors

Aspirin, the nonsteroidal anti-inflammatory drugs (NSAIDs), and the cyclooxygenase-2 (COX-2) inhibitors are used for the management of joint pain and serositis in SLE. Extensive human data suggest that aspirin and NSAIDs are not teratogenic and may be used during the first two trimesters. During the third trimester, NSAIDs can cause premature closure of the ductus arteriosus and should be therefore discontinued. Aspirin is used for the management of the antiphospholipid syndrome and is often continued until shortly before delivery. There is less data on the safety of COX-2 inhibitors during pregnancy, and therefore, it is probably best to discontinue these medications during pregnancy. The COX-2 inhibitory effect of both traditional NSAIDs and the selective COX-2 inhibitors can theoretically inhibit implantation; thus, I recommend that patients discontinue these medications during a potential conception cycle and resume the medication either at the time of a confirmed pregnancy test or at the start of menses. The American Academy of Pediatrics considers aspirin and most nonsteroidals to be compatible with breast-feeding. Shorter acting NSAIDs such as ibuprofen may be preferable to minimize accumulation in breast milk.

Antimalarials

The antimalarial agents, hydroxychloroquine and chloroquine, are used part of the mainstay of treatment of SLE. For many years, these medications were thought to be incompatible with pregnancy. This was based on animal studies that demonstrated ocular toxicity and one human case report of a woman who took chloroquine during several pregnancies and had infants with congenital defects including mental retardation and pigment deposition. Several studies have shown that antimalarials are compatible with pregnancy with no untoward effects. Surveys of American rheumatologist revealed that close to 69 % of practitioners were continuing these medications during pregnancy. Moreover, data suggest that maintenance of antimalarials may decrease flares during pregnancy and improve outcome. Therefore, current recommendations are to continue antimalarials during pregnancy. Consensus opinion of expert rheumatologists concluded that antimalarials are compatible with nursing.

Glucocorticoids

Glucocorticoids are frequently used in the management of SLE. Prednisone and prednisolone, the preparations most commonly used, are not readily metabolized by the placenta and reach the fetus at very low concentration. In contrast, betamethasone and dexamethasone reach the fetus at higher concentration. For this reason, these latter forms are used to hasten lung maturity in fetuses with imminent premature delivery. Glucocorticoids increase the incidence of cleft palate formation in animals. In humans, large case series including those treated with a mean dose of 8 mg a day of glucocorticosteroids during pregnancy have not shown an increased incidence of anomalies. However, a meta-analysis of pregnancy exposures of glucocorticoid exposure demonstrated a 3.4-fold increased risk of cleft palate formation in fetuses exposed to this medication in utero. Later in pregnancy, glucocorticoids contribute to premature rupture of the membranes and small for gestational age babies in addition to increasing maternal risk of gestational diabetes, hypertension, and osteoporosis. Nonetheless, glucocorticoids remain a reasonable management choice for disease flares. Clinicians should try to use the minimal dose possible to relieve symptoms. For patients who are treated with steroids during pregnancy, stress dose steroids should be given during labor or when a cesarean section is performed. Glucocorticoids are compatible with breast-feeding. At doses greater than 20 mg a day, I recommend pumping and discarding breast milk the first 4 h after ingestion.

Azathioprine

The purine analogue, azathioprine, is used for the management of renal disease, skin disease, and as a steroid-sparing agent in SLE. Trophoblastic damage after in utero exposure to azathioprine occurs in murine pregnancy models. In humans, azathioprine is metabolized minimally by the placenta so that limited amounts of the active ingredient reach the fetus. While case reports of craniofacial malformations and chromosomal abnormalities have been reported in offspring exposed to azathioprine in utero, larger case series have failed to substantiate this increased risk of congenital anomalies. In 142 transplant recipients who were given azathioprine during pregnancy, there were some anomalies seen, but this was thought not to be above the background rate of congenital anomalies. While small for gestational age infants and premature rupture of the membranes were reported in some of these pregnancies, there have been no reports of increased number of congenital anomalies above the background rate. Although the FDA considers this medication a class D, the transplant literature suggests that azathioprine may be used in pregnant patients who require immunosuppression. Azathioprine can cause immunosuppression in the newborn and should not be used in nursing mothers.

Cyclosporine

In rodents, cyclosporine crosses the placenta in very low concentrations. In humans, there are differing opinions on whether or not cyclosporine crosses the placenta in significant concentrations. Regardless, there seems to be no increased risk of teratogenicity over background rates. In one study of 154 pregnancies in renal transplant patients in which the mothers were taking cyclosporine, there was no higher rate of complications or congenital anomalies in babies exposed to cyclosporine in utero. Other transplant series and registries have confirmed these findings. In a report of 500 pregnancies in which mothers were taking cyclosporine, there was no increased risk of congenital anomalies. Live birth rates were lower, but this might reflect the sicker patient population being maintained on cyclosporine A. Finally, a meta-analysis concluded that cyclosporine does not appear to be a major teratogen, although it may be associated with increased rates of premature delivery. The literature suggests that cyclosporine may be used for immunosuppression during pregnancy. Cyclosporine is not compatible with nursing because of the risk of immunosuppression in the offspring.

Mycophenolate Mofetil (CellCept®)

Mycophenolate mofetil is a purine synthesis inhibitor that is one of the mainstays of therapy in the treatment of lupus nephritis. There have been several case reports of congenital anomalies in humans exposed to mycophenolate mofetil in utero. This medication is considered a category D by the FDA. Given the existing information, this medication should be discontinued before pregnancy and avoided in nursing mothers.

Methotrexate

Methotrexate is a folate antagonist that is sometimes used in the management of SLE. In both rodent models and in humans, this medication is both profoundly teratogenic and abortogenic. The majority of toxicity occurs during the first trimester. The FDA considers this medication a category X. Patients who are on this medication should use a reliable form of birth control. Women should wait at least one ovulatory cycle after stopping methotrexate before trying to get pregnant. Some providers recommend waiting three conception cycles after discontinuing this medication prior to conception. This medication is not compatible with breast-feeding.

Cyclophosphamide

Cyclophosphamide is a cytotoxic agent that is used to treat SLE renal disease and CNS manifestations. Cyclophosphamide causes chromosomal damage in murine embryos. In humans, limb and cardiac anomalies have been reported after in utero cyclophosphamide exposure. There have been case reports of pregnant women being treated in the late second and third trimesters with cyclophosphamide for Wegener's granulomatosis and Hodgkin's lymphoma without fetal compromise. Nonetheless, cyclophosphamide should only be used during pregnancy in life-threatening situations. Cyclophosphamide is not compatible with nursing.

IVIG

IVIG is used for the management of ITP and refractory antiphospholipid syndrome during pregnancy. Case reports suggest that it is safe.

Tumor Necrosis Factor-Alpha Blockade and Inhibitors

Biologics that are directed against the tumor necrosis factor-alpha are rarely used in the treatment of SLE in particular because early studies suggest that these medications may induce the production of anti-dsDNA antibodies. While these medications are rated category B for use during pregnancy, there have been 41 cases of possible anomalies related to in utero exposure to these medications reported to the FDA. The significance of this finding is unclear as the actual number of exposed pregnancies is unknown. Given their limited use in SLE, TNF-blocking medications should be avoided during pregnancy

Leflunomide

Leflunomide is used to treat skin and joint manifestations in SLE. This extremely teratogenic (risk category is X) medication is absolutely contraindicated in pregnancy. In general, I try to avoid this medication in women of childbearing potential. In those women who are taking this medication and who desire pregnancy, they must discontinue the medication 2 years prior to conception or undergo drug elimination with cholestyramine (8 g three times a day be given for 11 days).

Rituximab and Other Biologics

Current recommendations are to avoid these medications during pregnancy as there are limited data on the safety of these medications during pregnancy. Prolonged B cell depletion in offspring exposed to rituximab during pregnancy can occur. How long before conception these medications can be safely given is unclear. There is insufficient data to conclude anything regarding the safety of other newer biologics such as abatacept and belimumab. Given this paucity of information, these medications should be discontinued during pregnancy.

Miscellaneous

The antihypertensives angiotensin-converting enzyme inhibitors, angiotensin receptor antagonists, and many diuretics are contraindicated during pregnancy. Beta blockers and methyldopa may be used for the management of blood pressure during pregnancy. For anticoagulation, low-dose aspirin and unfractionated and low molecular weight heparin are recommended. Heparins should be held for 12–24 h prior to delivery. Calcium and vitamin D supplementation should be given to those on glucocorticoids or heparin.

Medication Recommendations

SLE patients should be maintained on their antimalarials during pregnancy. Mild flares can be managed with NSAIDs and low-dose prednisone. More severe flares can be treated with higher dose glucocorticoids, azathioprine, and cyclosporine. Life-threatening disease should be treated with pulse steroids and in rarely cytotoxic agents. Methotrexate, leflunomide, mycophenolate mofetil, and the biologics should be avoided.

Conclusions

Fortunately, most SLE patients can consider pregnancy if they so desire. Fertility issues are predominantly related to prior cyclophosphamide use and the antiphospholipid syndrome. For those patients who choose to become pregnant, disease needs to be under control, in particular in those with a history of renal disease. While many patients can be managed with their rheumatologist and obstetrician, patients with a history of moderate or severe disease or poor prior pregnancy outcome ought to be managed by a high-risk obstetrician. In all cases, good communication between the patient and her providers with careful monitoring of disease and fetal development is crucial. Prepregnancy labs or early pregnancy labs are helpful for reference later during pregnancy to gage disease activity. Differentiating SLE flare from preeclampsia can be challenging, although laboratory studies can be helpful. Those with anti-Ro and anti-La monitoring require additional evaluation for CCHB. Patients should remain on their antimalarials during pregnancy as ample evidence suggests that these medications may improve pregnancy outcome. NSAIDs can be used up to the third trimester for disease symptoms. Low-dose steroids can be used for mild symptoms of flare, although patients should be aware that there is a three- to fourfold increased incidence of cleft palate formation in fetuses exposed during the first trimester. Later in pregnancy, glucocorticoids can contribute to the increased incidence of gestational diabetes, pregnancy-induced hypertension, osteopenia, and premature rupture of the membranes. For moderate disease flares, high dose glucocorticoids, azathioprine, and cyclosporine can be given. Patients need to understand that in addition to the risks of glucocorticoids described above, the FDA considers azathioprine and cyclosporine as potential teratogens despite significant evidence to the contrary. For severe disease, pulse steroid therapy and IVIG are safe. Only life-threatening situations should be managed with cytotoxic agents. Mycophenolate mofetil, leflunomide, and methotrexate are teratogenic and should be avoided. There is insufficient data in regard to the use of the biologics during pregnancy. Most importantly, careful conversations between the patients and their treating physician(s) should occur so that potential hazards to the fetus and the mother are fully disclosed prior to the initiation of therapy during pregnancy.

Sources

1. Slater CA, Liang MH, McCune JW, Christman GM, Laufer MR. Preserving ovarian function in patients receiving cyclophosphamide. Lupus. 1999;8(1):3–10.
2. Bermas BL. Oral contraceptives in systemic lupus erythematosus—a tough pill to swallow? N Engl J Med. 2005;353:2602–4.
3. Van Nieuwenhoven ALV, Heineman MJ, Faas MM. The immunology of successful pregnancy. Hum Reprod Update. 2003;9(4):347–57.
4. Lund CJ, Donovan JC. Blood volume during pregnancy. Significance of plasma and red cell volumes. Am J Obstet Gynecol. 1967;98(3):394–403.
5. Marik PE, Plante LA. Venous thromboembolic disease and pregnancy. N Engl J Med. 2008;359(19):2025–33.
6. Heckman JD, Sassard R. Current concepts review. Musculoskeletal considerations in pregnancy. J Bone Joint Surg Am. 1994;76(11):1720–30.
7. Van den Broe NR, Letsky EA. Pregnancy and the erythrocyte sedimentation rate. BJOG. 2001;108(11):1164–7.
8. Ruiz-Irastorza G. Evaluation of systemic lupus erythematosus activity during pregnancy. Lupus. 2004;13(6):679–82.
9. Petri M, Howard D, Repke J, Goldman DW. The Hopkins Lupus Pregnancy Center: 1987–1991 update. Am J Reprod Immunol. 1992;28(3–4):188–91.
10. Izmirly PM, Kim MY, Llanos C, et al. Evaluation of the risk of anti-SSA/Ro-SSB/La antibody-associated cardiac manifestations of neonatal lupus in fetuses of mothers with systemic lupus erythematosus exposed to hydroxychloroquine. Ann Rheum Dis. 2010;69:1827–30.
11. Sibai BM. Imitators of severe pre-eclampsia. Semin Perinatol. 2009;33(3):196–205.
12. Al Arfaj AS, Khalil N. Pregnancy outcome in 396 pregnancies in patients with SLE in Saudi Arabia. Lupus. 2010;19(14):1665–73.
13. Smyth A, Oliveira HM, Lahr BD, et al. A systematic review and meta-analysis of pregnancy outcomes in patients with systemic lupus erythematosus and lupus nephritis. Clin J Am Soc Nephrol. 2010;5:2060–8.
14. Marker-Hermann E, Fischer-Betz R. Rheumatic diseases and pregnancy. Curr Opin Obstet Gynecol. 2010;22:458–65.
15. Ruiz-Irastorza G, Khamashta MA. Managing lupus patients during pregnancy. Best Pract Res Clin Rheumatol. 2009;23:575–82.
16. American Academy of Pediatrics Committee on Drugs. Transfer of drugs and other chemicals into human milk. Pediatrics. 2001;108(3):924–36.
17. Clouse ME, Magder L, Witter F, Petri M. Hydroxychloroquine in lupus pregnancy. Arthritis Rheum. 2006;54(11):3640–7.
18. Ostensen M, Khamashta M, Lockshin M, et al. Anti-inflammatory and immunosuppressive drugs and reproduction. Arthritis Res Ther. 2006;8(3):209.
19. Briggs GG, Freeman RK, Yaffe SJ. Drugs in pregnancy and lactation. Baltimore: Williams and Wilkins; 2001.
20. Pyllie L, Mazzotta P, Pastuszak A, et al. Birth defects after maternal exposure to corticosteroids: prospective cohort study and meta-analysis of epidemiological studies. Teratology. 2000;62(6):385–92.
21. Amenti VT, Ahlswede KM, Ahlswede BA, Jarrell BE, Moritz MJ, Burke JF. National transplantation pregnancy registry-outcomes of 154 pregnancies in cyclosporine-treated female kidney transplant recipients. Transplantation. 1994;57(4):502–6.
22. Donnenfeld AE, Pastuszak A, Noah JS, Schick B, Rose NC, Koren G. Methotrexate exposure prior to and during pregnancy. Teratology. 1994;49(2):79–81.
23. Koren G, Inoue M. Do tumor necrosis factor inhibitors cause malformations in humans? J Rheumatol. 2009;36(93):665–6.

Chapter 15
Antiphospholipid Syndrome

Bonnie L. Bermas

The antiphospholipid syndrome (APS) is a disorder that is characterized by the presence of antibodies directed against phospholipid moieties in conjunction with venous and/or arterial thromboembolic events and/or obstetrical complications. There are other associated features including but not limited to seizures, thrombocytopenia and autoimmune hemolytic anemia, livedo reticularis, and renal disease. Rare complications include the catastrophic APS in which multiple clotting events occur simultaneously or in rapid succession. The antiphospholipid antibody syndrome can be seen by itself; primary APS, or in conjunction with other diseases such as systemic lupus erythematosus (SLE); secondary APS. This chapter will discuss the clinical manifestations and the management of the APS.

For many years, it was known that some women with SLE were prone to thromboembolic events and recurrent obstetrical losses. Subsequently, there were case reports published of SLE patients presenting with thromboembolic disorders in the presence of a circulating anticoagulant as measured by in vitro coagulation assays (lupus anticoagulant). It was later, however, after the discovery of anticardiolipin (aCL) antibodies, that Graham Hughes and others described the clinical association of these antibodies, both the lupus anticoagulant and the aCL antibodies, with thromboembolic events. Initially called "Hughes' syndrome," it is now referred to as the APS.

B.L. Bermas, M.D. (✉)
Division of Rheumatology, Director, Lupus and Antiphospholipid Center,
Brigham and Women's Hospital, 75 Francis Street, Boston, MA 02115, USA

Harvard Medical School, Boston, MA, USA
e-mail: bbermas@partners.org

Clinical Manifestations

Thromboembolic events and obstetrical complications are the signature findings of this disorder (Table 15.1). Venous thromboembolic events are the most common manifestation. In particular deep vein thrombosis affecting the calf are the most frequent location seen but the renal veins, the hepatic, axillary, subclavian, and retinal veins, the cerebral sinuses, and the vena cavae may also be involved. Calf deep vein thromboses may result in pulmonary emboli. Superficial thrombophlebitis can also occur.

Arterial events can occur in any major artery in the body. In particular, cerebral arterial thrombosis are seen (resulting in CVAs, TIAs), but coronary, renal, and mesenteric arteries and arterial bypass graft occlusions have also been reported. Cerebral vascular accidents and TIAs and myocardial infarctions in patients under the age of 40 with no apparent cause should trigger an investigation for antiphospholipid antibodies (aPLs).

Recurrent thrombotic events are common. In general venous events are followed by a subsequent venous event and arterial events are associated with subsequent arterial events.

Obstetrical events include recurrent first trimester miscarriages, second or third trimester pregnancy losses, and pre-eclampsia. There is some controversy regarding whether early (before 10 weeks of gestation) spontaneous abortions are truly part of this syndrome. Many experts maintain that it is the later first trimester pregnancy losses, after 9–10 weeks of gestation, at the time the embryo becomes a fetus and is more dependent upon placental circulation that reflects this disorder. Pre-eclampsia is also thought to be more common in individuals with antiphospholipid antibodies as is HELLP syndrome.

Valvular heart disease, also referred to as Libman Sacks endocarditis, can be caused by verruccae that form near the edge of cardiac valves. These verruccae consist of accumulations of immune complexes, fibrin, and platelet thrombi. The mitral, aortic, and tricuspid valves are most commonly involved. While usually

Table 15.1 Clinical manifestations in the diagnosis of antiphospholipid syndrome

Venous thrombotic events
- Deep vein thrombosis
- Renal vein thrombosis
- Pulmonary embolic

Arterial thrombotic events
- Any major arterial clot
- Cerebral vascular accidents
- Myocardial infarctions

Obstetrical complications
- Three or more first trimester spontaneous abortions
- Second or third trimester pregnancy loss

asymptomatic, if the verrucal lesions are extensive, the healing process can produce damage leading to valvular regurgitation occasionally severe enough to necessitate surgical repair of the valve. These verrucae can also fragment and produce systemic emboli, and damaged valves may be a target for infective endocarditis.

Individuals with the APS may also have immune mediated thrombocytopenia. Those with what is sometimes referred to as Evan's syndrome, ITP and autoimmune hemolytic anemia, have a high frequency (approaching 80 %) of antiphospholipid antibodies.

Catastrophic Antiphospholipid Syndrome

Fewer than 1 % of individuals with APS will develop widespread thromboembolic disease with multi-organ failure. When this does occur, it is referred to as "catastrophic APS" or CAPs. Patients with catastrophic APS may have laboratory features such as elevated fibrin degradation products, depressed fibrinogen levels, or elevated D-dimer concentrations that are more typically found with disseminated intravascular coagulation (DIC). This disorder has a high mortality rate (approaching 50 %). It is diagnosed when three or more organs or tissues develop thrombi within the course of a week. It must be confirmed by histopathology of the occluded vessels and the presence of an antiphospholipid antibody.

Common Clinical Associations

Migraine headaches are found in individuals with APS. Livedo reticularis, a lacey venous pattern found on the skin is also found in APS. Less common clinical features are listed in Table 15.2.

Diagnostic Criteria

A panel of clinical experts created diagnostic and classification criteria known as the Sapporo criteria and revised Sapporo criteria. According to the more recent Sapporo criteria, the APS is defined as the presence on two separate occasions 12 weeks apart of either an IgM or IgG aCL antibody, an anti-B2-glycoprotein I antibody, or an accepted confirmed lupus anticoagulant test, in the presence of a venous clot, an arterial clot or an obstetrical complication (defined as three or more first trimester spontaneous abortions, or second or third trimester intrauterine fetal demise).

Table 15.2 Less frequently found clinical features of APS

Neurological
- Seizures
- Cognitive impairment
- White matter lesions
- Transverse myelopathy
- Sensorineural hearing loss

Hematological
- Hemolytic anemia
- Thrombocytopenia
- TTP/HUS

Cutaneous
- Digital necrosis
- Splinter hemorrhages
- Superficial venous thrombosis
- Post-phlebitic ulcers
- Circumscribed cutaneous necrosis
- Thrombocytopenic purpura
- Pseudovasculitis
- Extensive cutaneous necrosis

Pulmonary
- Pulmonary arterial thrombosis
- Alveolar hemorrhage

Ocular
- Amaurosis fugax
- Retinal venous and arterial occlusion
- Anterior ischemic optic neuropathy

Other
- Adrenal infarct/hemorrhage leading to adrenal insufficiency
- Avascular necrosis

Differential Diagnosis

Other conditions, in particular those associated with recurrent thrombi and obstetrical complications can be confused with APS. Moreover, APS can coexist with other diseases that may result in a synergistic effect to cause thromboembolic and/or obstetric complications (Table 15.3).

Pathogenesis

The pathogenesis of this disorder is not completely understood. What is known is that some antiphospholipid antibodies can interfere with the normal pathways of coagulation causing procoagulant activity of protein C, annexin V, and platelets amongst

Table 15.3 Differential diagnosis

Recurrent venous thrombosis etiology
- Inherited and acquired coagulation/anticoagulation factors
  - Protein C deficiency
  - Protein S deficiency
  - Factor V Leiden deficiency
- Defective clot lysis
- Cancer and myeloproliferative disorders
- Nephrotic syndrome

Arterial thrombosis
- Atherosclerosis
- Embolic disease
- Atrial fibrillation, atrial myxoma
- Endocarditis
- Cholesterol emboli
- Paradoxical emboli
- TTP/HUS
- Vasculitis
- Hyperviscosity syndrome

Recurrent pregnancy losses
- Endocrinopathies
- Anatomic abnormalities
- Genetic etiologies
- Age related
- Idiopathic

other factors. These antibodies may also impair fibrinolysis and increase vascular tone. Nonetheless, the antibodies themselves are probably not sufficient for the manifestations of clotting. Rather, a second "hit" such as surgery, pregnancy, prolonged immobilization, genetic disorders of clotting (see above), and smoking may be required for the full thromboembolic and obstetrical manifestations to occur.

One of the most interesting and potentially fruitful areas of investigation in this disorder has to do with the role of complement activation in this syndrome. Several murine and human studies have shown that at least as far as the obstetrical complications go, the clinical events appear to be mediated through the complement system

Laboratory Testing

There are three major types of antiphospholipid (aPL) antibodies: aCL antibodies; B-2 glycoprotein I antibodies; and lupus anticoagulants. The false-positive VDRL, a reaction of sera against the cardiolipin used in the VDRL assay, is of historical interest only. This test's lack of sensitivity and specificity prevent it from being clinically useful.

Anticardiolipin Antibodies

The development of the enzyme-linked immunosorbent assays (ELISA) for aCL antibodies occurred in the early 1980s. At that time, standardize sera was used to create international units. IgG and IgM aCL are the most commonly tested and are one of the tests that can be used to make the diagnosis of APS. IgG aCL are thought to be the most clinically significant, and risk of an event is related to titer. Many in this field will divide aCL into low titer, less than 40 international units, and moderate titer–high titer antibodies, greater than 40 international units. IgM aCL are not as clinically specific. These antibodies (IgM aCL) can occur after bacterial and viral infections.

Lupus Anticoagulant

The lupus anticoagulant test is a misnomer. Fewer than half of the individuals with this antibody have SLE. Moreover, the antibody that causes the lupus anticoagulant test positivity it is a procoagulant in vivo. The test is performed using an in vitro clotting test such as the dilute Russell viper venom time, a kaolin clotting time, or an activated partial thromboplastin time. If the test is prolonged, a two step confirmatory process must be employed to demonstrate true positivity. In the first step, sera from healthy controls needs to be added back to see if the prolongation is due to a factor deficiency. If after the first step the test is still prolonged then phospholipids need to be added back to make certain that the prolongation is due to an antiphospholipid antibody. If the patient is already anticoagulated, testing for an anticoagulant can be tricky.

When evaluating a patient for APS, one should test for the presence of both an aCL antibody and a lupus anticoagulant as these are separate classes of antibodies and one can be positive while the other is negative.

B-2 Glycoprotein I Antibodies

B2-glycoprotein I inhibits platelet activation and coagulation. Antibodies to this substance can cause thrombophilia. Antibodies to B2-glycoprotein I can be found in isolation (11 % of patients) but generally are found in association with other antiphospholipid antibodies. Although testing for the presence of these antibodies is not recommended as a screening tool, when clinical suspicion is high, testing for this antibody is indicated.

Other Tests

While IgA, IgD, and other antiphospholipid antibodies such as anti-phosphatidyl serine have been described in case reports, they are not uniformly accepted as part of the diagnostic criteria.

Management of Antiphospholipid Syndrome

The management of this disorder is the same whether it is primary or secondary APS. Treatment options include unfractionated heparin, low molecular weight heparin, warfarin, antiplatelet therapies, and hydroxychloroquine. Below we will discuss treatment approaches depending on clinical presentation.

Venous or Arterial Clotting Events

Venous events thromboembolic events in this disorder include deep vein thrombosis, renal vein thrombosis, pulmonary emoboli amongst other findings, while arterial events encompass clots of any artery and can include cerebral vascular accidents and myocardial infarctions. When patients first present with a clinical thromboembolic event and the etiology is determined to be APS, the patients should be anticoagulated as per standard protocol with unfractionated heparin or low molecular weight heparin with bridging to warfarin therapy. The one exception is in the case of coexisting pulmonary hemorrhage, a rare manifestation of APS, where it is preferable to use unfractionated heparin because its anticoagulant activity is more readily acutely reversed. After initial anticoagulation, the patient should be transitioned to long-term warfarin therapy.

Warfarin Therapy

The targeted INR for warfarin therapy in the APS has been a subject of debate. Two separate studies in the 1990s suggested that maintaining an INR between 3.0 and 4.0 minimized the risk or recurrent thrombotic events while maintaining a tolerable risk of bleeding complications. Subsequently, data suggested that targeting the INR to a level between 2.0 and 3.0 may be adequate to prevent recurrent thrombotic events while reducing the risk of bleeding complications. Therefore, the current recommendation is to target the INR to the 2.0–3.0 range. However, in the setting of an arterial thrombotic event or recurrent thrombotic event, I, as do others, will often target the INR to a level of 3.0.

While the majority of the existing literature focuses on warfarin therapy for long-term management, there is some evidence that low molecular weight heparin may also be used to prevent subsequent clotting events. These medications are easier to use in the sense that they are not subject to the vicissitudes of the INR level that many APS patients on warfarin therapy experience. However, there is currently insufficient data to conclude absolutely that these medications are as effective as warfarin therapy.

Duration of therapy. Currently, the recommendation is that warfarin therapy should be used indefinitely as the risk of subsequent thrombotic events remains in patients with APS. In some circumstances, when a clear coexisting risk factor has been identified and removed, this recommendation may be modified.

Inferior vena cava filters. In patients with an absolute contraindication to anticoagulation or in whom anticoagulation has failed, inferior vena cava filters may be used when clinically warranted.

Antiplatelet Therapy

Antiplatelet therapy is of limited utility in the management of full-blown APS. Neither low-dose aspirin nor clopidogrel are effective in preventing subsequent clotting events. The one exception is in the case of cerebral vascular accidents where there is some evidence that low-dose aspirin therapy is adequate to prevent future events. Low-dose Aspirin is also often used in the setting of high titer aPL in the absence of clinical events although there is really no objective data to support this approach.

Newer Agents

Currently, the newer anticoagulant agents have not been studied in this disorder. However, if they can be shown to be effective, they will be advantageous in this population as warfarin therapy is particularly difficult to administer and monitor, and is contraindicated in pregnant women.

Drug Interactions and Dietary Interactions

As in other conditions, certain medications including NSAIDs, acetaminophen, and others, and foods high in Vitamin K (leafy vegetables) can interfere with warfarin therapy. Therefore, patients should be counseled accordingly.

Special Clinical Circumstances

Catastrophic Antiphospholipid Syndrome

The prognosis for patients with CAPs is quite poor with standard anticoagulation. It is important to treat any underlying disorder such as infection that may have precipitated this clinical entity. Acutely, patients should be anticoagulated with heparin with ultimate bridging to warfarin therapy. High-dose steroids (e.g., methylprednisolone 1 g intravenously for daily for 3 days followed by 1 mg/kg prednisone equivalent per day) and, plasma exchange with or without intravenous immunoglobulin (0.4 mg/kg intravenously for 5 days) in combination with anticoagulation can improve outcome redundent as is.

Valvular Heart Disease

Valvular heart disease or Libman Sacks endocarditis can be seen in the APS. While some case series have suggested a higher rate of valvular involvement than previous thought (approaching 70 % by TTE in those with SLE), current recommendations are to refer for ECHO only when clinically indicated by either change in symptoms or change in cardiac exam. For those with valvular thickening, low-dose aspirin is recommended. In those with documented vegetations, and/or thromboembolic events, anticoagulation with warfarin to an INR or 2.0–3.0 is advised although whether this prevents future events is unclear. The use of glucocorticoids for this syndrome is controversial.

Renal Disease

Renal insufficiency and even renal failure can result from microthrombi in the renal vasculature and impact renal function. While evidence is not conclusive, some clinicians will treat with redundent as written either aspirin or warfarin if there is not a contraindication.

Cerebral Vascular Accidents

Cerebral vascular accidents with no other clinical manifestation of this disorder in the setting of antiphospholipid antibodies are a special circumstance. Recent guidelines from the neurologic literature suggest that low-dose aspirin therapy is sufficient to prevent future ischemic events; however, controversy remains. Many of the patients in the study used to justify this approach had significant comorbidity for cerebral vascular accidents including hypertension, diabetes, and older age. Thus, this approach may not apply to the younger patient who has no clear risk factors and who presents with a cerebral vascular accident and/or TIA in the setting of antiphospholipid antibodies. In this latter situation this author, as do many rheumatologists, recommends full anticoagulation with either warfarin or low molecular weight heparin in conjunction with aspirin for an indefinite period of time.

Thrombocytopenia

Autoimmune thrombocytopenia has been described in the APS. In general, standard management with glucocorticoids (in particular dexamethasone) and in some cases splenectomy are indicated. Rituximab, danizol, dapsone, and IVIG have also been used in case series.

Positive Antiphospholipid Antibodies or Lupus Anticoagulant in the Absence of a Clinical Event

The management of these patients remains controversial. However, recent studies did not demonstrate the benefit of prophylactic low-dose aspirin in these patients with the exception of those individuals who have coexisting SLE. This latter group may benefit from both low-dose aspirin and hydroxychloroquine therapy.

Management of Obstetrical Complications

Obstetrical complications of the APS include recurrent spontaneous miscarriages during the first trimester. While three or more miscarriages at any point during the first trimester can be used to diagnose this disorder, individuals with APS are particularly prone to pregnancy losses after 10 weeks of gestation at the time that the embryo enters the fetal phase. Second or third trimester intrauterine fetal demise, intrauterine growth retardation, and pre-eclampsia are also found. For the purposes of diagnosis only fetal loss is considered part of the classification criteria.

Recurrent miscarriages. Women who have had recurrent pregnancy losses or second and third trimester losses thought to be secondary to the APS should be managed with a combination of antiplatelet therapy and anticoagulation during a subsequent pregnancy. There are some studies that suggest that antiplatelet therapy adds little to anticoagulation with heparin, but most studies have been performed with both low-dose aspirin and heparin being used simultaneously.

Low-dose aspirin (81 mg a day) should be started at the time of conception. In general, this medication should be discontinued a week prior to delivery with the exception of those women who have a high risk of thromboembolic disease.

Subcutaneous low molecular weight heparin at doses of 5,000–10,000 units subcutaneously twice a day should also be used for treatment. While most of the randomized trials have been done with unfractionated heparin, case series suggest that low molecular weight heparin is as beneficial, and therefore may be preferable given the ease of dosing compared with unfractionated heparin.

The timing of the initiation of therapy is somewhat controversial. Some practitioners advocate waiting until an intrauterine pregnancy is documented prior to the initiation of heparin therapy. However, in circumstances of coexisting clotting issues or significant obstetrical losses it may be preferred to begin therapy at or before the time of conception. Therapy should be continued up until the time of delivery and resumed following delivery for a period of 4–6 weeks as the postpartum period is one of high risk for clotting events.

Treatment Failure

The majority of women treated with anticoagulation will go on to have a successful pregnancy. However, there are some patients who will fail anticoagulation therapy. For these patients, IVIG at a dosing of (0.4 g/kg/day for 5 days each month) starting with a conception cycle had been used with some success. There have also been reports of plasmapheresis being used also with limited success.

Hydroxychloroquine. Hydroxychloroquine is thought to be of benefit in the APS in general. Whether or not it is beneficial for obstetrical complications is unknown but certainly in those patients who have coexisting SLE it should be used and maintained throughout pregnancy.

Pregnant Patients with a History of Venous or Arterial Thrombosis

For patients who have had a history of thromboembolic events and the APS, higher doses of unfractionated or low molecular weight heparin is advised during pregnancy.

Positive Antiphospholipid Antibodies in the Absence of Clinical Events

Management of women who have either not had a clinical event or have had one or two miscarriages during the first 10 weeks of gestation in the presence of antiphospholipid antibodies remain a treatment predicament. There are no data that suggest that prophylactic treatment with full anticoagulation is indicated. Some clinicians advocate using a baby aspirin in this situation although there are no data that suggest this treatment prevents pregnancy complications.

Pre-eclampsia

Pre-eclampsia occurs in greater frequency in individuals who have APS and aPLs. There is some evidence that baby aspirin may prevent pre-eclampsia. Therefore, in those patients with a prior history of pre-eclampsia, baby aspirin may be of benefit. Some clinicians will advocate full anticoagulation for these patients although there are no evidence that this therapy works.

Other Antiphospholipid Antibodies

While IgA and IgD aCL antibodies, and other antiphospolipid antibodies have been described in individuals with recurrent miscarriage, there is no clear evidence to support the use of anticoagulation to prevent obstetrical complications in a subsequent pregnancy in individuals with these antibodies.

Labor and Delivery

In general, low molecular weight heparin should be discontinued 24–48 h prior to delivery. In patients for whom the risk of clotting is high, it is helpful to switch to unfractionated heparin as the delivery date approaches so that treatment can continue as long as possible.

Prednisone. There is no evidence that glucocorticoids add additional benefit to the treatment recommendations noted above. Therefore, empiric use of glucocorticoids in the absence of other indications is unnecessary.

Experimental therapy. Anti-complement therapy and biologics are currently being investigated for utility in this syndrome. Thus far, there is no conclusive evidence that these medications are of benefit in pregnant women.

Conclusion

In conclusion, the APS remains a clinically challenging entity with both clotting and obstetrical complications. Given the current state of evidence, lifelong anticoagulation with either warfarin or low molecular weight heparin is indicated for the thromboembolic manifestations and heparin (either unfractionated or low molecular weight heparin) in conjunction with aspirin is indicated for the treatment of obstetrical complications. Current investigations into targeted therapy or anti-complement therapy may prove to be the mainstays of management in the future.

Sources

1. Miyakis S, Lockshin MD, Atsumi T, et al. International consensus statement on an update of the classification criteria for definite antiphospholipid syndrome (APS). J Thromb Haemost. 2006;4:295.

2. Cervera R, Piette JC, Font J, et al. Antiphospholipid syndrome: clinical and immunologic manifestations and patterns of disease expression in a cohort of 1,000 patients. Arthritis Rheum. 2002;46:1019.
3. Asherson RA, Khamashta MA, Ordi-Ros J, et al. The "primary" antiphospholipid syndrome: major clinical and serological features. Medicine (Baltimore). 1989;68:366.
4. Mandreoli M, Zucchelli P. Renal vascular disease in patients with primary antiphospholipid antibodies. Nephrol Dial Transplant. 1993;8:1277.
5. Goodnight SH. Antiphospholipid antibodies and thrombosis. Curr Opin Hematol. 1994;1:354.
6. Asherson RA, Lioté F, Page B, et al. Avascular necrosis of bone and antiphospholipid antibodies in systemic lupus erythematosus. J Rheumatol. 1993;20:284.
7. Tektonidou MG, Varsou N, Kotoulas G, et al. Cognitive deficits in patients with antiphospholipid syndrome: association with clinical, laboratory, and brain magnetic resonance imaging findings. Arch Intern Med. 2006;166:2278.
8. Sanna G, Bertolaccini ML, Khamashta MA. Unusual clinical manifestations of the antiphospholipid syndrome. Curr Rheumatol Rev. 2006;2:387.
9. Muscal E, Brey RL. Neurologic manifestations of the antiphospholipid syndrome: integrating molecular and clinical lessons. Curr Rheumatol Rep. 2008;10:67.
10. Rosove MH, Brewer PM. Antiphospholipid thrombosis: clinical course after the first thrombotic event in 70 patients. Ann Intern Med. 1992;117:303.
11. Tektonidou MG, Laskari K, Panagiotakos DB, Moutsopoulos HM. Risk factors for thrombosis and primary thrombosis prevention in patients with systemic lupus erythematosus with or without antiphospholipid antibodies. Arthritis Rheum. 2009;61:29.
12. Ruffatti A, Del Ross T, Ciprian M, et al. Risk factors for a first thrombotic event in antiphospholipid antibody carriers. A multicentre, retrospective follow-up study. Ann Rheum Dis. 2009;68:397.
13. Asherson RA, Cervera R, Piette JC, et al. Catastrophic antiphospholipid syndrome: clues to the pathogenesis from a series of 80 patients. Medicine (Baltimore). 2001;80:355.
14. Santoro SA. Antiphospholipid antibodies and thrombotic predisposition: underlying pathogenetic mechanisms. Blood. 1994;83:2389.
15. Wisløff F, Jacobsen EM, Liestøl S. Laboratory diagnosis of the antiphospholipid syndrome. Thromb Res. 2002;108:263.
16. Harris EN, Gharavi AE, Boey ML, et al. Anticardiolipin antibodies: detection by radioimmunoassay and association with thrombosis in systemic lupus erythematosus. Lancet. 1983; 2:1211.
17. Ichikawa K, Khamashta MA, Koike T, et al. Beta 2-glycoprotein I reactivity of monoclonal anticardiolipin antibodies from patients with the antiphospholipid syndrome. Arthritis Rheum. 1994;37:1453.
18. Forastiero R, Martinuzzo M. Prothrombotic mechanisms based on the impairment of fibrinolysis in the antiphospholipid syndrome. Lupus. 2008;17:872.
19. Girardi G, Berman J, Redecha P, et al. Complement C5a receptors and neutrophils mediate fetal injury in the antiphospholipid syndrome. J Clin Invest. 2003;112:1644.
20. Girardi G, Redecha P, Salmon JE. Heparin prevents antiphospholipid antibody-induced fetal loss by inhibiting complement activation. Nat Med. 2004;10:1222.
21. Shamonki JM, Salmon JE, Hyjek E, Baergen RN. Excessive complement activation is associated with placental injury in patients with antiphospholipid antibodies. Am J Obstet Gynecol. 2007;196:167.e1.
22. Giles IP, Isenberg DA, Latchman DS, Rahman A. How do antiphospholipid antibodies bind beta2-glycoprotein I? Arthritis Rheum. 2003;48:2111.
23. Oku K, Atsumi T, Bohgaki M, et al. Complement activation in patients with primary antiphospholipid syndrome. Ann Rheum Dis. 2009;68:1030.
24. Goldberg SN, Conti-Kelly AM, Greco TP. A family study of anticardiolipin antibodies and associated clinical conditions. Am J Med. 1995;99:473.
25. Segal JB, Streiff MB, Hofmann LV, et al. Management of venous thromboembolism: a systematic review for a practice guideline. Ann Intern Med. 2007;146:211.

26. Crowther MA, Ginsberg JS, Julian J, et al. A comparison of two intensities of warfarin for the prevention of recurrent thrombosis in patients with the antiphospholipid antibody syndrome. N Engl J Med. 2003;349:1133.
27. Finazzi G, Marchioli R, Brancaccio V, et al. A randomized clinical trial of high-intensity warfarin vs. conventional antithrombotic therapy for the prevention of recurrent thrombosis in patients with the antiphospholipid syndrome (WAPS). J Thromb Haemost. 2005;3:848.
28. Moll S, Ortel TL. Monitoring warfarin therapy in patients with lupus anticoagulants. Ann Intern Med. 1997;127:177.
29. Erkan D, Harrison MJ, Levy R, et al. Aspirin for primary thrombosis prevention in the antiphospholipid syndrome: a randomized, double-blind, placebo-controlled trial in asymptomatic antiphospholipid antibody-positive individuals. Arthritis Rheum. 2007;56:2382.
30. Alarcón-Segovia D, Boffa MC, Branch W, et al. Prophylaxis of the antiphospholipid syndrome: a consensus report. Lupus. 2003;12:499.
31. Erkan D, Merrill JT, Yazici Y, et al. High thrombosis rate after fetal loss in antiphospholipid syndrome: effective prophylaxis with aspirin. Arthritis Rheum. 2001;44:1466.
32. Ruiz-Irastorza G, Khamashta MA. The treatment of antiphospholipid syndrome: a harmonic contrast. Best Pract Res Clin Rheumatol. 2007;21:1079.
33. Ruiz-Irastorza G, Hunt BJ, Khamashta MA. A systematic review of secondary thromboprophylaxis in patients with antiphospholipid antibodies. Arthritis Rheum. 2007;57:1487.
34. Sacco RL, Adams R, Albers G, et al. Guidelines for prevention of stroke in patients with ischemic stroke or transient ischemic attack: a statement for healthcare professionals from the American Heart Association/American Stroke Association Council on Stroke: co-sponsored by the Council on Cardiovascular Radiology and Intervention: the American Academy of Neurology affirms the value of this guideline. Stroke. 2006;37:577.
35. Durand JM, Lefevre P, Kaplanski G, et al. Correction of thrombocytopenia with dapsone in the primary antiphospholipid syndrome. J Rheumatol. 1993;20:1777.
36. Erkan D, Asherson RA, Espinosa G, et al. Long term outcome of catastrophic antiphospholipid syndrome survivors. Ann Rheum Dis. 2003;62:530.
37. Lockshin MD, Erkan D. Treatment of the antiphospholipid syndrome. N Engl J Med. 2003;349:1177.
38. Zar T, Kaplan AA. Predictable removal of anticardiolipin antibody by therapeutic plasma exchange (TPE) in catastrophic antiphospholipid antibody syndrome (CAPS). Clin Nephrol. 2008;70:77.
39. Kasthuri RS, Roubey RA. Warfarin and the antiphospholipid syndrome: does one size fit all? Arthritis Rheum. 2007;57:1346.
40. Ruiz-Irastorza G, Khamashta MA, Hunt BJ, et al. Bleeding and recurrent thrombosis in definite antiphospholipid syndrome: analysis of a series of 66 patients treated with oral anticoagulation to a target international normalized ratio of 3.5. Arch Intern Med. 2002;162:1164.
41. Kumar D, Roubey RA. Use of rituximab in the antiphospholipid syndrome. Curr Rheumatol Rep. 2010;12(1):40–4.
42. Cervera R, Khamashta MA, Shoenfeld Y, et al. Morbidity and mortality in the antiphospholipid syndrome during a 5-year period: a multicentre prospective study of 1000 patients. Ann Rheum Dis. 2009;68:1428.

Chapter 16
Lupus-Like Syndromes Related to Drugs

Joseph F. Merola

Introduction

A wide variety of agents have been implicated in the development of autoimmunity including pharmacologic, chemical, environmental, dietary, herbal, and infectious agents. Certain drugs, for example, may lead to the development of autoantibodies and, in some cases, a clinical autoimmune syndrome. In systemic lupus erythematosus (SLE), a drug might (a) exacerbate underlying idiopathic SLE, (b) induce SLE in a predisposed patient, or (c) cause the distinct syndrome of drug-induced lupus (DIL). Causality of potential inciting agents is hard to prove, with many associations based upon case report and observational data. However, several controlled studies have been conducted to implicate a number of drugs in the development of drug-related lupus. It is important to note that there is a greater likelihood of an individual producing autoantibodies in the presence of a given drug than showing signs of a clinical lupus-like syndrome.

The number of medications causing drug-induced autoimmunity is increasing. The use of biologics, many of which are meant to be immunomodulatory in activity, has broadened the clinical spectrum of autoantibody production and clinical manifestations of drug-induced autoimmune syndromes. Outside of a small group of medications for which properly controlled studies have demonstrated causality, it can be difficult to know how strongly associated a medication or other exposure might be with an incident autoimmune syndrome as most literature is usually in the form of case reports and case series. There should be a temporal relationship between

---

J.F. Merola, M.D. (✉)
Department of Medicine, Division of Rheumatology and Department of Dermatology,
Brigham and Women's Hospital, 75 Francis Street, Boston, MA 02115, USA

Harvard Medical School, Boston, MA, USA
e-mail: jmerola@partners.org

the drug in question and the clinical findings. Further confirmation may come with inadvertent reexposure to the same drug or similar drug in its class. With a few exceptions, the drug dosage does not appear to correlate with development of autoimmunity, but instead cumulative dose.

Environmental agents have been associated with a variety of autoimmune syndromes. Examples include exposure to hydrazines, aromatic amines, silica, and polyvinyl chloride. The toxic oil syndrome and the eosinophilic-myalgia syndrome, with similarities to systemic sclerosis and muscle disorders, are related to the ingestion of denatured rapeseed oil and L-tryptophan ingestion, respectively. Chronic heavy metal exposure such as mercury, gold, and cadmium has been implicated in immune-complex-mediated renal disease and other lupus-like disorders.

Drug-Induced Lupus

Epidemiology

DIL was first reported in 1953 in patients taking hydralazine. There are an estimated 15,000–30,000 cases of DIL per year, equal in males and females, and it is more common in older people and Caucasians. DIL represents 10 % of all lupus cases in the USA. The risk of developing DIL is quite different among medication exposures. For example, 15–20 % taking procainamide, 7–13 % taking hydralazine, 2 per 1,000 taking anti-TNF, and 5 per 10,000 taking minocycline.

Associated Drugs

A variety of drugs have been identified as being definite, probable, or possible/unlikely causes of DIL (Table 16.1). It should be noted, however, that due to a lack of analytical studies, "risks" are currently assigned largely based on number of case reports published in the literature.

A lupus-like syndrome is most common with the drug procainamide. Nearly all patients given this medication will, after 2 years, have a positive antinuclear antibody (ANA) titer. Importantly, however, symptoms will develop in about one-third of these patients. Therefore, in patients exposed to procainamide, a negative ANA test has a very good negative predictive value for DIL due to this agent. A reactive metabolite of procainamide, procainamide-hydroxylamine, has been implicated in the development of DIL. There is little or no antibody formation, however, with administration of the N-acetylprocainamide metabolite of procainamide (not commercially available). Typical clinical manifestations are described below.

The incidence of disease with administration of hydralazine is 5–10 %. Risk factors of DIL with hydralazine include drug dose (more than 200 mg/day and/or cumulative dose of more than 100 g), female gender, slow acetylation, HLA-DR4

Table 16.1 Drugs associated with drug-induced lupus

Class of drug	Definite association	Probable association	Possible association
Antiarrythmic	Procainamide (high risk), quinidine	Amiodarone	
Antibiotics	Isoniazid, minocycline	Sulfonamides, rifampin, nitrofurantoin	Penicillin, tetracycline
Anticonvulsant		Phenytoin, mephenytoin, trimethadione, ethosuximide, carbamazepine	Valproate
Antidepressants		Lithium carbonate	
Antifungal		Terbinafine (SCLE)	Griseofulvin
Antihistaminic			Cimetidine, promethazine
Antihypertensive	Diltiazem (SCLE[a])		Clonidine, prazosin
Antihypertensives—ACE inhibitors		Captopril	Enalapril
Antihypertensives—diuretics	Hydralazine (high risk)	Hydrochlorothiazide	Chlorthalidone, spironolactone
Antihypertensives—beta blockers	Practolol	Acebutolol, atenolol, labetalol, metoprolol, oxprenolol, pindolol, propranolol	
Antimigraine			Methysergide
Anti-Parkinson	Methyldopa		
Antipsychotics	Chlorpromazine		Reserpine
Biologics	Antitumor necrosis factor alpha therapy (adalimumab, etanercept, infliximab), interferon-alpha	Interferon-gamma	
Cholesterol-lowering agent			Statins (including lovastatin, simvastatin, atorvastatin), gemfibrozil
Hormonal			Danazol, leuprolide acetate, aromatase inhibitors
NSAID		Para-aminosalicylate, sulfasalazine	5-aminosalicylate, diclofenac, Ibuprofen, mesalamine, sulindac, tolmetin

(continued)

Table 16.1 (continued)

Class of drug	Definite association	Probable association	Possible association
Other	Penicillamine (antirheumatic)	Glyburide (diabetes), ticlopidine (antiplatelet), docetaxel (chemotherapeutic)	Gold-salts (antirheumatic), timolol (ophthalmic)
Thyroid medication		Methimazole, methylthiouracil, propylthiouracil, thionamide	
Xanthine oxidase inhibitor			Allopurinol

SCLE subacute cutaneous lupus erythematosus

genotype, and low levels of the fourth complement component. The commonest clinical features are described below.

Minocycline causes a DIL syndrome classically in young women being treated for acne vulgaris. The antibody profile of these patients is interesting in that a positive ANA is frequently encountered as well as a p-ANCA. About one-half of affected patients have laboratory evidence of liver involvement. One should avoid the use of minocycline in patients with idiopathic SLE as it has been associated with flare of idiopathic SLE as well as the drug-induced syndrome associated with this medication. Clinical features include ANA positivity (92 %), p-ANCA positivity (83 %), antihistone positivity (0–13 %), and positive anti-dsDNA along with fever, arthralgia/myalgia, symmetric arthritis, and elevated transaminases. A pneumonitis may occur as well as cutaneous vasculitis. Genetic susceptibility is implied, particularly HLA-DQB1 and either HLA-DR2 or HLA-DR4.

Clinical Features

DIL shares many clinical features with idiopathic SLE but with some notable differences. The demographics of the affected populations differ with idiopathic SLE developing in a female to male ratio of 9:1 and an almost equal occurrence in males and females in DIL. The population that develop DIL closely relates to the type of diseases for which the particular drug is being prescribed, for example, young females with acne for minocycline exposure versus a more elderly population with a coronary artery disease medication-related exposure. Common presentations include generalized malaise, weakness, arthralgias, myalgias, and serositis, and occasionally, a frank symmetric polyarthritis develops. It is important to recognize, however, that clinical and serologic features cluster with the specific drug exposure in question. For instance, pleuritis occurs in 50 % of patients with DIL from procainamide, in 22 % exposed to quinidine, and <1 % exposed to minocycline, whereas

Table 16.2 Comparison of features of idiopathic and drug-induced lupus

Clinical feature	Idiopathic SLE	Drug-induced lupus
Gender predisposition (F:M)	9:1	1:1
Usual age	20–40	Drug-dependent, tends to be older population than idiopathic
Fever/malaise	40–85 %	40–50 %
Arthralgias/arthritis	75–95 %	80–95 %
Rash (all)	50–70 %	10–30 %
Rash (discoid)	20 %	Rare[a]
Rash (subacute cutaneous)[b]	58 %	20–40 %
Rash (malar/acute cutaneous)	42 %	2 %
Raynaud's	35–50 %	<25 %
Pleuritis/pleural effusion	16–60 %	10–50 % (Procainamide predom)
Pulmonary infiltrates	0–10 %	5–40 % (Procainamide predom)
Pericarditis	6–45 %	2–18 %
Hepatomegaly/splenomegaly	10–45 %	5–25 %
Renal involvement	30–50 %	0–5 %
CNS/neurologic involvement	25–70 %	0–2 %
Hematologic	Common	Unusual

[a]Discoid lesions may be seen rarely with use of biologic agents, such as anti-TNF-alpha inhibitors
[b]High percentage of drug-induced variants than thought in the past, 70–90% anti-SSA/Ro positive

transaminase abnormalities in the minocycline group occur in 32–54 % and are not a common feature of procainamide- or quinidine-induced DIL.

Pleuropulmonary/cardiac manifestations may include pleuritis, pericarditis, pleural effusions, and pulmonary infiltrates, particularly in patients exposed to procainamide. Coexisting conditions can make diagnosis a challenge, such as the heart failure patient with pleural effusion. DIL related to procainamide is milder than idiopathic SLE. Fever is less common, and skin and renal involvement is often absent. A case of primary antiphospholipid antibody syndrome to procainamide has been reported.

Hydralazine-induced DIL most typically produces musculoskeletal symptoms although has been associated with more severe and even fatal outcomes. Serositis, namely pericarditis, occurs in <5 % of patients.

Nonspecific drug rashes may occur, such as the morbilliform drug eruption; however, DIL rashes, such as a subacute cutaneous lupus rash from exposure to diltiazem, will be considered separately (see below). One helpful diagnostic clue may be the presence of discoid lupus lesions, which are found almost exclusively in idiopathic SLE as opposed to DIL (rare exceptions include the use of newer biologic agents such as anti-TNF-alpha drugs). In many cases, the only way to make the diagnosis of DIL is to stop the potentially offending agent and monitor the patient for improvement.

Other clinical features of idiopathic SLE, such as overt nephritis, hematologic, neurologic disease, and chronic cutaneous discoid lupus are rarely seen in DIL syndromes as described in case reports. It is important to note that more overlap is seen with SLE as the use of newer immunomodulatory biologic agents increases (see Table 16.2).

Table 16.3 Comparison of laboratory features of drug-induced lupus and SLE

Laboratory feature	Idiopathic SLE (%)	Drug-induced lupus
ANA	95–98	95–100 %
Anti-dsDNA	50–80	<5 % (rare)
Anti-Smith	20–30	<5 % (rare)
Anti-RNP	40–50	20%
Antihistone[a]	60–80	90–95 %
Low complement levels	40–65	0 %
Anemia	30–90	0–46 %
Leukopenia	35–66	2–33 %
Positive Coombs' test	18–65	0–33 %[b]

[a] "Overall" presence in DIL; varies markedly between drug exposures, see text
[b] Most commonly with methyldopa exposure

Laboratory Features (see Table 16.3)

Antihistone antibodies are said to be present in more than 95 % of DIL overall. However, this figure most accurately represents their occurrence following procainamide and quinidine exposure as antihistone antibodies have been detected in only 32 % of minocycline-exposed, 42 % of propylthiouracil-exposed, and <50 % of statin-exposed patients who develop DIL. Importantly, up to 80 % of Individuals with idiopathic systemic lupus also have antihistone antibodies. However, patients with idiopathic systemic lupus also have a variety of other autoantibodies, such as those to extractable nuclear antigens, which is an important piece of evidence in differentiating these groups. In particular, antibodies to double-stranded DNA have historically been thought rare in DIL and helpful in distinguishing from idiopathic systemic lupus, where the antibodies are more commonly found.

The antihistone antibody antigenic target may be different in DIL as opposed to the antihistone antibody found in patients with idiopathic systemic lupus (i.e., antibody directed against a complex of the histone dimer H2A-H2B/DNA complex and H1/H3-H4 complex with a drug-induced etiology, antibody directed against a complex of H1/H2B histone subunits in idiopathic systemic lupus).

Induction of antibodies to double-stranded DNA is typically absent in DIL due to procainamide, hydralazine, and isoniazid; however, these antibodies may be seen with cytokine/anti-cytokine therapies such as anti-TNF therapies.

Diagnosis

Unfortunately, no definitive criteria, diagnostic test, or procedure exists for the diagnosis of DIL. The presence of clinical symptoms of systemic lupus, serologic data including a positive ANA, ingestion of a suspected culprit drug over a period of 3 weeks to 2 years prior to the development of clinical signs/symptoms, rapid improvement with drug withdrawal, and recurrence of symptoms with rechallenge have been proposed as diagnostic criteria. In the majority of cases, cessation of symptoms after withdrawal of the offending drug will confirm suspicion.

Drug-Induced Lupus due to Anti-TNF-Alpha Agents

Despite the high number of patients exposed to this class of medications which includes infliximab, etanercept, adalimumab, golimumab, and certolizumab, DIL from anti-TNF-alpha agents remains relatively rare. The most typical clinical features are similar to those described above; however, several differences are noteworthy. Well-described is the development of skin lesions of subacute cutaneous lupus and, more recently, chronic cutaneous lupus (discoid variant) with the use of anti-TNF agents. These reactions may occur slightly more frequently with etanercept than infliximab. The development of serositis is another clinical manifestation, more frequently observed in those treated with infliximab than etanercept or adalimumab. Renal disease has been observed in case reports. Anti-dsDNA antibodies are commonly seen with exposure to anti-TNF agents while antihistone antibodies occur less frequently. It is important to state that the development of autoantibodies during treatment with this class of medication is exceedingly common (elevated ANA 79–100 %, anti-dsDNA 72–92 %, antihistone 17–57 % of patients treated with anti-TNF drug), while clinical signs and symptoms of a DIL syndrome is rare.

Herbal Medicines as a Cause of Rheumatologic Disease

Alfalfa (L-canavanine) was identified as an agent that can cause a lupus-like illness in primates and possibly exacerbate lupus in humans. Yohimbine has also been implicated as a cause of a lupus-like syndrome. Kava-kava as well as the alga *Spirulina platensis* has been reported to cause a dermatomyositis-like illness, while Echinacea has been implicated in flares of other autoimmune skin diseases. With the increasing use of herbal medications, it is of increasing importance to obtain a medication history to include over-the-counter and herbal supplements in patients as it is likely that more reports will emerge of associated autoimmune conditions.

Drugs Causing or "Unmasking" Underlying Idiopathic Systemic Lupus Erythematosus

Distinct from the syndrome of "drug-induced-lupus" is the concept of unmasked or exacerbated idiopathic underlying SLE. Drugs implicated include sulfonamide antibiotics, namely trimethoprim-sulfamethoxazole, penicillins, antiepileptic drugs, minocycline, cimetidine, hydralazine, and hydrochlorothiazide. While no strong data exists to deem these agents as absolutely contraindicated in patients with systemic lupus, one may consider alternative agents or have a heightened suspicion of symptoms of a flare when using these agents. There are some data to support an increased incidence of adverse drug reactions, namely rash, with the use of trimethoprim-sulfamethoxazole in lupus patients compared to controls and overall higher incidence of allergy to sulfonamide moiety–containing compounds among lupus patients particularly with anti-Ro and anti-RNP positivity.

Drug-Induced Cutaneous Lupus

Interestingly, newer data suggests that many more cases of subacute cutaneous lupus erythematosus (SCLE) may be drug-induced than previously thought. Of note, in both idiopathic and drug-induced forms, 70–90 % of patients with SCLE are anti-Ro/SSA positive. Drug-induced etiology should now be considered in any case of subacute cutaneous lupus. The skin changes usually occur 4–20 weeks after starting the offending agent and may cause a more widespread involvement than idiopathic SCLE. Patients rarely experience systemic symptoms although serositis is reported. Many of the drugs implicated are cardiac drugs, being used with more frequency in an aging population. In addition to the commonly implicated medications including hydrochlorothiazide, calcium channel blockers (diltiazem, nifedipine, verapamil), a number of angiotensin-converting enzyme inhibitors (captopril, enalapril, lisinopril), and statin medications (pravastatin, simvastatin), some newer reports include terbinafine (as an oral antifungal), proton-pump inhibitors (omeprazole, pantoprazole, lansoprazole), leflunomide, bupropion, acebutolol, and capecitabine. TNF-alpha inhibitor medications are also implicated with reports of SCLE developing in patients receiving etanercept, adalimumab, and infliximab. Distinguishing between idiopathic and drug-induced SCLE may be difficult clinically, but a few clues may be the extent of cutaneous involvement as well as the presence of eosinophils present on skin biopsy, favoring a drug-induced variant (see Fig. 16.1).

Although very rare, there are reports of drug-induced chronic cutaneous lupus erythematosus—"discoid" lupus in the setting of TNF-alpha inhibitor use. The mean duration of onset is 8 months and has been reported with infliximab and etanercept as well as several fluorouracil agents including tegafur and uracil-tegafur.

Pathogenesis

The mechanisms underlying the development of DIL seem to be diverse although many appear to involve drug metabolism and the interaction of drug metabolites with an altered immune system. Broadly, genetic predisposition (i.e., HLA allele

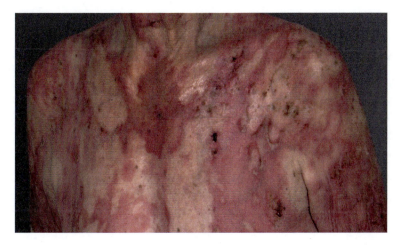

Fig. 16.1 Drug-induced subacute cutaneous lupus (courtesy of the Joseph F. Merola, MD collection)

associations, metabolic enzyme variants), epigenetic phenomena (i.e., inhibition of DNA methylation), drug metabolism (i.e., acetylator status, differences in oxidative drug metabolism as in P450 enzyme polymorphisms), drug activation of lymphocytes (i.e., nonspecific activation, drug as hapten, mimicry, disruption of central immune tolerance), sex hormone modulation, and TNF-alpha inhibition may play varying roles based on the specific drug metabolite. A host of other mechanisms still remain to be worked out in order to fully explain the phenomenon of DIL.

Formation of "reactive metabolites" with similar characteristics may help to explain why chemicals with diverse structure can induce similar clinical outcomes. Acetylation of drugs leads to their elimination, and therefore, rapid acetylation is protective against reactive metabolite formation. In some patients, labeled "slow acetylators," a genetically mediated decrease in the hepatic synthesis of *N*-acetyltransferase increases the likelihood of developing a DIL syndrome. Procainamide, propylthiouracil, isoniazid, hydralazine, quinidine, and chlorpromazine are readily oxidized to reactive cytotoxic species by activated leucocytes. The metabolites of these drugs are likely involved in the induction of DIL, possibly via hapten-like reactions with nucleoproteins or direct interaction with HLA molecules. Furthermore, these metabolites (specifically procainamide-hydroxylamine) have been shown to interfere with T-cell maturation in the thymus, resulting in the passage of autoreactive T cells into peripheral circulation. Administration of procainamide-hydroxylamine (PAHA) into the thymus of normal adult mice leads to the development of anti-chromatin antibodies and has been found to disrupt the induction of anergy of mature T lymphocytes. Procainamide may further act via DNA demethylation activity as described below.

DNA demethylation leads to increasing activation of a number of promoter regions with resultant expression of several pro-inflammatory cytokines and therefore enhanced lymphocyte responsiveness. Hydralazine, for example, via inhibition of the ERK pathway, prevents induction of DNA methyltransferase, thereby stimulating T-cell activity. Similar activities have been described with procainamide metabolites where treatment of T helper 2 cells in vitro makes them autoreactive.

Anti-TNF therapies may lead to DIL by downregulating mechanisms controlling B-cell hyperactivity and via inhibition of a normal feedback loop which instead produces increased type I interferon (i.e., interferon-alpha).

Genetic disposition includes both HLA alleles and drug metabolism-affecting factors. Emphasis has largely focused on HLA allele associations historically. Sulfasalazine- and 5-aminosalicylate-induced lupus includes risk factors in the HLA DRB1*0301 haplotype. HLA-DR4, HLA-DR2, and HLA-DQB1 alleles have been implicated in DIL secondary to minocycline.

Treatment

Recognizing and discontinuing the offending agent is a more important aspect of treatment. Constitutional and musculoskeletal symptoms may be controlled with nonsteroidal anti-inflammatory agents (NSAIDs) alone. Low-dose prednisone may be required for refractory symptoms. Higher doses of prednisone may be necessary to treat more serious disease manifestations such as rare hematologic, renal, neurologic complications. In the patient in whom prolonged treatment is required to control symptoms, idiopathic SLE should be suspected. Autoantibody serologies may persist for a long while after discontinuation of the offending agent.

Conclusions

A number of medications and environmental exposures have been described that lead to DIL—a constellation of clinical signs, symptoms, and serologic abnormalities distinct from, but with many similarities to, idiopathic SLE. The exact manifestations of this syndrome vary by specific drug exposure, and with the increasing use of newer agents (in particular immune-modulatory therapies), the clinician needs to have heightened awareness of this entity.

Sources

1. Aloush V, Litinsky I, Caspi D, Elkayam O. Propylthiouracil-induced autoimmune syndromes: two distinct clinical presentations with different course and management. Semin Arthritis Rheum. 2006;36(1):4–9.

2. Bachmeyer C, Cadranel JF. Minocycline-induced lupus and autoimmune hepatitis: family autoimmune disorders as possible risk factors. Dermatology. 2002;205(2):185–6.
 3. Birnbaum B, Sidhu GS, Smith RL, Pillinger MH, Tagoe CE. Fulminating hydralazine-induced lupus pneumonitis. Arthritis Rheum. 2006;55(3):501–6.
 4. Borchers AT, Keen CL, Gershwin ME. Drug-induced lupus. Ann N Y Acad Sci. 2007;1108: 166–82.
 5. Callen JP. Drug-induced subacute cutaneous lupus erythematosus. Lupus. 2010;19(9): 1107–11.
 6. Cameron HA, Ramsay LE. The lupus syndrome induced by hydralazine: a common complication with low dose treatment. Br Med J (Clin Res Ed). 1984;289(6442):410–2.
 7. Dedeoglu F. Drug-induced autoimmunity. Curr Opin Rheumatol. 2009;21(5):547–51.
 8. Dunphy J, Oliver M, Rands AL, Lovell CR, McHugh NJ. Antineutrophil cytoplasmic antibodies and HLA class II alleles in minocycline-induced lupus-like syndrome. Br J Dermatol. 2000;142(3):461–7.
 9. Ferraro-Peyret C, Coury F, Tebib JG, Bienvenu J, Fabien N. Infliximab therapy in rheumatoid arthritis and ankylosing spondylitis-induced specific antinuclear and antiphospholipid autoantibodies without autoimmune clinical manifestations: a two-year prospective study. Arthritis Res Ther. 2004;6(6):R535–43. Epub 2004 Sep 23.
10. Hess E. Drug-related lupus. N Engl J Med. 1988;318(22):1460–2.
11. Jeffries M, Bruner G, Glenn S, Sadanandan P, Carson CW, Harley JB, Sawalha AH. Sulpha allergy in lupus patients: a clinical perspective. Lupus. 2008;17(3):202–5.
12. Kretz-Rommel A, Rubin RL. A metabolite of the lupus-inducing drug procainamide prevents anergy induction in T cell clones. J Immunol. 1997;158(9):4465–70.
13. Lee AN, Werth VP. Activation of autoimmunity following use of immunostimulatory herbal supplements. Arch Dermatol. 2004;140(6):723–7.
14. Margolis DJ, Hoffstad O, Bilker W. Association or lack of association between tetracycline class antibiotics used for acne vulgaris and lupus erythematosus. Br J Dermatol. 2007; 157(3):540–6. Epub 2007 Jun 26.
15. Mongey AB, Donovan-Brand R, Thomas TJ, Adams LE, Hess EV. Serologic evaluation of patients receiving procainamide. Arthritis Rheum. 1992;35(2):219–23.
16. Mor A, Pillinger MH, Wortmann RL, Mitnick HJ. Drug-induced arthritis and connective tissue disorders. Semin Arthritis Rheum. 2008;38(3):249–64. Epub 2007 Dec 31. Review.
17. Muramatsu M, Nakajima M, Mori M, Sobashima H, Sano H, Katao K. A case of primary antiphospholipid antibody syndrome associated with procainamide induced systemic lupus erythematosus. Nihon Naika Gakkai Zasshi. 1995;84(10):1736–8.
18. Noël B. Lupus erythematosus and other autoimmune diseases related to statin therapy: a systematic review. J Eur Acad Dermatol Venereol. 2007;21(1):17–24.
19. Reidenberg MM, Drayer DE. Procainamide, N-acetylprocainamide, antinuclear antibody and systemic lupus erythematosus. Angiology. 1986;37(12 Pt 2):968–71.
20. Schoonen WM, Thomas SL, Somers EC, Smeeth L, Kim J, Evans S, Hall AJ. Do selected drugs increase the risk of lupus? A matched case-control study. Br J Clin Pharmacol. 2010; 70(4):588–96.
21. Schur PH, Rose BD. Drug-induced lupus. In: Pisetsky DS, Greene JM, editors. UpToDate. Waltham: UpToDate; 2011.
22. Speirs C, Fielder AH, Chapel H, Davey NJ, Batchelor JR. Complement system protein C4 and susceptibility to hydralazine-induced systemic lupus erythematosus. Lancet. 1989;1(8644): 922–4.
23. Vasoo S. Drug-induced lupus: an update. Lupus. 2006;15(11):757–61.

Chapter 17
New and Emerging Therapies

Elena M. Massarotti

The advent of biotechnology combined with an increasing understanding of the immunopathogenesis of rheumatic diseases has led to an explosion of new biological therapies that have been approved or are in development. Examples of these include anti-TNF inhibitors, B-cell-depleting agents, costimulatory modulators, and anti-IL-6 therapy for the treatment of rheumatoid arthritis, the most common inflammatory rheumatic disease, affecting about 1 % of the North American population. While the understanding of the pathogenesis of lupus has evolved over the last decades, the identification of a single, targetable molecule whose inhibition would mitigate the myriad manifestations of this relatively rare, heterogeneous disease remains elusive. However, several trials, including those that failed to meet primary endpoints, offered rheumatologists important lessons regarding pathogenesis and treatment that help to inform present and future drug development. This chapter summarizes these new and emerging therapies for lupus.

Biological Therapy

Biological therapies are directed against specific components of the immune system. Examples of biological therapies include antitumor necrosis factor (anti-TNF) inhibitors currently in widespread use for rheumatoid arthritis and inflammatory bowel disease. Over the last decade, numerous molecules have been investigated as potential targets for the treatment of lupus with disappointing

---

E.M. Massarotti, M.D. (✉)
Division of Rheumatology, Center for Clinical Therapeutics,
Brigham and Women's Hospital,
75 Francis Street, Boston, MA 02115, USA

Harvard Medical School, Boston, MA, USA
e-mail: emassarotti@partners.org

results, and many other immunological targets are being tested as potential new avenues for treatment.

In March 2011, the FDA approved belimumab for the treatment of lupus patients with active symptoms of lupus while taking "standard therapy." Belimumab is a monoclonal antibody directed against soluble B-cell-activating factor (BAFF), which is a critical factor involved in B-cell development. Animal models of lupus and preclinical studies showed that BAFF levels were elevated in patients with active lupus, and autoantibody production is increased in lupus patients—autoantibodies are manufactured by B cells. These observations led to the development of this novel molecule, the first biological therapy for the treatment of lupus.

The overall positive benefits of belimumab were shown in two large phase III trials done involving over 1,600 patients with active lupus despite taking "standard therapy" including nonsteroidal anti-inflammatory agents, antimalarials, immunosuppressive therapies, and corticosteroids. Subjects who had been treated with any B-cell-depleting therapy at any time in the past, or with intravenous cyclophosphamide 6 months before study entry, were excluded from participation. The primary outcome measure was a novel systemic lupus responder index, or SRI, that combined the BILAG, physician global assessment, and the SELENA-SLEDAI. Most subjects had mucocutaneous or musculoskeletal disease, and subjects with severe kidney or central nervous system disease were excluded. In both phase III studies, subjects treated with belimumab 10 mg/kg had a statistically significant improvement in the SRI compared with placebo. The effect size was small for both phase III studies, and the clinical response was not maintained at 76 weeks for the US/Western Europe study. A reduction in steroids and reduced number of flares was observed. Treatment was continued for a year, and the adverse event rate in treatment groups as compared with placebo-treated subjects was comparable, with an overall favorable safety profile for belimumab.

Resistant Disease and Investigational Therapy

Anti-B-Cell Therapy

Rituximab

Rituximab is a chimeric monoclonal antibody directed against anti-CD20-bearing B cells. The approval of belimumab came on the heels of two large placebo-controlled trials of rituximab in global lupus and lupus nephritis that failed to show benefit of this agent. Favorable results noted in uncontrolled observational studies of rituximab with cyclophosphamide led to these two large international, multicenter studies. The EXPLORER study compared the safety and efficacy of rituximab versus placebo in patients with active lupus despite taking background immunosuppressive therapy and used improvement in the BILAG as the primary outcome measure. No demonstrable benefit was seen. In the LUNAR study, subjects with biopsy-proven class III or IV lupus nephritis were randomized to receive mycophenolate mofetil (MMF) alone or MMF with rituximab and used a predefined measure of complete renal response that incorporated creatinine, urinary protein excretion, and urinary sediment as the primary outcome measure. No additional benefit of rituximab to MMF was seen.

Patients with severe organ involvement who are resistant to cyclophosphamide therapy generally do poorly. The optimal approach to such patients is uncertain including use of the new FDA-approved agent, belimumab, as the phase III studies of belimumab excluded subjects with severe kidney or CNS disease, and those subjects treated with intravenous cyclophosphamide for 6 months prior to study entry.

Atacicept

Atacicept is a recombinant fusion protein comprised of a portion of the transmembrane activator and calcium modulator and an immunoglobulin chain (TACI-Ig). Atacicept targets two molecules that otherwise promote B-cell survival when they interact with TACI on the B-cell surface. These are B-cell-activating factor of the tumor necrosis family (BAFF, also known as B-lymphocyte stimulator or BLyS®) and a proliferation-inducing ligand (APRIL).

A dose-dependent decrease in peripheral blood lymphocytes and in immunoglobulin levels was observed when atacicept was given to 32 patients with SLE in a safety and dose-ranging study. In this open-label study, there was a suggestion of clinical improvement and few adverse effects. A study of atacicept in patients with lupus nephritis study was halted due to an unacceptable incidence of infections in patients who were concurrently given mycophenolate. A study of atacicept in subjects with non renal manifestations of lupus has just completed enrollment. This multicenter, international study examined whether treatment with atacicept prevented lupus flares.

Epratuzumab

Epratuzumab, a humanized monoclonal antibody that binds to CD22 on B-cell surfaces, is another anti-B-cell agent being tested in patients with lupus. CD22 is a member of the Ig superfamily, which binds to sialic acid-bearing molecules on other hematopoietic and nonhematopoietic cells. Epratuzumab has been used to treat non-Hodgkin lymphoma. Favorable results with epratuzumab were noted in a 12-week phase IIb study of moderate to severe lupus subjects and prompted the initiation of a large multicenter phase III study that is currently enrolling subjects.

T-Cell Inhibition

Abatacept blocks the activation of T cells and was approved by the FDA for use in treating rheumatoid arthritis in 2005. A study that randomly assigned 118 patients to abatacept or placebo found that it did not improve cardiovascular, musculoskeletal, or cutaneous lupus. The protocol was hampered by the administration of high-dose steroids to both arms for 3 months along with immunosuppressive agents. The flare rates did not differ in part because abatacept takes 6 months to become optimally effective and most of the flares occurred between months 3 and 6. A large phase III study of abatacept in combination with cyclophosphamide in lupus nephritis is being conducted by the immune tolerance network (ITN).

Cyclosporine

Cyclosporine inhibits the transcription process that is normally associated with T cell activation. Addition of cyclosporine may allow a reduction in use of glucocorticoids. As an example, an unblinded study randomly assigned 89 patients with SLE who were taking ≥15 mg of prednisolone per day, and who required the addition or change of a glucocorticoid-sparing drug, to receive either cyclosporine or azathioprine. Both cyclosporine and azathioprine allowed for a reduction in prednisone at the end of 1 year of study. There was no statistically significant difference between cyclosporine and azathioprine in the reduction in dose (mean decrease in daily prednisolone dose of 9.0 and 10.7 mg, respectively, a difference of −1.7 mg) (95 % CI −4.4 to +0.9).

Similar rates of study drug discontinuation were noted for each group. Discontinuations due to lack of efficacy and for side effects were also similar. In this study, neither severe hypertension nor irreversible renal injury occurred in the cyclosporine-treated subjects. However, hypertension was noted more frequently in patients who received cyclosporine (49 % vs. 14 %), as was an increase in the serum creatinine (13 % vs. 2 %). When cyclosporine is used in clinical practice, these side effects must be anticipated. Frequent monitoring of blood pressure and renal function is necessary for appropriate dose titration.

Other Agents in Clinical Trials

A number of other therapeutic approaches have been tried or are under investigation in SLE. These include intravenous immunoglobulin, thalidomide, bromocriptine, zileuton, cyclosporine, sirolimus, anti-CD40, LJP 394, anti-C5 complement monoclonal antibody, anti-IL-10, B-cell depletors, mizoribine, immunoadsorption (via perfusion of patients' blood through a column of immobilized C1q or polyclonal sheep antihuman immunoglobulin), use of recombinant human interleukin-1 receptor antagonist (anakinra), anti-IL-6, spliceosomal peptide P140, noncoding (micro) RNA molecules, interferon alpha inhibitors, and an anti-TNF monoclonal antibody (infliximab) tocilizumab. Trials involving humanized monoclonal antibodies directed against interferon-α are also under way.

Hematopoietic Stem Cell Transplantation

The proposed mechanism of action of hematopoietic stem cell transplantation is that it provides a period free from memory T-cell influence, during which maturation of new lymphocyte progenitors can occur without recruitment to anti-self-activity.

Results from this approach are limited and include:

- High-dose chemotherapy followed by autologous stem cell transplantation administered to 50 patients with glomerulonephritis, cerebritis, transverse myelitis, autoimmune cytopenia, catastrophic antiphospholipid syndrome, and/or vasculitis despite intravenous cyclophosphamide. The overall 5-year survival was 84 %, and the probability of disease survival at 5 years was 50 %. Treatment-related mortality, in an intention to treat analysis, was 4 %.
- Results from the European Registry of autologous stem cell transplantation for SLE were notable for induction of remission of disease activity in 33 of 50 cases. However, one-third of the patients relapsed at a median of 6 months; survival was 62 % at 48 months, with treatment-related mortality of 12 %.

Stem cell transplantation remains complex, costly, and, despite improvements in treatment-related mortality, risky. Additional study, including direct comparison to more conventional treatment approaches in randomized controlled trials, is needed before any recommendation can be made regarding the role of stem cell transplantation in the treatment of SLE.

Immunoablation Alone

Immunoablation without bone marrow or stem cell support has also been effective in some patients with moderate to severe SLE refractory to glucocorticoids and immunosuppressive therapy. However, safety concerns caused the US National Institutes of Health to halt their trial that was examining the effectiveness of immunoablation alone.

Sources

1. Tyndall A. Cellular therapy of systemic lupus erythematosus. Lupus. 2009;18:387.
2. Merrill JT, Neuwelt CM, Wallace DJ, et al. Efficacy and safety of rituximab in moderately-to-severely active systemic lupus erythematosus: the randomized, double-blind, phase II/III systemic lupus erythematosus evaluation of rituximab trial. Arthritis Rheum. 2010;62:222.
3. Wallace DJ, Stohl W, Furie RA, et al. A phase II, randomized, double-blind, placebo-controlled, dose-ranging study of belimumab in patients with active systemic lupus erythematosus. Arthritis Rheum. 2009;61:1168.

4. Navarra SV, Guzmán RM, Gallacher AE, Hall S, Levy RA, Jimenez RE, Li EK, Thomas M, Kim HY, León MG, Tanasescu C, Nasonov E, Lan JL, Pineda L, Zhong ZJ, Freimuth W, Petri MA, BLISS-52 Study Group. Efficacy and safety of belimumab in patients with active systemic lupus erythematosus: a randomised, placebo-controlled, phase 3 trial. Lancet. 2011;377(9767):721–31.
5. Merrill JT, Burgos-Vargas R, Westhovens R, Chalmers A, D'Cruz D, Wallace DJ, Bae SC, Sigal L, Becker JC, Kelly S, Raghupathi K, Li T, Peng Y, Kinaszczuk M, Nash P. The efficacy and safety of abatacept in patients with non-life-threatening manifestations of systemic lupus erythematosus: results of a twelve-month, multicenter, exploratory, phase IIb, randomized, double-blind, placebo-controlled trial. Arthritis Rheum. 2010;62(10):3077–87.
6. Cardiel MH, Tumlin JA, Furie RA, Wallace DJ, Joh T, Linnik MD, LJP 394-90-09 Investigator Consortium. Abetimus sodium for renal flare in systemic lupus erythematosus: results of a randomized, controlled phase III trial. Arthritis Rheum. 2008;58(8):2470–80.
7. Merrill JT, Wallace DJ, Petri M, Kirou KA, Yao Y, White WI, Robbie G, Levin R, Berney SM, Chindalore V, Olsen N, Richman L, Le C, Jallal B, White B, Lupus Interferon Skin Activity (LISA) Study Investigators. Safety profile and clinical activity of sifalimumab, a fully human anti-interferon alpha monoclonal antibody, in systemic lupus erythematosus: a phase I, multicentre, double-blind randomised study. Ann Rheum Dis. 2011;70(11):1905–13.
8. Up to Date: Many articles in UpToDate in rheumatology

Chapter 18
Co-morbidities in Systemic Lupus Erythematosus

Mary Gayed, Chee-Seng Yee, Sasha Bernatsky, and Caroline Gordon

Cardiovascular Disease

This is increasingly recognised as a cause of considerable morbidity and mortality in lupus patients. In addition to reviewing the magnitude of cardiovascular risk in terms of events such as myocardial infarction and stroke due to atherosclerosis, the ability to assess preclinical disease using surrogate markers will be discussed. Risk factors and mechanisms involved in the development of atherosclerosis will be considered and finally strategies for reducing the risk of cardiovascular complications will be outlined.

M. Gayed, M.B.Ch.B.
Rheumatology Department, City Hospital, Sandwell
and West Birmingham Hospitals, NHS Trust,
Birmingham B18 7QH, UK

C.-S. Yee, Ph.D. • C. Gordon, M.D. (✉)
Rheumatology Department, City Hospital, Sandwell
and West Birmingham Hospitals, NHS Trust,
Birmingham B18 7QH, UK

Rheumatology Research Group, East Wing, School of Immunity and Infection,
College of Medical and Dental Sciences, University of Birmingham,
Birmingham B15 2TT, UK
e-mail: p.c.gordon@bham.ac.uk

S. Bernatsky, Ph.D.
Royal Victoria Hospital, 687 Pine Avenue West, V-Building,
Montreal, QC, Canada H3A 1A1

Magnitude of Cardiovascular Risk in SLE

Cardiovascular Events and Mortality

Systemic lupus erythematosus (SLE) is associated with a two to fivefold increase of death compared to the general population, although many advances have been made since the 1950s when the 5 year survival was only 50 %. A bimodal pattern of mortality has been reported in SLE patients with early mortality (less than 5 years since diagnosis) more likely to be due to severe disease activity and/or sepsis, and late mortality often associated with the complications of atherosclerosis.

The international study by the Systemic Lupus International Collaborating Clinics (SLICC) group with 9,547 patients showed that the all-cause standardised mortality rate (SMR) was 2.4 and the SMR for circulatory diseases (heart disease, arterial disease and cerebrovascular disease) was 1.7 (95 % CI: 1.5–1.9) as compared to normals. Studies have shown that the overall prevalence of myocardial infarction in lupus cohorts around the world is 6–10 %, and, that lupus patients are five to ten times more likely to suffer than the general population from symptomatic ischaemic heart disease (IHD). Autopsy studies have shown that over 50 % of lupus patients have moderate to severe atherosclerosis.

Ischaemic cardiovascular disease usually occurs in post-menopausal women over the age of 60 years. However premature atherosclerotic disease has been observed in SLE, with women aged 35–44 being shown to have a risk of myocardial infarction (MI) 50 times higher than women in the Framingham cohort, and women with SLE in older age groups having a risk 2.5–4 times higher than expected. In a Canadian cohort the relative risk for MI attributed to SLE was 10.1 and for stroke was 7.9 after controlling for traditional risk factors for atherosclerosis suggesting disease-related predisposing factors.

Surrogate Markers for Cardiovascular Disease

Various non-invasive techniques have been investigated as surrogate markers of cardiovascular disease. These techniques may be both helpful for demonstrating increased risk and response to interventions designed to reduce the number of cardiovascular events. Carotid ultrasound is a validated surrogate marker for cardiovascular disease risk, as there is a strong correlation between carotid and coronary atherosclerosis in the general population. B-mode carotid ultrasound can be used to demonstrate both carotid plaque due to atherosclerosis (with or without stenosis) and increased carotid intima-media thickness (IMT) as a marker of subclinical atherosclerosis and predictor of myocardial infarction and stroke.

An alternative non-invasive method is electron beam computed tomography (EBCT), which has previously been demonstrated to be a sensitive method of detecting the risk of future coronary vascular disease in asymptomatic patients. Studies comparing lupus patient with no history of coronary artery disease with age and sex matched controls have demonstrated statistically significant two to threefold increases in the frequency of patients with coronary artery calcification on EBCT.

Table 18.1 Cardiovascular risk factors in SLE

Modifiable traditional risk factors
Hypertension
Dyslipidaemia (hypercholesterolaemia)
Diabetes
Obesity
Smoking
Lack of exercise

Disease related
Autoantibodies (including antiphospholipid antibodies)
Inflammation (pro-inflammatory cytokines, elevated CRP)
Disease activity and renal involvement
Imbalance of vascular damage and repair
Drugs (corticosteroids)

In addition there was an increased frequency of lupus patients with plaques and increased number of plaques on carotid ultrasonography. EBCT imaging results are most dramatic for female patients under 55 years of age in whom rates of subclinical atherosclerosis in controls are low (<5 %) but may be increased over fourfold in SLE (>20 %). Furthermore accelerated plaque and IMT progression has been demonstrated by carotid ultrasound in SLE patients compared with controls (27 % versus 10 % over a mean of 4.2 years).

Other non-invasive methods used to assess cardiovascular disease include flow-mediated dilatation which can be used to screen for endothelial dysfunction and pulse wave velocity which assesses arterial stiffness. These techniques have been less well studied than carotid ultrasound in lupus. Carotid IMT is considered the best established surrogate marker of cardiovascular disease. In both lupus patients and the general population progression of cardiovascular disease measured by carotid IMT over time including the ability to predict cardiovascular events over 10 years has been demonstrated. The response to cardiovascular risk-reducing strategies has been shown in the general population by the reduction in IMT over time.

Risk Factors for Cardiovascular Disease

Traditional Risk Factors

Cohort studies have shown that the traditional cardiovascular risk factors defined by the Framingham studies (hypertension, hypercholesterolemia, diabetes, older age, and post-menopausal status) are more prevalent in lupus patients than in controls and accumulate over time, but these factors do not fully explain the increased risk of cardiovascular disease in SLE patients. It is increasingly clear that there are disease-related risk factors which are discussed in the next section. Lupus patients should be screened for the modifiable risk factors yearly (Table 18.1) and given advice on how to reduce these risks (Table 18.2 and see below).

Table 18.2 Management of modifiable cardiovascular risk factors

Risk factor	Target	Management
Dyslipidaemia	LDL levels <3.5 mmol/l	• Check once a year minimum • Lifestyle advice (low fat diet/exercise/weight loss) • Review steroid dose and aim for minimum • Hydroxychloroquine to be considered • Statin if conservative measures fail
Obesity	BMI<25 Waist circumference <35 in. in women <40 in. in men	• Lifestyle advice • Diet and exercise • Minimize steroid dose
Hypertension	BP<130/80	• Check at every clinic visit • Lifestyle modification (low-salt diet) • ACE inhibitor, particularly in diabetics and patients with renal disease • Add ARB and/or calcium channel blocker if insufficient • Add B blocker only to vasodilated patients if Raynaud's phenomenon • Minimize steroid dose
Diabetes/glucose intolerance	HbA1C<7 %	• Screen yearly and if abnormal review at every visit • Lifestyle advice (low sugar and fat diet/exercise/weight loss) • Minimize steroid dose • Aggressive management BP, lipids other risk factors • Annual glucose and HbA1C monitoring
Smoking	Cessation	• Enquire about smoking status at least yearly in "non-smokers" and at every clinic visit in smokers • Counsel regarding importance of cessation/not smoking (especially cardiovascular risk and lung cancer) • Refer to local smoking cessation clinic
Disease related		
Renal disease	BP≤130/80 Proteinuria<1g Normal renal function Normal serology (anti-dsDNA, C3, C4)	• Aggressive BP control • ACE inhibitor and/or ARB • Immunosuppressive agent and reducing course of steroids • Augment therapy if poor response
Antiphospholipid syndrome with thromboembolic events	Regular INR monitoring to ensure target achieved on warfarin Factor X level for low molecular weight heparin	• Warfarin • Heparin in pregnancy

(continued)

Table 18.2 (continued)

Risk factor	Target	Management
SLE disease activity	Review disease activity and medications at all visits	• Minimum possible steroid dose • Consider steroid sparing agents • Hydroxchloroquine in most • Cytotoxics if necessary

SLE patients have an increased prevalence of hypertension and dyslipidaemia, discussed further in the next section. Hypertension is particularly common in patients with lupus nephritis and in those on corticosteroids. There is little data assessing the prevalence of diabetes in lupus patients (3–5 %) but steroid-induced diabetes may develop. Furthermore there is increasing evidence for insulin resistance and metabolic syndrome in non-diabetic SLE patients, with 18 % affected in one study. This syndrome is discussed further below.

Other modifiable factors that are well recognised to increase the risk of atherosclerosis include smoking and lack of exercise (Table 18.1). SLE patients do not smoke more than the general population but there is evidence that some lupus patients take up smoking after the diagnosis of lupus. SLE patients usually have a sedentary lifestyle and low physical activity has been demonstrated to be associated with increased subclinical atherosclerosis and pro-inflammatory high-density lipoprotein (HDL).

Lipid Abnormalities

Dyslipidaemia is one of the most important modifiable risk factors for cardiovascular disease and in SLE patients is characterised by a reduced HDL level, raised total cholesterol and triglycerides, unchanged or elevated low-density lipoprotein (LDL), raised very low-density lipoproteins (VLDL) and elevated lipoprotein(a). The mechanisms resulting in dyslipidaemia may involve pro-inflammatory cytokines such as TNF-α and interferon-α and other mechanism including the effects of corticosteroids and renal disease especially nephrotic syndrome. TNF-α is associated with low HDL levels and may reduce the effect of lipoprotein lipase resulting in elevated levels of VLDL, due to reduced conversion to LDL, and high triglyceride levels. The development of anti-lipoprotein lipase antibodies that correlate with high triglyceride levels and low LDL levels may enhance cardiovascular risk.

HDL cholesterol is usually considered an anti-inflammatory molecule that prevents the formation of oxidised LDL (ox-LDL) and the development of foam cell which is critical for the formation of atherosclerotic plaque. In lupus, there is evidence that HDL function may be disordered and that a pro-inflammatory HDL (piHDL) is formed that is less able to prevent the formation of ox-LDL than normal HDL. Higher levels of piHDL and ox-LDL have been observed in SLE patients compared with rheumatoid arthritis patients and elevated piHDL is associated with established cardiovascular disease, carotid plaque, increased IMT and with low physical activity in women with SLE.

Paraoxonase 1 (PON1) is an anti-oxidant component of HDL that inhibits oxidation of lipoproteins and reduces ox-LDL. PON1 levels are reduced in lupus patients and this has been associated with an increased risk of atherosclerotic events. This may be due to autoantibodies directed against HDL and apolipoprotein A-1, a lipoprotein associated with HDL.

Metabolic Syndrome

The metabolic syndrome comprises a cluster of factors including abdominal obesity, atherogenic dyslipidaemia and insulin resistance that increase the risk for type two diabetes, cardiovascular and cerebrovascular disease. An increased prevalence of metabolic syndrome with insulin resistance has been observed in up to one-third of SLE patients compared to the general population in whom it occurs in about 10 %. The relationship between SLE and insulin resistance had been studied and found to be associated with increased C-reactive protein (CRP), ox-LDL, homocysteine, thrombomodulin but not disease activity or damage. The association with glucocorticoid therapy has been variable with some studies showing no association with current or past therapy and one showing an association with prednisolone doses >7.5 mg daily over the last 4 months.

Homocysteine

In the general population elevated homocystinuria is associated with atherosclerotic disease and in SLE patients elevated levels of homocysteine correlate with coronary calcification, carotid plaque progression and cardiovascular events. The molecular basis of the relationship between atherosclerosis and hyperhomocystinuria is poorly understood. Although homocysteine is thought to exert its effect through oxidative damage of the endothelial membrane and lipid peroxidation, there is no strong evidence that the genes involved in homocysteine metabolism contribute to atherosclerosis.

Disease-Related Risk Factors

Disease Activity

Several studies have shown that ongoing or increasing lupus disease activity is associated with an increased risk of subsequent cardiovascular events, rises in systolic blood pressure, glucose and triglycerides, and a fall in HDL. Renal disease is associated with an increased risk of hypertension, dyslipidaemia, atherosclerosis and deaths due to cardiovascular and cerebrovascular events in lupus cohorts and in general. Renal biopsies from patients with chronic renal disease have demonstrated ox-LDL in sclerotic and mesangial regions. However further work is needed to ascertain whether enhanced LDL oxidisation has a role in the development of renal disease in SLE patients or is a secondary occurrence with nephritis. The exact mechanisms involved in these associations between disease activity, renal involvement, dyslipidaemia and cardiovascular disease remain uncertain and are likely to be multifactorial involving both disease-related and therapy-related factors.

Inflammation and the Development of Atherosclerotic Plaques

Inflammation plays a key role in the development of atherosclerosis in the general population and is characterised by a variety of mechanisms that overlap with those involved in chronic autoimmune/inflammatory conditions such as SLE. Multiple inflammatory mediators involved in the initiation and progression of atherosclerotic plaques include various cytokines, chemokines and complement, resulting in an increased expression of cell adhesion molecules on leucocytes and endothelial cells that stimulate leucocyte adhesion and recruitment to the vessel wall. Systemic inflammation may activate the coagulation cascade, in addition to generating thrombin and activating platelets which may play a role in atherosclerosis formation.

Atherosclerotic plaques consist of three histological components: a large lipid core, many inflammatory cells and a thin fibrous cap. The risk of acute cardiovascular events with high morbidity and mortality is linked to atherosclerotic plaque vulnerability, rather than progressively increasing plaque size leading to haemodynamically significant stenosis and ischemia as previously thought. Inflammation causes the fibrous cap to be thinned, with reduced smooth muscle synthesis and increased collagen breakdown. The upregulation of cytokines in SLE, causing endothelial activation, has been implicated as a cause of vulnerable plaque rupture due to plaque destabilisation. Upregulation of interferon alpha may initially stimulate atherosclerotic development, commencing endothelial damage and abnormal vascular repair. Several pro-inflammatory cytokines have been implicated in accelerating atherosclerosis, including TNF-α, interleukin-1, and interleukin-12, in addition to autoantigens such as heat-shock proteins. Levels of TNF-α and adhesion molecules have been shown to be associated with coronary atherosclerosis independently of the Framingham risk score and with insulin resistance in SLE patients.

Epidemiological studies established that CRP, which is induced by pro-inflammatory cytokines, is an independent risk factor for myocardial infarction and stroke in men with no other risk factors. In the Framingham heart study and in lupus studies an association between CRP and carotid atherosclerosis and IMT has been demonstrated, and higher levels of CRP have predicted cardiovascular events. CRP is thought to contribute to endothelial damage and is probably involved in mediating the effects of immune complexes and complement activation.

Atherosclerotic lesions have been found to contain immune complexes, and immune complexes have been identified as a risk factor for atherosclerosis in the general population with studies demonstrating a correlation between the level of circulating immune complexes and the future development of a myocardial infarction. Autoantibody production and binding to target cells or proteins can induce inflammatory mediators (including cytokines), formation of atherogenic immune complexes and loss of atheroprotective components in lupus patients. Antibodies to endothelial cells, ox-LDL, lipoprotein lipase, HDL, apolipoprotein-A1 and heat-shock protein 60/65 have been reported but their role in premature atherosclerosis in lupus remains uncertain.

Antibodies to Endothelial Cells and Antiphospholipid Syndrome

A significant proportion of SLE patients have autoantibodies to endothelial cells and antiphospholipid antibodies that may promote endothelial damage in vivo and in vitro. Endothelial cell antibodies have been associated with cardiovascular disease in the general population but although they can be associated with lupus disease activity, they are not necessarily more raised in SLE patients with cardiovascular disease.

Antiphospholipid antibodies are present in 30–50 % of patients with SLE, and approximately one-third to half of these patients will develop the antiphospholipid syndrome. The presence of antiphospholipid antibodies has been associated with cardiovascular disease in the general population and SLE patients in some, but not all, studies. An association between serum levels of anti-cardiolipin antibodies and both the incidence and severity of acute coronary syndrome, stroke and myocardial infarction has been reported. Anti-cardiolipin antibodies cross react with other autoantibodies, such as anti-oxidised-LDL neoepitopes, promoting an increase in uptake of ox-LDL by macrophages, particularly in the presence of piHDL, antibodies to B2-glycoprotein-I and immune complexes. These macrophages subsequently develop into foam cells resulting in the formation of fatty streaks and atheromatous plaques. A novel mechanism proposed for cardiovascular disease in these patients is the inhibition of binding of the anti-thrombotic plasma protein annexin V by antiphospholipid antibodies. Annexin V has been found in abundance in atherosclerotic plaques, particularly at sites prone to rupture, leading to the suggestion that this protein may stabilise plaques and inhibit plaque rupture.

Imbalance of Vascular Damage and Repair

Endothelial damage is a key event in atherosclerosis. Several factors may contribute to this injury in SLE patients including; shear stress, viruses, homocysteine, autoantibodies, immune complexes, complement activation and oxidative stress and endothelial damage in turn may promote cytokine stimulation such as TNF-α. It has been proposed that an additional mechanism that may drive premature atherosclerosis is an imbalance between vascular damage and repair, characterised by accelerated endothelial cell apoptosis, generation of apoptotic microparticles that induce endothelial dysfunction and inappropriate repair of the endothelium. Bone marrow derived endothelial progenitor cells and circulating angiogenic cells of myelomonocytic origin are important in maintaining endothelial integrity but may be dysfunctional in lupus due to exposure to IFN-alpha, a cytokine that is increasingly being recognised as playing an important role in the aetiopathogenesis of this disease in many patients.

Endothelial progenitor cells have been reported to be reduced in both number and functional capability in SLE patients. SLE patients with no history of cardiovascular events or low Framingham cardiovascular risk have significantly reduced endothelial progenitor cells and impaired ability to differentiate into mature endothelial progenitor cells compared with matched controls. Disease activity is associated inversely with levels of endothelial progenitor cells but no relationship has been found with any specific lupus manifestations.

Effect of Immunosuppressive Drugs on Cardiovascular Risk

Corticosteroids

Prednisolone exposure and cumulative dose are positively associated with atherosclerotic plaque, but it is unclear whether this is resultant from higher lupus activity or the steroid itself. Steroids in themselves can induce hypertension, insulin resistance, lipid disturbance and obesity which all contribute to cardiovascular disease. Prednisolone may exert a bimodal action as it is atherogenic but on the other hand it is also anti-inflammatory. The greatest risk probably comes from higher doses since there is a direct association between dose and total cholesterol, blood pressure, and weight but the duration of exposure also appears to be important.

Hydroxychloroquine

It has been suggested that hydroxychloroquine may have a beneficial effect on lipid levels, reducing total cholesterol, LDL, triglycerides, markers of insulin resistance, and subclinical atherosclerosis. Some studies have suggested anti-malarials may inhibit platelet aggregation and the thrombogenic effects of antiphospholipid syndrome but a recent systematic review found very little evidence for this view.

Cyclophosphamide

Previous studies found an association between cyclophosphamide and atherosclerosis in SLE patients, but it is now considered that cyclophosphamide may be a surrogate marker for more active and severe SLE disease, which in itself is associated with increased cardiovascular risk. In one study cyclophosphamide exposure was associated with a reduction in cardiovascular risk.

Methotrexate

Several studies have reported that folate antagonism due to methotrexate may increase serum homocysteine levels in RA patients. A small study looking at nine lupus patients with lupus, demonstrated an association between methotrexate use and elevated levels of homocysteine, but this was of marginal significance after adjusting for sex, age, and disease activity score (SLEDAI). However a larger sample is needed to evaluate this further, particularly as lupus patients are at increased risk of hyperhomocystinuria independent of methotrexate therapy.

Mycophenolate Mofetil

Treatment with mycophenolate mofetil, has been suggested to be vasculoprotective, but this requires further investigation to establish this relationship. Mycophenolate has been suggested reduce cardiovascular events in transplant patients treated with this drug, as it suppresses glycosylation of adhesion molecules, blocks leukocyte adhesion and inhibits smooth muscle proliferation and pro-inflammatory cytokines.

Prevention and Treatment of Cardiovascular Disease

Cardiovascular risk factors must be addressed in addition to the treatment of lupus with disease modifying drugs if morbidity and mortality due to cardiovascular events are to be reduced (Table 18.2). There has been some improvement in this aspect of management but there is still room for further improvement. For example in one study, hypertension was adequately treated in 96 % of patients in the 1996–2000 time period compared to 88 % of patients in the 1990–1995 period. However, hypercholesterolemia was treated in a minority (9 %) of patients in the 1990–1995 time period but still only 28 % of the patients in 1996–2000 time period. These results suggest that more emphasis need to be placed on appropriate management of cardiovascular risk factors in SLE patients.

EULAR has recently recommended that although there are currently no validated guidelines, modifiable risk factors for cardiovascular disease should be monitored and treated according to the existing guidelines for the general population. They have suggested more frequent assessments for patients in certain situations, for example on corticosteroid therapy. However as the traditional risk factors do not fully account for the increased incidence of cardiovascular disease in SLE, there is an argument for treating SLE as an independent risk factor for cardiovascular disease somewhat like diabetes, with aggressive assessment and management of blood pressure and cholesterol. In addition SLE disease activity should be managed aggressively, with the addition of other disease modifying agents to reduce steroid dose, as inflammation plays a significant role in cardiovascular disease. Table 18.2 summarises treatment strategies that should be considered in lupus patients to reduce cardiovascular risk.

Lifestyle Advice

Lifestyle advice should be provided, so patients who smoke should be encouraged to stop and their body mass index (BMI) should be kept between 20 and 25 kg/m^2. As waist circumference is an important marker of visceral or intra-abdominal fat, waist circumference should be <40 in. in men and <36 in. in women. Prevention of obesity should be encouraged by educating patients regarding the importance of a healthy diet and regular exercise for at least 30 min three to four times per week, for example walking, cycling, or swimming.

Lipid-Lowering Treatment

Lipid profile (cholesterol, LDL, HDL, and triglycerides) should be checked annually. If LDL is raised a cholesterol-lowering diet should be initiated, with reduction in glucocorticoid dosage if possible and commencement of anti-malarial treatment unless contraindicated. Treatment with a statin should be considered, unless the patient is planning pregnancy in the next year, if LDL does not fall to levels between 2.6 and 3.4 mmol/l with these measures. Statins in the general population, when used as primary or secondary prevention, reduce cardiovascular morbidity and mortality. In animal models statins demonstrated immunomodulating effects and improve SLE but this has yet to be shown in human lupus. Fibrates should be considered for patients with hypertriglyceridaemia.

Anti-hypertensives

Hypertension should be aggressively managed. The target blood pressure should be 130/80 mmHg or less. Initially lifestyle advice should be given, except in those patients with IHD where a beta blocker should be initiated unless there is Raynaud's phenomenon. In diabetics and patient with lupus nephritis an angiotensin-converting enzyme (ACE) inhibitor or angiotensin receptor blocker (ARB) should be commenced. Calcium channel blockers may also be helpful, particularly in patients with severe Raynaud's phenomenon. In addition to aggressive blood pressure control in all patients as advised by local or national guidelines, corticosteroid therapy should be kept as low as possible by the addition of anti-malarials and/or cytotoxic agents.

Aspirin

The use of aspirin for secondary prevention of cardiovascular events in the general population has been established. Although there are no specific trials in lupus to support this recommendation in lupus, low-dose aspirin should be used in SLE patients with a previous history of angina/MI or TIA/stroke, and in addition some suggest that it be offered to those without a history of these events, but who have at least one risk factor other than SLE (hypertension, diabetes, or hypercholesterolemia) and in unreformed smokers. Low-dose aspirin use has also been advocated for patients with antiphospholipid antibody positivity, but who have not had an event requiring anti-coagulation. A caveat is that some advocate that aspirin should be avoided in those under 18 years of age due to the risk of Reye's syndrome and in those with antiphospholipid syndrome already on warfarin, as combination therapy does not usually confer any extra advantage and does increase the risk of bleeding. But aspirin and warfarin may be considered in patients with thromboembolic events despite warfarin therapy with INR 3–4.

Metabolic Bone Disease in SLE

The most recognised disorder of the bone in SLE patients is osteoporosis with fragility fractures; this is due in part to the widespread usage of corticosteroids in the treatment of SLE. Other contributory treatment-related factors are cyclophosphamide and depot medroxyprogesterone acetate and other mechanisms as discussed below including early onset menopause with and without cyclophosphamide, other drugs such as anti-epileptic drugs, smoking and physical inactivity (Table 18.3). However, there are other metabolic bone disorders that require consideration in SLE patients, particularly vitamin D deficiency as lupus patients are advised to avoid the UV light that is needed for vitamin D metabolism. This section will therefore discuss osteoporosis and vitamin D deficiency. There are other metabolic bone disorders which are far less common in lupus patients and these will not be discussed here, such as renal osteodystrophy.

Osteoporosis and Fragility Fractures

Magnitude of Osteoporosis Risk

Osteopaenia, osteoporosis and fragility fractures are prevalent in SLE patients. Cross sectional studies of large SLE cohorts have reported the prevalence of osteopaenia to be 40–50 %, osteoporosis to be 10–15 % and fragility fractures to be

Table 18.3 Important risk factors for osteoporosis in SLE

Increasing age
Menopause
Vitamin D deficiency
Systemic glucocorticoids
Cyclophosphamide (with resultant premature menopause)
Depot medroxyprogesterone acetate
Anti-epileptic drugs
Physical inactivity

9–15 %, respectively. It should be born in mind that the majority of the patients in the cohorts were pre-menopausal.

Risk Factors for Osteoporosis (Table 18.3)

Demographic Factors

The main predictors of osteoporosis and fragility fractures are increasing age and post-menopausal status as in the normal population. Reduced bone mineral density (BMD) is associated with increased risk of fragility fractures and reduced BMD, classified as osteopenia or osteoporosis according to WHO criteria, is more common in patients of non-African origin. Another factor that may contribute to reduced BMD that needs to be considered in lupus patients is reduction in UV light exposure causing vitamin D deficiency which will be discussed in the next section.

Glucocorticoids

One of the main reasons for the high prevalence of osteoporosis in lupus is due to the fact that oral glucocorticoids remain widely used in the treatment of SLE disease activity. Although disease activity may have a direct effect on BMD, there is no doubt that glucocorticoids have wide-ranging effects on bone metabolism (both directly and indirectly) resulting in reduced bone formation and enhanced bone resorption. The rate of glucocorticoid-related bone loss is most rapid in the first 6 months of treatment, but it has to be borne in mind that the bone loss rate remains two to three times the normal, even after the initial rapid phase of bone loss. There is evidence to suggest that glucocorticoid-related fractures occur at a higher BMD as compared to age-related and post-menopausal osteoporosis. Furthermore, there is a dose-dependent increase in risk of fractures, with no safe dose, although patients given more than 10 mg prednisolone daily are at greatest risk and pre-menopausal patients are at much less risk of fractures than post-menopausal women.

Cyclophosphamide

The use of cyclophosphamide may result in premature menopause and the risk is increased with older age at the start of therapy (especially 35 years and older) and higher cumulative dose of exposure (especially greater than 7 g). The Eurolupus protocol (500 mg given 2 weekly for 6 doses) results in significantly less risk of premature menopause than the traditional NIH regime for lupus nephritis.

Progestogens

Although oestrogen-based contraception has been shown to be relatively safe for use in SLE patients, it is not recommended in severe disease and in those at risk of

Table 18.4 Treatment of osteoporosis

General measures
Weight-bearing exercises
Falls prevention
Correction of nutritional deficiencies (especially calcium and vitamin D)
Smoking cessation
Reduction in alcohol consumption
Specific measures
Calcium and vitamin D supplementation
Bisphosphonates
Parathyroid hormone
Denosumab
Strontium
Raloxifene

thrombosis (including those with antiphospholipid antibodies). In these patients, progesterone-only contraception is recommended and depot medroxyprogesterone acetate is a popular method of contraception as it is given by intramuscular injection every 3 months. However, there is evidence to show that long-term use of depot medroxyprogesterone acetate contraception can result in up to 5 % reduction in the bone density as compared to age-matched controls. Whether similar effects will be seen with other progesterone-only contraception remains uncertain as they have not been well studied.

Prevention and Treatment of Osteoporosis

Although BMD threshold (T score cut-off of −2.5 or less) is used for diagnosis of osteoporosis, it is less useful as an intervention threshold as some of the clinical risk factors (such as age and glucocorticoids) act independently of BMD to increase the risk of fragility fractures. As a result, algorithms based on clinical risk factors have been developed to calculate the probability of fracture in the future to help inform the decision on when to initiate treatment. The most widely used algorithm is the FRAX calculator which provides a 10 year probability of a hip or major osteoporotic fracture. The intervention threshold does vary between countries as different countries use different guidelines as to when treatment should be initiated. The other limitations of FRAX are that it is not applicable to those under 40 years of age and it does not differentiate between high-dose and low-dose glucocorticoids.

General Management

The general management of osteoporosis includes weight-bearing exercise, correction of nutritional deficiencies (especially calcium and vitamin D), smoking cessation and reduction in alcohol consumption (Table 18.4). There is evidence that supplementation with calcium and vitamin D reduces risk of non-vertebral and hip fractures. Prevention of falls is also important. As SLE often affects pre-menopausal women, special consideration has to be given to women who are considering future pregnancy, as none of the agents used in the treatment of osteoporosis are safe in pregnancy apart from calcium and vitamin D supplementation.

Drug Treatment (Table 18.4)

Bisphosphonates are the most widely used pharmacological agents in the treatment of osteoporosis. Alendronate, risedronate and zoledronate have been shown to be effective in the treatment of glucocorticoids-induced osteoporosis. In women who may be considering pregnancy in the future, agents with short half-lives are recommended (e.g. risedronate) if such treatment is felt to be essential. The main limitation to the use of bisphosphonates in pre-menopausal women is the prolonged skeletal half-life of some agents (particularly Alendronate). They should be discontinued at least a year before conception due to animal studies suggesting a risk of congenital bone abnormalities if exposure to high doses occurs in utero.

Teriparatide is a recombinant form of a portion of the human parathyroid that stimulates new bone formation. In glucocorticoid-induced osteoporosis, it has been shown to be superior to alendronate. Denosumab, a humanised monoclonal antibody targeting receptor activator of nuclear factor-kappa B ligand (RANKL), is the latest pharmacological agent that has been approved for treatment of post-menopausal osteoporosis. It is an anti-resorptive agent as it inhibits osteoclast activity. However, it has not been assessed in glucocorticoid-induced osteoporosis. Other agents that are effective in post-menopausal osteoporosis are strontium ranelate and raloxifene but they have not been studied in glucocorticoid-induced osteoporosis. None of these agents can be recommended in pre-menopausal women planning pregnancy.

Vitamin D Deficiency

Magnitude of the Risk of Vitamin D Deficiency

Vitamin D deficiency is defined as serum 25-hydroxyvitamin D level of less than 20 ng/ml (50 nmol/l). Osteomalacia is the severe end of the spectrum of vitamin D deficiency which results in defective mineralisation of the bone matrix. There is a further category considered to be vitamin D insufficiency, defined by serum 25-hydroxyvitamin D levels of between 20 and 30 ng/ml (50 and 75 nmol/l), which is associated with elevated serum parathyroid hormone and decreased intestinal calcium absorption. The main source of vitamin D is from conversion of 7-dehydrocholesterol into vitamin D in the skin through exposure to ultraviolet light from sunlight. Dietary intake of vitamin D is often inadequate as few foods contain sufficient quantity of vitamin D.

Vitamin D deficiency and insufficiency are common in lupus cohorts with reported prevalence of around 20 and 50–75 %, respectively. This is not surprising due to the avoidance of ultraviolet light and the use of sunscreen to prevent flares of the disease. Inadequate vitamin D results in decreased intestinal absorption of calcium leading to increased parathyroid hormone. Parathyroid hormone increases osteoclastic activity causing osteopaenia and osteoporosis, with increased risk of fractures. Apart from that, vitamin D is required for optimal muscle function and reduced level of vitamin D is associated with increased risk of falls. Furthermore, there is some evidence to indicate that low serum vitamin D is associated with increased SLE disease activity.

Vitamin D Treatment

In the situation where there is inadequate sun exposure, the daily requirement of vitamin D is approximately 800–1,000 IU of vitamin D_3 to maintain vitamin D sufficiency. If vitamin D_2 is used instead, doses up to three times that of vitamin D_3 will be required as it is about 30 % in equivalence to vitamin D_3. There is considerable variation in the preparations of Vitamin D that are available for oral or intramuscular use and the regimes used vary depending on local availability. A loading regimen may be required in vitamin D insufficiency and deficiency to rapidly replete vitamin D (see Further Reading). It should be noted that there is often poor adherence to combined oral calcium/vitamin D_3 preparations as they are not very palatable and that vitamin D_3 alone is not widely available.

Cancer Risk in SLE

It has been demonstrated clearly that individuals with SLE have specific patterns in terms of cancer susceptibility. The recent published data suggest a relatively small (10–15 %) increase in cancer in SLE overall, compared to the general population. A heightened risk is most notable for hematologic cancers, especially non-Hodgkin's lymphoma (NHL), where a threefold increased risk is seen in SLE, compared with the general population. However, recent data have emphasised that persons with SLE may also have a decreased risk of certain cancers including breast, endometrial and ovarian cancers. The risk related to non-melanoma skin cancer in SLE has not been well studied, due to limitations in cancer registries regarding the documentation of these cancers.

Specific Types of Cancer with Increased Risk in SLE

Hematologic Cancers

The greatest risk is of lymphoma in SLE patients and this has been replicated in many studies. Persons with SLE do have an increased risk not only of developing

NHL but also of dying from it. An increased risk has also been demonstrated for other types of hematological malignancies, including Hodgkin's lymphoma (HL) and leukemia. Multiple myeloma is not itself clearly increased, although one study has shown an increased risk of monoclonal gammopathy in SLE compared to the general population.

The etiology of the increased risk for hematologic cancers in SLE remains under study; the key question is the extent to which immunosuppressive exposures play a role, compared to other factors, including disease activity itself. One of the general mechanisms for lymphoma development involves juxtaposition of an oncogene beside a gene important for immune cell function. The dysregulated lymphocyte proliferation that may occur in persons with SLE could potentially lead to translocation like this, and favours development of a lymphoma. In a case–cohort study of malignancy in SLE, multivariate models demonstrated that the presence of lupus damage (on modified SLICC/ACR damage index scores) was associated with overall cancer risk in SLE (adjusted HR 3.1, 95 % CI 2.0, 4.8). Although the SLICC/ACR Damage Index is *not* a measure of disease activity itself, damage scores have been shown to reflect the impact of cumulative disease activity and correlate with clinical severity. Further work in progress will hopefully determine the extent to which SLE activity may drive risk of lymphoma in SLE.

Lung Cancer

Several cohort studies have showed an increased risk of lung cancer in patients with SLE. A recent study reported that although the histological distribution of cancers in the SLE group and general population were comparable, there was a potential increase in the incidence of rare cancers (such as bronchoalveolar and carcinoid). In that sample, not surprisingly, a large number of the SLE patients who developed lung cancer were smokers; interestingly, only a small number had been previously exposed to immunosuppressive drugs. Further case–cohort analyses have confirmed smoking as an important predictor of lung cancer in SLE, which provides physicians with another reason to counsel SLE patients to stop smoking.

Cervical Cancer and Dysplasia

Invasive cervical cancer is not a common malignancy (occurring in about 6 per 100,000 women in North America), but there is evidence that women with SLE are at increased risk. A recent review indicated that cervical cancer was not shown to be increased in SLE in many single-centre studies, but in fact because this is a relatively rare cancer, single-centre studies are usually not able to demonstrate the risk of this malignancy with precision. In updated analyses of the multi-centre SLE cohort, the SIR for cervical cancer was consistent with increased risk (SIR 1.65, 95 % CI 1.09–2.41).

The importance of cervical dysplasia as a concern in women with SLE should be recognised by the rheumatology community as it is increasingly acknowledged that this risk may be particularly driven by exposure to immunosuppressants. At least some individuals with SLE appear to have a particularly high risk of HPV infection which predisposes to cervical dysplasia, and this risk of HPV infection may be associated with immune dysfunction and/or immunosuppressant use.

Routine screening for this complication, according to general population guidelines, is important, but unfortunately may be neglected; in one study, patients with SLE with the most severe disease (based on SLE/ACR damage index scores) were the least likely to have undergone cervical screening. Cervical screening is particularly important in women who have had a previous abnormal pap result and/or risk factors for HPV infection.

Do Drugs Cause Cancer in SLE?

Based largely on studies of increased cancer risk in renal transplant patients, who are also treated with immunosuppressant agents, there exists concern that much of the excess cancer risk in SLE is due to immunosuppressive use. Contrary to this view, other studies have found that many of the patients with SLE diagnosed with (and/or dying from) malignancies had not been exposed to immunosuppressive drugs.

Some preliminary case–control analyses have been performed in an SLE sample from Sweden. However, with only 16 cases of NHL arising in SLE, the study was not able to produce precise estimates of the effects of azathioprine or cyclophosphamide exposures, and did not focus on other drug exposures. Moreover, they were unable to produce estimates adjusted for disease activity. Similarly, descriptive analyses of a small number of myeloid leukemia cases from the same population revealed that only a small minority (2/18) had never received azathioprine or cyclophosphamide. A larger, multi-centre, case–cohort study produced adjusted drug-specific hazard ratio (HR) estimates for hematological cancer, using a lag period of 5 years post-exposure. With adjustment for demographics, disease duration and lupus damage, the hazard ratio for cyclophosphamide was 3.55 (95 % CI 0.94–13.37): for azathioprine 1.02 (95 % CI 0.34–3.03) and for methotrexate, 2.57 (95 % CI 0.80–8.27). The lack of precise results has lead to further attempts to differentiate the effects of lupus activity versus treatment in an ongoing case–control study of lymphoma risk in SLE.

There are actually hypotheses suggesting that drug exposures could decrease the incidence of certain cancers, but in the case–cohort analyses indicated above, antimalarials showed no definite protective effects against cancer risk, either overall or with respect to hematological malignancies. Still, in the oncology world, antimalarial drugs have been suggested to have potential applications in cancer treatment, possibly through a cell death process called autophagy. Given the known role of inflammation in cancer, it is possible that even more potent immunosuppressive drugs could decrease the risk of certain types of solid cancer. To further study this intriguing hypothesis in SLE will require concerted efforts.

Hormone-Sensitive Cancers with Decreased Risk in SLE

Breast, Endometrial and Ovarian Cancer

In recent updates of data from the largest study of cancer in SLE to date a significant decreased risk was seen for hormone-sensitive cancers, including breast cancer (standardized incidence ratio, SIR 0.70, 95 % CI 0.58, 0.85), endometrial cancer (SIR 0.49, 95 % CI 0.27, 0.83), and ovarian cancer (0.56, 95 % CI 0.28, 0.97). This lower risk of several hormone-sensitive cancers may invoke the possibility of alterations in the metabolism of estrogen and/or other hormones in women with SLE. On the other hand, as mentioned above, it is possible that some drug exposures in SLE may actually be beneficial with respect to cancer risk. And of course it is known that aspirin and non-steroid anti-inflammatory drugs may be protective for a number of cancers and corticosteroids may also mediate cancer risk. Finally, decreased incidence of certain cancers in SLE could be related to specific genetic factors that put an individual at risk for SLE, but protect against things like breast cancer; again, this hypothesis remains to be tested.

Cancer Risk in SLE: Summary

Though much has been learnt in the past 10 years with respect to cancer risk in SLE, much remains unknown. At the present time there is evidence that both SLE activity itself, and some of the drugs used to treat it (specifically, cyclophosphamide) may be risk factors for hematologic malignancies. This provides additional motivation for the development of more effective and safer lupus drugs.

At the same time, a decreased risk of certain non-hematologic cancers is good news for lupus patients. Regardless, patients with SLE should continue to undergo preventative measures such as smoking cessation and engagement in regular cancer screening programs, particularly for cervical cancer.

Sources

Cardiovascular Disease

1. Ahmad Y, Shelmerdine J, Bodill H, et al. Subclinical atherosclerosis in systemic lupus erythematosus (SLE): the relative contribution of classic risk factors and the lupus phenotype. Rheumatology (Oxford). 2007;46(6):983–8.
2. Bruce IN. Cardiovascular disease in lupus patients: should all patients be treated with statins and aspirin? Best Pract Res Clin Rheumatol. 2005a;19(5):823–38.
3. Bruce IN. 'Not only…but also': factors that contribute to accelerated atherosclerosis and premature coronary heart disease in systemic lupus erythematosus. Rheumatology (Oxford). 2005b;44(12):1492–502.

4. Chung CP, Avalos I, Oeser A, et al. High prevalence of the metabolic syndrome in patients with systemic lupus erythematosus: association with disease characteristics and cardiovascular risk factors. Ann Rheum Dis. 2007;66(2):208–14.
5. Elliott JR, Manzi S. Cardiovascular risk assessment and treatment in systemic lupus erythematosus. Best Pract Res Clin Rheumatol. 2009;23(4):481–94.
6. Frostegard J. Atherosclerosis in patients with autoimmune disorders. Arterioscler Thromb Vasc Biol. 2005;25(9):1776–85.
7. Kaplan MJ. Premature vascular damage in systemic lupus erythematosus. Autoimmunity. 2009;42(7):580–6.
8. McMahon M, Grossman J, Skaggs B, et al. Dysfunctional proinflammatory high-density lipoproteins confer increased risk of atherosclerosis in women with systemic lupus erythematosus. Arthritis Rheum. 2009;60(8):2428–37.
9. Ruiz-Irastorza G, Ramos-Casals M, Brito-Zeron P, Khamashta MA. Clinical efficacy and side effects of antimalarials in systemic lupus erythematosus: a systematic review. Ann Rheum Dis. 2010;69(1):20–8.
10. Mosca M, Tani C, Aringer M, et al. European League Against Rheumatism recommendations for monitoring patients with systemic lupus erythematosus in clinical practice and in observational studies. Ann Rheum Dis. 2010;69(7):1269–74.
11. Parker B, Bruce IN. The metabolic syndrome in systemic lupus erythematosus. Rheum Dis Clin North Am. 2010;36(1):81–97. viii.
12. Volkmann ER, Grossman JM, Sahakian LJ, et al. Low physical activity is associated with proinflammatory high-density lipoprotein and increased subclinical atherosclerosis in women with systemic lupus erythematosus. Arthritis Care Res (Hoboken). 2010;62(2):258–65.

Metabolic Bone Disease

1. Yee CS, Crabtree N, Skan J, Amft N, Bowman S, Situnayake D, et al. Prevalence and predictors of fragility fractures in systemic lupus erythematosus. Ann Rheum Dis. 2005;64(1):111–3.
2. Bultink IE, Lems WF, Kostense PJ, Dijkmans BA, Voskuyl AE. Prevalence of and risk factors for low bone mineral density and vertebral fractures in patients with systemic lupus erythematosus. Arthritis Rheum. 2005;52(7):2044–50.
3. Holick MF. Vitamin D deficiency. N Engl J Med. 2007;357(3):266–81.
4. Kanis JA, Oden A, Johansson H, Borgstrom F, Strom O, McCloskey E. FRAX and its applications to clinical practice. Bone. 2009;44(5):734–43.
5. Toloza SM, Cole DE, Gladman DD, Ibanez D, Urowitz MB. Vitamin D insufficiency in a large female SLE cohort. Lupus. 2010;19(1):13–9.
6. Amital H, Szekanecz Z, Szucs G, Danko K, Nagy E, Csepany T, et al. Serum concentrations of 25-OH vitamin D in patients with systemic lupus erythematosus (SLE) are inversely related to disease activity: is it time to routinely supplement patients with SLE with vitamin D? Ann Rheum Dis. 2010;69(6):1155–7.

Cancer Risk

1. Bernatsky S, Boivin JF, Joseph L, et al. An international cohort study of cancer in systemic lupus erythematosus. Arthritis Rheum. 2005;52(5):1481–90.
2. Bernatsky S, Joseph L, Boivin JF, et al. The relationship between cancer and medication exposures in systemic lupus erythematosus: a case cohort study. Ann Rheum Dis. 2008;67:74–9.

3. Nath R, Mant C, Luxton J, Hughes G, Raju KS, Shepherd P, Cason J. High risk of human papillomavirus type 16 infections and of development of cervical squamous intraepithelial lesions in systemic lupus erythematosus patients. Arthritis Rheum. 2007;57(4):619–25.
4. Lofstrom B, Backlin C, Sundstrom C, Ekbom A, Lundberg IE. A closer look at non-Hodgkin's lymphoma cases in a national Swedish systemic lupus erythematosus cohort: a nested case-control study. Ann Rheum Dis. 2007;66:1627–32.
5. King JK, Costenbader KH. Characteristics of patients with systemic lupus erythematosus (SLE) and non-Hodgkin's lymphoma (NHL). Clin Rheumatol. 2007;26(9):1491–4.

Index

A
Abatacept, 223, 224
Acitretin, 87, 88
Acute cutaneous LE (ACLE)
 bullous, 67
 generalized rash, 66, 67
 histology, 67
 lupus band test, 67, 68
 malar rash, 66, 67
 TEN-like, 66, 67
Acute lupus pneumonitis (ALP), 115–116
Acute respiratory distress syndrome (ARDS), 117
Airways disease, 119
Alcohol, 7
Alopecia, 77–78
Alveolar hemorrhage, 34
American College of Rheumatology (ACR) criteria
 evolution, for SLE, 1, 2
 for lupus diagnosis, 27
ANA induction. *See* Antinuclear antibodies (ANA) induction
Anemia
 anemia of chronic inflammation (ACI), 130
 aplastic anemia, 132
 autoimmune hemolytic anemia (AIHA), 130–132
 iron deficiency, 130
 pure red cell aplasia, 132
 sickle cell anemia, 132
Annular subacute cutaneous LE, 68
Anti B cell therapy
 atacicept, 223
 cyclosporine, 224
 epratuzumab, 223
 hematopoietic stem cell transplantation, 225
 immunoablation, 225
 rituximab, 222–223
 T-cell inhibition, 223–224
Anticardiolipin (aCL) antibodies, 195, 200
Anti-DNA antibodies, 14, 15, 17, 18
Anti-double stranded DNA antibodies (anti-dsDNA), 3, 7
Antihistone antibodies, in drug-induced lupus, 214
Anti-hypertensives, for cardiovascular disease, 237
Anti-La antibodies, 185
Antimalarials, 189
 for cutaneous LE, 83–84
Antinuclear antibodies (ANA) induction
 anti-DNA antibodies, 17, 18
 cytosine-guanosine dinucleotide repeats (CpG motifs), 17
 expression, stages of, 16
 nuclear antigens, features, 16
 RNA binding proteins (RBPs), 16, 17
Antiphospholipid syndrome (APS), 3, 47–48, 129, 195
 in cardiovascular disease, 234
 catastrophic, 197, 202–203
 cerebral vascular accidents, 203
 clinical features, 198
 clinical manifestations, 196–197
 definition, 197
 diagnostic criteria, 197
 differential diagnosis, 198, 199
 labor and delivery, 206
 laboratory testing, 199–200
 management, 201

Antiphospholipid syndrome (APS) (cont.)
  obstetrical complications, management of, 196, 204–205
  pathogenesis, 198–199
  positive antibodies, in absence of clinical events, 204, 205
  pre-eclampsia, 205–206
  renal disease, 203
  Sapporo criteria, 197
  thrombocytopenia, 204
  treatment failure, 205
  valvular heart disease, 196, 203
  venous/arterial clotting events, 196
    antiplatelet therapy, 202
    drug interactions and dietary interactions, 202
    warfarin therapy, 201–202
Antiplatelet therapy, APS, 202
Anti-Ro antibodies, 3, 185
Anti-Sm antibodies, 14, 15
Anti-TNF-alpha agents, 215
Anxiety disorders, 174
Aplastic anemia, 132
Apoptosis, 20, 21
APS. *See* Antiphospholipid syndrome (APS)
ARDS. *See* Acute respiratory distress syndrome (ARDS)
Arthralgias, 94
Arthritis, 94
  erosive, 98–99
Aspirin, 188, 189, 202, 204, 205
  for cardiovascular disease, 237–238
Atacicept, 223
Atherosclerotic plaques development and inflammation, in cardiovascular disease, 233–234
Autoantibodies testing
  pattern of immunofluorescence, 29
  titer, 29
Autoimmune hemolytic anemia (AIHA), 130–132
Avascular necrosis (AVN). *See* Osteonecrosis (ON)
Azathioprine, 44, 86, 148, 153, 190, 244

B

Belimumab, 88, 222, 223
B-2 glycoprotein I antibodies, 200
Biological therapy, 221–222
Bisphosphonates, for osteoporosis, 241
Breast cancer risk, 245

Bronchiolitis obliterans organizing pneumonia (BOOP). *See* Cryptogenic organizing pneumonia (COP)
Bronchoscopy, 114, 116, 118

C

Cancer risk, 61
  cervical cancer, 243
  drugs, 244–245
  dysplasia, 244
  hematologic cancers, 242–243
  hormone-sensitive cancers, with decreased risk, 245
  lung cancer, 243
Cardiovascular disease (CVD), 33, 47–48
  events and mortality, 228
  prevention and treatment
    anti-hypertensives, 237
    aspirin, 237–238
    lifestyle advice, 237
    lipid lowering treatment, 237
  risk factors for
    disease activity, 232–233
    dyslipidaemia, 230, 231
    endothelial cells and antiphospholipid syndrome, antibodies to, 234
    homocysteine, 232
    hypertension, 230, 231
    immunosuppressive drugs, 235–236
    inflammation and atherosclerotic plaques development, 233–234
    lipid abnormalities, 231–232
    metabolic syndrome, 232
    modifiable, management of, 230–231
    vascular damage and repair, imbalance of, 234–235
  surrogate markers
    EBCT, 228, 229
    intima-media thickness (IMT), 229
    ultrasound, 228, 229
Catastrophic antiphospholipid syndrome (CAPs), 197, 202–203
CCHB, 185
CCLE. *See* Chronic cutaneous lupus erythematosus (CCLE)
Celiac disease, 159
Cellcept®. *See* Mycophenolate mofetil (MMF)
Cellular immune disturbances, in SLE, 19–20
Cerebral vascular accidents, APS and, 203
Cerebrospinal fluid (CSF) analysis, 178
Cerebrovascular system
  conduction system disease, 108

Index

coronary artery disease, 108–110
disease, 110, 169–170
   management of, 170
myocarditis, 107
pericarditis, 105–106
peripheral vascular disease, 110–111
valvular heart disease, 106–107
Cervical cancer, 243
Chilblain LE, 75–76
Chloroquine (CQ), 44, 83, 84
Chronic cutaneous lupus erythematosus (CCLE)
   Chilblain LE, 75–76
   discoid LE (DLE), 71–73
   hypertrophic/verrucous LE, 76
   lupus panniculitis/profundus, 73, 74
   tumid lupus erythematosus, 73–75
Chronic inflammatory demyelinating polyradiculopathy (CIDP), 175
Cigarette smoking, 7
CLE. *See* Cutaneous lupus erythematosus (CLE)
Cognitive dysfunction, 172
Cognitive impairment, 46
Complement, 141, 143, 144
Conduction system disease, 108
Contraception, 57–58, 181–182
Coronary artery disease
   antibodies, 109
   care for, 109
   causes for, 108
   prevalence of, 108
   steroids, 108, 109
Corticosteroids
   for cardiovascular disease, 235
   in cutaneous LE treatment
      intralesional, 82
      topical, 82
      systemic, 153
Cosmetics and hair products, 56
Cranial neuropathies, 176
C-reactive protein (CRP), 233
Crohn's disease, 159
Cryptogenic organizing pneumonia (COP), 119
Crystalline silica, as risk factor for SLE, 8
Cutaneous lesions, 31
Cutaneous lupus, drug-induced, 216, 217
Cutaneous lupus erythematosus (CLE)
   CLASI, 89
   nonspecific skin disease
      alopecia, 77–78
      cutaneous vasculitis, 79–80
      livedo reticularis and racemosa, 79
      mucosal ulceration, 80
      periungal telangiectasias and palmar erythema, 80
      photosensitivity, 77
      Raynaud's phenomenon, 78–79
      urticaria, 81
      urticarial vasculitis, 80
   specific skin disease
      acute cutaneous LE (ACLE), 66–68
      chronic, 71–76
      neonatal LE (NLE), 70–71
      subacute cutaneous LE (SCLE), 68–70
   treatment of, 90
      antimalarials, 83–84
      azathioprine, 86
      biologics, 88–89
      corticosteroids, 82
      cyclophosphamide, 86
      dapsone, 87
      intravenous immunoglobulin (IVIG), 88
      methotrexate, 84–85
      mycophenalate mofetil (MMF), 85–86
      photoprotection, 81
      retinoids, 87–88
      smoking cessation, 81–82
      thalidomide, 86–87
      topical calcineurin inhibitors, 82–83
Cutaneous Lupus Erythematosus Disease Area and Severity Index (CLASI), 89
Cutaneous vasculitis, 79–80
CVD. *See* Cardiovascular disease (CVD)
Cyclophosphamide, 44, 182, 191
   for cardiovascular disease, 235
   in cutaneous LE treatment, 86
   for osteoporosis, 239
   proliferative lupus nephritis, 145, 148
Cyclosoxygenase (COX-2) inhibitors, 188, 189
Cyclosporine, 190–191, 224
Cytosine-guanosine dinucleotide repeats (CpG motifs), 17

D

Dapsone, in cutaneous LE treatment, 87
Delirium, 172–173
Dementia, 177
Depression, 173–174
Diabetes, 48
Diarrhea, 161–162
Diet and nutrition, 55–56

Diffuse alveolar hemorrhage (DAH), 116–117
Discoid LE (DLE)
　generalized, 71, 73
　localized, 73
　scarring, 72
　scarring alopecia, 72
Disseminated intravascular coagulation (DIC), 129
Double-stranded DNA (dsDNA) antibodies, 29–30
Drug-induced lupus (DIL)
　anti-TNF-alpha agents, 215
　associated drugs, 210–212
　autoimmune syndromes, 209, 210
　clinical features, 212–213
　cutaneous lupus, 216, 217
　diagnosis, 214–215
　epidemiology, 210
　herbal medicines, rheumatologic disease, 215
　hydralazine, 210, 218
　idiopathic SLE, 215–216
　laboratory features, 214
　minocycline, 212
　pathogenesis, 216–218
　procainamide, 210, 213
　treatment, 218
Dyskinesias, 175, 176
Dyspepsia, 156–157
Dysphagia, 155–156
Dysplasia, 244
Dyspnea, 113–114

E
Echocardiography, valvular heart disease, 106
Efalizumab, 89
Electroencephalography (EEG), 179
　neuropsychiatric SLE, 46
Electron beam computed tomography (EBCT), cardiovascular disease, 228, 229
Endometrial cancer risk, 245
Endothelial cell antibodies, 234
Epidemiology, of SLE
　classification, 1–3
　disease activity/flare, 10
　heterogeneity and subtypes, 3–4
　incidence and prevalence
　　age, sex, race and ethnicity, 4
　　genes and environment, in pathogenesis, 5
　　worldwide epidemiology, 4–5
　risk factors for
　　alcohol, 7
　　breast implants, hair dyes, and lipstick, 8
　　cigarette smoking, 7
　　crystalline silica, 8
　　early life factors, 6
　　environmental contaminants, 7
　　Epstein Barr virus (EBV), 9
　　hormonal/reproductive factors, 5–6
　　immunizations, 9
　　incidence of, 6
　　nutritional factors, 9
　　pesiticides, 7–8
　　socioeconomic position, 8–9
　　solvents, 8
　　ultraviolet (UV) light, 9–10
Epratuzumab, 89, 223
Epstein Barr virus (EBV), 9
Erosive arthritis, 98–99
Esophageal hypomotility, 155
Eye disease, 35

F
Fasciitis, 99–100
Fertility, 182–183
Fractures, 102–103
　fragility, 238–241

G
Gastro-esophageal reflux disease (GERD), 155
Gastrointestinal (GI) manifestations, 33
　esophagus and stomach
　　dyspepsia, 156–157
　　dysphagia, 155–156
　liver, 163
　oral cavity, 154–155
　pancreas, 162
　small and large intestines
　　celiac disease, 159
　　infectious diarrhea, 161–162
　　inflammatory bowel disease, 159
　　intestinal pseudo-obstruction, 160–161
　　lupus mesenteric vasculitis, 157–158
　　peritonitis, 161
　　pneumatosis cystoides intestinalis, 162
　　protein-losing gastroenteropathy, 159–160
　symptoms
　　drugs, 152
　　hydroxychloroquine, 153
　　immunosuppressive medications, 153
　　NSAIDs, 151–153

Index

systemic corticosteroids, 153
viral hepatitis reactivation, 154
Glomerulonephritis, 21, 22
Glucocorticoids, 59, 60, 189–190, 224
lupus nephritis, 147–148
for osteoporosis, 239
Gluten sensitive enteropathy.
See Celiac disease

H
Headaches, 171
Helicobacter pylori infection, 157
Hematologic abnormalities, 35–36
Hematologic cancers, 242–243
Hematologic manifestations, of SLE
anemia, 130–132
antiphospholipid antibody syndrome, 129
leukopenia, 132–134
lymphadenopathy, 135
lymphoproliferative disorders, 135
macrophage-activation syndrome (MAS), 134–135
thrombocytopenia
immune thrombocytopenic purpura, 126–128
thrombotic thrombocytopenic purpura, 128–129
Hematopoietic stem cell transplantation, 225
Hemophagocytic lymphohistiocytosis (HLH), 134
Heparin, 204, 206
Hepatitis, 154, 163
Hepcidin, 130
Herbal medicines, rheumatologic disease, 215
Homocysteine, in cardiovascular disease, 232, 235, 236
Hormone-sensitive cancers, 245
Hughes' syndrome. *See* Antiphospholipid syndrome (APS)
Hydralazine, 210, 218
Hydroxychloroquine (HCQ), 44, 83–85, 153
APS, 205
for cardiovascular disease, 235
Hypercoagulable state (thrombophilia), 35–36
Hypertrophic/verrucous LE, 76
Hypoalbuminemia, 159, 160

I
Idiopathic SLE, 215–216
Imaging
lupus diagnosis, 30
neuropsychiatric SLE, 46, 178–179

Immune thrombocytopenic purpura (ITP)
hypoproduction, 126
intravenous immunoglobulin (IVIG), 127
novel therapies, 128
prednisone, 127
splenectomy, 127, 128
steroids, 127
Immunoablation, 225
Immunopathogenesis and immunopathology, in SLE
ANA induction
anti-DNA antibodies, 17, 18
cytosine-guanosine dinucleotide repeats (CpG motifs), 17
expression, stages of, 16
nuclear antigens, features, 16
RNA binding proteins (RBPs), 16, 17
autoantibodies production, 11, 12
cellular immune disturbances
affinity maturation, 20
B and T cells, 20
DNA and RNA, immunostimulatory activity, 19, 20
interferon, 19
plasma cells, 20
disease susceptibility, determinants of
in female, effects of hormones, 12
genetic factors, 12, 13
multigenic, 14
murine studies, 13
self antigen role, 20–21
serological disturbances, in lupus
anti-DNA and anti-Sm, 14, 15
antiphospholipid syndrome, 15
clinical associations of autoantibodies, 16
Ro and La antigens, 15
tissue inflammation and damage, mechanisms of
atherosclerosis, 22, 23
glomerulonephritis, 21, 22
immune complexes, role of, 22, 23
Immunosuppressive drugs
for cardiovascular disease, 235–236
GI manifestations, 153
Infertility, 183
Inflammatory bowel disease, 159
Interferons, 19
International Society of Nephrology/Renal Pathology Society (ISN/RPS), 142
Interstitial lung disease (ILD), 117–118
Intestinal pseudo-obstruction (IPO), 160–161
Intestines, manifestations of, 157–162

Intravenous immunoglobulin (IVIG), 88, 127, 191
Iron deficiency anemia, 130
Isotretinoin, 87, 88
ITP. *See* Immune thrombocytopenic purpura (ITP)

J

Jaccoud arthropathy, 95–98
   MTP joints, valgus angulation, 97
   multiple reducible swan-neck deformities, 96

L

Labor and delivery, antiphospholipid syndrome and, 206
Large granular lymphocyte leukemia (LGL), 133
Leflunomide, 192
Leukocytoclastic vasculitis, 79
Leukopenia, 132–134
Libman Sacks endocarditis. *See* Valvular heart disease
Lipid abnormalities, in cardiovascular disease, 231–232
Lipid lowering treatment, for cardiovascular disease, 237
Livedo racemosa, 79
Livedo reticularis, 79
Liver, 163
LN. *See* Lupus nephritis (LN)
Lung cancer, 243
Lung disease, 34
Lupus
   anticoagulant, 200
   diagnosis
      ACR criteria for, 27, 28
      autoantibodies, 29
      dsDNA and Sm antibodies, 29–30
      imaging, 30
      laboratory testing for, 28–31
      questionnaire for, 26
      symptoms, 26
   differential diagnosis
      cardiovascular disease, 33
      cutaneous lesions, 31
      eye disease, 35
      GI system, 33
      hematologic abnormalities, 35–36
      lung disease, 34
      lymphadenopathy, 32
      mucosal lesions, 32
      neuropsychiatric (NP) symptoms, 35
      polyarthritis/polyarthralgia, 32
      pulmonary hypertension, 34
      Raynaud's phenomenon, 32
      renal disease, 33
      systemic symptoms, 31
   treatment (*see* Treatment of lupus)
Lupus Foundation of America (LFA), 52
Lupus mesenteric vasculitis (LMV), 157–158
Lupus nephritis (LN), 45
   clinical manifestations, 139
   diagnosis of, 140
   differential diagnosis of, 143
   epidemiology, 140
   immune complexes deposition, 140, 141
   ISN/RPS classification, 142
   laboratory findings
      for diagnosis, 141
      for monitoring, 143–144
   pathogenesis, 140–141
   progressive renal failure, risk factors for, 146
   renal biopsy
      indications for, 142
      significance of, 141–142
      silent nephritis, 141, 142
      transformation of, 143
   renal failure, 147
   repeat biopsy, guidelines for, 143
   treatment
      adjunctive, 144
      induction, 147–148
      maintenance, recommendations, 148
      membranous, 148
      proliferative lupus nephritis, 145–146
      of relapses, 147
      of SLE nephritis, 144
Lupus panniculitis/profundus, 73, 74
Lymphadenopathy, 32, 135
Lymphoma, 242, 243
Lymphopenia, 132, 133
Lymphoproliferative disorders, 135

M

Macrophage-activation syndrome (MAS), 134–135
Magnetic resonance imaging (MRI), neuropsychiatric SLE, 46
Medroxyprogesterone acetate, 238, 240
Membranous lupus nephritis, therapy for, 148
Meningitis, 177
Metabolic bone disease
   osteoporosis and fragility fractures

magnitude of risk, 238–239
  prevention and treatment, 240–241
  risk factors, 238–240
  vitamin D deficiency, 241–242
Metabolic syndrome, in cardiovascular disease, 232
Methotrexate, 44, 84–85, 191
  for cardiovascular disease, 235–236
Minocycline, 212
Miscarriages, recurrent, 204–205
MMF. *See* Mycophenolate mofetil (MMF)
Monitoring SLE, in clinic/bedside
  baseline and repeat laboratory monitoring, 40
  with blood tests, caveats on, 43
  clinical symptoms, signs and laboratory tests, 41–42, 44
  frequency of, 40
  in-hospital patient, 43, 45
  outcome measure for, 43
  treatment effects, 44, 45
  treatment related co-morbidities and situations in
    anti-phospholipid syndrome, 47–48
    neuropsychiatric, 46–47
    during pregnancy, 47
    renal disease, 45–46
Movement disorders, 175–176
Mucosal lesions, 32
Musculoskeletal manifestations, of SLE
  arthralgias, 94
  arthritis, 94
  erosive arthritis, 98–99
  fasciitis, 99–100
  fibromyalgia, 93
  fractures, 102–103
  Jaccoud arthropathy, 95–98
  myositis, 102
  nodules, 98
  osteonecrosis (ON), 100–102
  spine, 100
  synovium, 95
  tendon involvement, 98
Mycophenolate mofetil (MMF), 44, 85–86, 145, 148, 191
  for cardiovascular disease, 236
Myocarditis, 107
Myositis, 102

N

Necrotizing fasciitis (NF), 99–100
Neonatal LE (NLE), 70–71

Neuropathies, 175
  cranial, 176
Neuropsychiatric aspects, of lupus
  clinical syndromes
    cerebrovascular disease, 169–170
    cognitive dysfunction, 172
    headaches, 171
    seizure disorders, 170–171
  evaluation
    CSF analysis, 178
    electroencephalography, 179
    imaging studies, 178–179
    serologic testing, 178
  history, in identification of, 168
  pathophysiology, 168–169
  peripheral nervous system in, 175
  psychiatric manifestations, 172–175
    anxiety disorders, 174
    delirium, 172–173
    depression, 173–174
    psychosis, 173
    rare, 174–175
  symptoms, 35
    cranial neuropathies, 176
    dementia, 177
    meningitis, 177
    movement disorders, 175–176
    transverse myelitis, 176–177
  syndromes in SLE, 168
Neuropsychiatric SLE, 46–47
Neutropenia, 132, 133
Nodules, 98
Non-scarring alopecia, 77, 78
Non-steroidal anti-inflammatory drugs (NSAIDs), 44, 188, 189, 193
  GI manifestations, 152, 153
Nutrition, 55–56
  factors, 9

O

Obliterative bronchiolitis (OB), 119
Ocular toxicity, antimalarials, 83, 84
Optic neuritis, 176
Oral cavity, 154–155
Osteonecrosis (ON), 100–102
Osteoporosis
  magnitude of risk, 238–239
  prevention and treatment, 240–241
  risk factors, 238–240
Ovarian cancer risk, 245

P

Pancreatitis, 162
Paraoxonase 1 (PON1), 232
Parenchymal disease
  acute, 114–117
  chronic, 117–118
Patient–doctor relationship, in treatment of lupus, 51–52
Pericarditis, 105–106
Peripheral nervous system, in lupus, 175
Peripheral vascular disease, 110–111
Peritonitis, 161
Pesticides, as risk factor for SLE, 7–8
PET scanning, neuropsychiatric SLE, 46, 47
Photoprotection, cutaneous LE treatment, 81
Photosensitivity, cutaneous LE, 77
Pimecrolimus, 83
Pleura, in SLE, 119–120
Pleural effusion, 116, 120
Pleuritis, 120
PLGE. *See* Protein-losing gastroenteropathy (PLGE)
Pneumatosis cystoides intestinalis, 162
Pneumonitis, 34
Polyarthritis/polyarthralgia, 32
Prednisone, 44
Preeclampsia, 186, 205–206
Pregnancy and SLE
  antimalarials, 189
  anti-Ro and anti-La antibodies, 185
  aspirin, 188, 189
  azathioprine, 190
  contraception, 57–58, 181–182
  COX-2 inhibitors, 188, 189
  cyclophosphamide, 191
  cyclosporine, 190–191
  disease flares, 183, 184
  disease management, 187
  glucocorticoids, 189–190
  IVIG, 191
  leflunomide, 192
  lupus flare and preeclampsia, 186
  medication
    management, 188
    recommendations, 193
  methotrexate, 191
  monitoring, 47, 185
  mycophenolate mofetil (cellcept), 191
  NSAIDs, 188, 189
  outcome, effect of, 187
  physiologic changes, 183
  prepregnancy
    counseling, 184
    screening, 184–185
  renal disease, 186
  rituximab, 192
  tumor necrosis factor-alpha blockade and inhibitors, 192
Procainamide, 210, 213
Progestogens, for osteoporosis, 239–240
Proliferative lupus nephritis, therapy for
  complete remission, 145
  cyclophosphamide, 145
  induction, 146
  maintenance, 146
Protein-losing gastroenteropathy (PLGE), 159–160
Psoriasiform subacute cutaneous LE, 68, 69
Psychiatric manifestations, 172–175
Psychosis, 35, 173
Pulmonary arterial hypertension (PAH), 120–121
Pulmonary function testing (PFT), 113–116, 118, 119
Pulmonary manifestations, of SLE
  acute parenchymal disease
    infections, 114
    non-infectious lung disease, 115–117
    prophylaxis, 114
  acute reversible hypoxemia, 122
  airways disease, 119
  antiphospholipid antibodies (APL), 121
  chronic parenchymal disease, 117–118
  dyspnea, 113–114
  high resolution CT scan, 117–119
  parenchymal vasculature, 120
  pleura, in, 119–120
  shrinking lung syndrome, 122
  vaccination, 114
  vascular disorders, 120–121
Pulmonary veno-occlusive disease (PVOD), 121

Q

Quinacrine, 83, 84

R

Radiation therapy, 57
Raynaud's phenomenon, 32, 78–79
  and esophageal dysmotility, 156
Recurrent miscarriages, 204–205
Renal biopsy, lupus nephritis, 141–143
Renal disease, 33
  pregnancy, 186
  SLE monitoring, treatment related co-morbidities, 45–46

Renal failure, lupus nephritis, 147
  progressive, risk factors for, 146
Retinoids, in cutaneous
  LE treatment, 87–88
Reversible hypoxemia, acute, 122
Rheumatic diseases, 221
Rheumatoid arthritis, 28, 29
Rituximab, 44, 88, 192, 222–223
RNA binding proteins (RBPs),
  ANA induction, 16, 17

S

Scarring alopecia, in discoid LE, 72
Seizures, 35, 170–171
Self antigen role, in SLE, 20–21
Serological disturbances, in SLE
  anti-DNA and anti-Sm, 14, 15
  antiphospholipid syndrome, 15
  Ro and La antigens, 15
Serologic testing, 178
Shrinking lung syndrome, 34, 122
Sickle cell anemia, 132
Sjögren's syndrome (SS), 3
Small and large intestines,
  manifestations of, 157–162
Smith antibodies, 29–30
Smoking cessation, 56
  cutaneous LE treatment, 81–82
Socioeconomic position, 8–9
Spine, 100
Steroid psychosis, 173
Steroids, for immune thrombocytopenic
  purpura, 127
Stroke, 110, 169
Subacute cutaneous lupus erythematosus
  (SCLE), 3
  annular, 68
  drug-induced, 216
  medications, 69–70
  psoriasiform, 68, 69
Sun protection, 55
Synovium, 95

T

Tacrolimus ointment, 82–83
T cell inhibition, 223–224
Tendonitis, 98
Thalidomide, in cutaneous LE treatment, 86–87
Thrombocytopenia, 204
  definition, 125

immune thrombocytopenic purpura, 126–128
  incidence and mortality, 126
  thrombotic thrombocytopenic
    purpura, 128–129
Thrombotic thrombocytopenic purpura (TTP)
  ADAMTS13, 128, 129
  disseminated intravascular coagulation
    (DIC), 129
  plasmapheresis, 129
Tissue inflammation and damage,
  mechanisms of, 21–23
Topical calcineurin inhibitors, 82–83
Transverse myelitis, 176–177
Treatment of lupus
  comorbid conditions, 58
  contraception and pregnancy, 57–58
  cosmetics and hair products, 56
  diet and nutrition, 55–56
  disease activity and severity,
    determination of
      activity indices, 53
      clinically useful markers, 53
      investigational markers, 54
      laboratory testing, frequency of, 54
  immunizations, 56–57
  medications, avoidance of, 58–59
  organ involvement
    cancer risk, 61
    clinical remission, 62
    death, causes of, 61
    drugs, 59
    immunosuppressive agents, 59
    morbidity, 62
    patient survival, 60
    prognosis, 60
    prognostic factors, 61–62
  patient–doctor relationship, 51–52
  radiation therapy, 57
  smoking cessation, 56
  sun protection, 55
TTP. See Thrombotic thrombocytopenic
  purpura (TTP)
Tumid lupus erythematosus, 73–75
Tumor necrosis factor-alpha blockade
  and inhibitors, pregnancy, 192

U

Ulcerative Colitis (UC), 159
Ultraviolet (UV) light, as risk factor
  for SLE, 9–10
Ultraviolet radiation (UVR), 77

Undifferentiated connective tissue disease (UCTD), 28
Urticarial vasculitis, 80

V

Valvular heart disease, 106–107, 196, 203
Vascular damage and repair imbalance, in cardiovascular disease, 234–235
Venous/arterial clotting events, APS and, 196, 201–202
Verrucous LE, 76

Vitamin D deficiency, in metabolic bone disease
    magnitude of risk, 241–242
    treatment, 242

W

Warfarin therapy
    duration of, 201–202
    inferior vena cava filters, 202
    INR for, 201
Worldwide epidemiology, 4–5

Printed by Publishers' Graphics LLC